Non-Neoplastic Cytology

Syed M. Gilani • Guoping Cai
Editors

Non-Neoplastic Cytology

A Comprehensive Guide

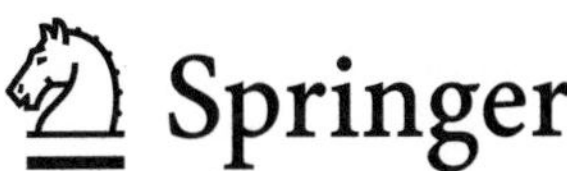 Springer

Editors
Syed M. Gilani
Department of Pathology
Albany Medical Center, Albany
Medical College
Albany, NY, USA

Guoping Cai
Department of Pathology
Yale School of Medicine
New Haven, CT, USA

ISBN 978-3-031-44291-9   ISBN 978-3-031-44289-6   (eBook)
https://doi.org/10.1007/978-3-031-44289-6

This Springer imprint is published by the registered company Springer Nature Switzerland AG
The registered company address is: Gewerbestrasse 11, 6330 Cham, Switzerland

Paper in this product is recyclable.

Preface

Cytology evaluates cellular details, and in contrast, histology relates to tissue assessment with rather preserved architecture. During daily cytology practice, we frequently encounter certain situations which are often challenging such as differentiating normal cytology components or nonneoplastic lesions from a neoplastic process, abnormality versus artifact, contaminants from lesional sampling, immunostain expression in unexpected cells, identifying/or characterizing infectious microorganisms, and use of special stains. In-depth knowledge about normal tissue cytology, the pattern of immunohistochemical expression in various organs, and recognizing diagnostic pitfalls would help to overcome diagnostically challenging situations.

This book is formatted to present a detailed and state-of-the-art approach to nonneoplastic cytology. High-yield content, mostly used in daily practice, is in tabular format. This book provides detailed information about cytomorphologic features of infectious microorganisms and the use of special stains, the use of immunohistochemistry along with expression in normal cell types, artifacts/contaminants or incidental findings, and cytomorphologic features of non-tumor-related lesions in an organ-based structure. There is a further elaboration of differential diagnosis and mimickers of cytologic material from normal parenchymal tissue, infectious/inflammatory conditions, and benign cystic lesions. The last chapter describes a quick overview of important reference material in tables, which is useful for daily anatomic pathology sign-out. This book provides all practical information about nonneoplastic cytology in one concise format using tables and images.

Albany, NY, USA   Syed M. Gilani
New Haven, CT, USA   Guoping Cai

Contents

1 Cytology Specimen Collection, Preparation, and Stains 1
Zoon Tariq and Syed M. Gilani

2 Urinary Tract Cytology 11
Guoping Cai

3 Cervical and Vaginal Cytology 35
Tong Sun and Syed M. Gilani

4 Peritoneal Washings and Ovary 51
Tong Sun and Syed M. Gilani

5 Body Cavity Fluid Cytology 57
Minhua Wang

6 Salivary Gland 73
Syed M. Gilani

7 Thyroid Gland 85
Syed M. Gilani

8 Neck Lesions 105
Syed M. Gilani

9 Lymph Node 113
Omar Al-Rusan and Saja Asakrah

10 Breast 141
Osvaldo Hernandez and Aylin Simsir

11 Respiratory Tract 189
Ruhani Sardana and Guoping Cai

12 Gastrointestinal Tract 217
Rita Abi-Raad

13 Pancreas 229
Xi Wang and Guoping Cai

14 Liver and Biliary Tract 247
Xi Wang and Guoping Cai

15 Kidney and Adrenal Gland 267
Khairya Fatouh and Syed M. Gilani

16 Soft Tissue 277
Juan Xing

17 Bone 301
Sigfred Lajara

18 Brain and Cerebrospinal Fluid 329
Armine Darbinyan, Anita Huttner, and Minhua Wang

19 Quick Review 341
Khairya Fatouh and Syed M. Gilani

Index 353

Chapter 1
Cytology Specimen Collection, Preparation, and Stains

Zoon Tariq and Syed M. Gilani

Specimen Collection Techniques [1]

- Slides preparation:
- The appropriate sample should be collected sufficiently for any cytology specimen to prepare slides (Table 1.1).
- Each slide should be labeled with at least two patient identifiers [2].
- A small amount of sample should be gently expelled onto a slide with the needle tip pointing down towards the slide near the frosted edge to give the most space for subsequent preparation [3].
- "Two-Slide Pull" method: a new clean slide can be used to spread the sample across the first slide to create a thin, evenly distributed smear with constant gentle pressure, or place the specimen close to the midpoint of the slide and place another slide on the top of the specimen and gently pull both slides on the opposite direction. This will generate two slides containing the specimen. One slide can be used for rapid onsite evaluation (ROSE) by airdrying first and then staining with Diff-Quik stain. In contrast, the other slide should rapidly be fixed using 95% ethyl alcohol or cytology spray fixative.
- For staining details, refer to *the specimen preparation section.*

Z. Tariq
Department of Pathology, George Washington University, Washington, DC, USA
e-mail: ztariq@mfa.gwu.edu

S. M. Gilani (✉)
Department of Pathology, Albany Medical Center, Albany Medical College,
Albany, NY, USA
e-mail: gilanis@amc.edu

S. M. Gilani, G. Cai (eds.), *Non-Neoplastic Cytology*,
https://doi.org/10.1007/978-3-031-44289-6_1

Table 1.1 Specimen collection techniques

Cytology technique	Procedure	Indications/uses	Preparation	Adequacy criteria	Contaminants
Fine needle aspiration (FNA)	Image guided: Endobronchial ultrasound (EBUS)	• Diagnosis, staging lung cancer • Mediastinal lymphadenopathy • Mediastinal mass • Parenchymal pulmonary nodules, endobronchial lesions	Direct smear, ThinPrep, cell block	Presence of lesional material	Bronchial cells, cartilage, upper respiratory tract epithelial cells
	Image guided: Endoscopic ultrasound (EUS)	• Primary diagnosis or staging of lesions of gastroesophageal, pancreaticobiliary, ampullary, intestinal or rectal area • Mass in pancreas, gallbladder, biliary tree, liver • Some retroperitoneal lesions		Presence of lesional cells	Oral and GI contaminants
	Image guided: Endoscopic retrograde cholangiopancreatography (ERCP)	• Strictures • Ampullary lesion		Epithelial cells or lesional cells	GI contaminants
	Thyroid	Thyroid lesion or nodule		≥6 groups of follicular cells with ≥10 cells/cluster with certain exception [4]	Gel material, skeletal muscle
	Salivary gland	Salivary gland lesion or nodule		Lesional cells Only normal salivary gland elements in context of mass may not represent lesional cells [5]	Skin
	Breast	Cystic or mass forming lesion		Presence of lesional cells (in correlation with clinical and imaging features)	Skin
	Superficial: Fat pad FNA	Amyloidosis		Fibroadipose tissue fragments and associated vessels	Skin, muscle

Exfoliative cytology	Cervical pap, anal pap	Screening for dysplasia or cancer infection	Liquid-based preparations (LBP: ThinPrep SurePath): Pap	Squamous cells [6]
				• Conventional: 8000–12,000
				  • LBP: ≥5000
				Anal
				  • Conventional: 2000–3000 nucleated squamous cells (NSC)
					–

	Urine	Screening, infection, neoplasia		Voided urine >30 mL [7]	–
	Cerebrospinal fluid	Infection, neoplasia/malignancy		–	Cartilage, blood elements
	Bronchial lavage	Infectious (pneumonia, TB, fungi) Malignancy		>10 alveolar macrophages or any abnormality [8]	Oral contaminants, upper respiratory epithelial cells
	Sputum	TB, *pneumocystis jirovecii* (PJP)		Preferably macrophages [8]	Oral contaminants (squamous epithelial cells)
	Brushings	Bronchial, biliary, esophageal		Lesional cells or epithelial cells	
	Washings	Bronchial, gastric, colonic, bladder, ureteral		Lesional cells or epithelial cells	
	Body cavities	Pleural, pericardial, peritoneal	LBP, cell block	Preferably >50–75 mL of fluid [9]	Skin, muscle
	Synovial fluid	Gout, pseudogout infection		–	–
	Vitreous fluid	Infection neoplasia	ThinPrep or direct smear	–	–
	Cyst fluid	Malignancy	LBP	–	–
	Nipple discharge	Malignancy	Direct smear	–	–

(continued)

Table 1.1 (continued)

Cytology technique	Procedure	Indications/uses	Preparation	Adequacy criteria	Contaminants
Touch prep or FNA procedure	Intraoperative consultation Intraoperative consultation and rapid on-site evaluation: Aims not only to improve diagnostic yield of the procedure but to also help ensure that adequate material is collected and allocated for ancillary tests based on the preliminary cytologic impression [10]	Infection, nonneoplastic, or neoplastic processes	Direct smear	Presence of lesional cells	–

- All specimens received directly into the cytopathology lab should be tightly secured in their respective containers, labeled, and accompanied by an appropriately completed patient requisition form.
- Fixation is in 95% alcohol (ethyl alcohol) for the majority of cases. Alcohol shrinks the cells making nuclear details clearer. 100% alcohol may be used in place of 95% ethyl alcohol.

Fine Needle Aspiration (FNA)

- This procedure is used to evaluate either superficial or deep-seated lesions. FNA of superficial lesions is with or without image guidance, while FNA of deep-seated lesions is performed under image guidance.
- Pathologists often perform FNA of superficial palpable lesions or fat-pad FNA.
- Superficial palpable lesions are generally aspirated with a 22–25 G needle attached to a 10–20 cc syringe.
- Some aspirated contents (2–3 drops) are placed onto a glass slide, and two direct smears are usually prepared using another clear slide. One slide is used for ROSE, while the other is fixed in alcohol for further evaluation.
- Needles should be rinsed in an appropriate solution or formalin to prepare a cell block that can be used for ancillary testing.

Exfoliative Cytology

- *Gynecologic cytology*: Liquid-based gynecological pathology specimens are collected using SurePath or Cytyc ThinPrep preparations for Pap tests.
- *Voided urine*: Discard first early morning urine; patient voids into specimen container; collect urine starting at midstream. Specimens must be submitted immediately to the lab to avoid cellular degeneration. Specimens can be submitted fresh or in 70% alcohol fixative for possible ancillary testing (FISH analysis). Cytology preparations of samples are examined for infections or malignancy.
- *CSF*: Aspirated CSF is evaluated for infection or malignancy.
- *Sputum*: Specimen is evaluated for infection or neoplastic process; complete series: early morning specimens each day for 3 days (if suspected tuberculosis).
- *Brushings*: Specimens are cellular, and mostly CytoLyt solution is used for preservation, but direct smears can also be prepared. The specimen is examined to evaluate for infection, nonneoplastic, or neoplastic processes.
- *Washings*: Bronchial washing is mostly used to evaluate for infection or malignancy. Peritoneal washing is to assess for a neoplastic process.
- *Body cavity fluids*: ThinPrep or cytospin preparations are commonly used. They are examined to determine the cause of fluid accumulation (nonneoplastic versus neoplastic).

  – Direct scrapings: Herpes virus detection: Tzanck test.

- Touch imprint: Touch imprint cytology is mostly used either for ROSE or during intraoperative frozen sections. The biopsy material is touched or scraped on the glass slide and is immediately fixed in alcohol with subsequent staining (Papanicolaou or rapid H&E) or air-dried and then stained with Diff-Quik stain. Squash preparations are also used (mostly in brain-frozen sections).

Specimen Preparation

- Cytology specimen received in the lab is processed based on the specimen site and volume. Direct smears from an FNA procedure usually have an air-dried preparation (Diff-Quik stained) and an alcohol-fixed preparation (Papanicolaou stain).
- Specimens may be concentrated by centrifugation to obtain a cell pellet.
- Papanicolaou (Pap) stain.

  - This staining technique is helpful for optimal visualization of cancer cells exfoliated from epithelial surfaces of the body.
  - The polychrome staining reaction is helpful in highlighting cytologic features, chromatin and cytoplasmic details.
  - Procedure.

    Fixation: Coplin jar with 95% ethyl alcohol (5–15 min).
    Hydration: running water.
    Nuclear staining: Harris hematoxylin (1–5 min).
    Rinse: running water.
    Scott's tap water/distilled water.
    Rinse: running water.
    Rinse: 95% ethyl alcohol, two changes (10 dips).
    Cytoplasmic staining: OG-6 for 30 s to a min.
    Rinse solution: 95% ethyl alcohol, three changes (10 dips).
    Cytoplasmic staining: EA-50 for 5 min.
    Rinse: 95% ethyl alcohol, three changes (10 dips).
    Final dehydration: 100% ethyl alcohol (10 dips).
    Clearing: xylene, three changes.
    Coverslip.

- Diff-Quik stain.

  - Use for ROSE, evaluate the cytoplasmic details, infectious organisms, and hematological elements.
  - Procedure.

    Fixative solution (methanol) for 30 s to 1 min.
    Solution I (eosinophilic) 10 dips.
    Solution II (basophilic) 10 dips.
    Rinse slides in running water.
    Coverslip.

- Rapid H&E stain.

  - The method is used mostly for intraoperative frozen sections and ROSE.
  - Nuclei stain blue; overstaining with hematoxylin results in dark nuclear staining and vice versa.

    Cytoplasm/other tissue elements, including RBCs, stain pink; overstaining with eosin results in dark cytoplasmic staining.

- Cell block.

  - A cell block may be prepared from any fluid, washing, brushing, or FNA, with the added benefit that this procedure obtains any tissue which may be present in the specimen. Cell block material can be used for ancillary testing if required.
  - Procedure.

    Centrifuge the specimen to obtain a pellet which includes the following procedure: Add 10 mL of absolute alcohol and centrifuge it, and gradually decant the supernatant. Add 15–20 mL formalin, again centrifuge it and pour supernatant. Add HistoGel drops to the pellet and then refrigerate it for a few minutes. Put the pellet in the cassette and submit it for processing.

Special Stains

Workup	Stain	Uses	Positive interpretation
Infectious organisms	Ziehl-Neelsen	Acid fast organisms	Red rod-shaped organisms on a blue background
	Modified Ziehl-Neelsen	Acid fast organisms	
	Kinyoun	Acid fast organisms	Red organisms on a blue-green background
	Fite	*Mycobacteria leprae*	Red organisms on a blue background
	Auramine-rhodamine	Acid fast organisms	Yellow-red fluorescence
	Grocott's methenamine silver (GMS)	Fungi especially PJP	Black organisms on pale green background
	Periodic acid Schiff (PAS)	Fungi; polysaccharides; neutral mucosubstances, basement membrane	Magenta-red organisms on blue-green background
	Brown-Hopps	Bacteria	Gram+: Blue Gram–: Red
	Brown-Brenn	Bacteria	Gram+: Purple-blue Gram–: Pink-red
	Warthin-starry	Spirochetes, *helicobacter pylori*	Dark brown-black organisms on pale yellow background

Workup	Stain	Uses	Positive interpretation
Other	Alcian blue	Acid mucopolysaccharides; for *Cryptococcus* spp.	Acid mucins: Blue
	Cresyl violet	Neurons (Nissl substance)	Granular purple-blue neuropil
	Fontana Masson	Melanin, argentaffin cell granules (of carcinoid tumor)	Melanin: Brown-black; on pale pink background
	PAS with diastase digestion	To differentiate mucin from glycogen, fungal infections, Whipple's disease	Light pink (replaces deep magenta of PAS only)
	Masson's trichrome	Connective tissue/vasculature, collagen, fibrosis	Collagen: Blue; nuclei: Brown/black; muscle: Red; cytoplasm: Pink
	Von Kossa	Calcium deposits	Gray-black calcium deposits on light pink background
	Reticulin	Reticulin fibers (tumor architecture)	Black fibers on gray-pink background
	Luxol fast blue	Myelin in nerves	Myelin: Blue-green Neuropil: Pink
	Verhoeff's elastic stain	Elastic fibers	Elastic fibers: Black Collagen: Red
	Bielschowsky silver stain	Nerve fibers (neurofibrillary tangles in Alzheimer's disease)	Black nerve fibers
	Oil red O	Lipid, lipid laden macrophages	Red
	Prussian blue	Iron (hemosiderin)	Bright blue on pink background
	Congo red	Amyloid	Salmon-pink and green birefringence under polarized light
	Thioflavin-T	Amyloid	Bright yellow-green fluorescence on black background
	Mayer Mucicarmine	Acid mucopolysaccharides; epithelial mucin; for *Cryptococcus* spp.	Red on yellow background
	Bile	Bilirubin	Emerald green
	Rhodanine	Copper	Bright red
	Myeloperoxidase (MPO)	Myeloid lineage, MPO deficiency	Blue-green or brown, if present
	Sudan black B	Neutral lipids	Black granular
	Leukocyte alkaline phosphatase	Alkaline phosphatase activity	Brown-black granules
	Toluidine blue	Mast cells	Dark rose-violet on a blue background
	Movat pentachrome	Collagen, elastic fibers, muscle, and mucin	Elastic fibers-black Collagen-yellow Mucin- blue Muscle-red

Immunohistochemistry

- An important development in cytopathology is the application of immunohistochemical staining (IHC) techniques on direct smears and ThinPrep slides, along with the traditional use on cell block material.
- Specimens with limited material or with no cell block can further be evaluated by performing stain on additional ThinPrep slide (such as PTH stain for parathyroid, calcitonin stain for medullary thyroid carcinoma).
- On cytology preparation (direct smear or ThinPrep), interpretation of IHCs with nuclear staining pattern is more straightforward.

Limitation

- Polyclonal antibodies are more sensitive and bind with more epitopes. Titration should be done cautiously to avoid overstaining (false positives).
- Monoclonal antibodies are more homogeneous and specific against a single epitope.
- Cytoplasmic or membranous staining interpretation on ThinPrep or direct smear slides is often challenging.
- Fixative-related issues: Alcohol fixative versus formalin fixative.

Acknowledgments None.

Conflict of Interest None.

References

1. VanderLaan PA. Molecular markers: implications for cytopathology and specimen collection. Cancer Cytopathol. 2015;123(8):454–60.
2. Al-Abbadi MA. Basics of cytology. Avicenna J Med. 2011;1(1):18–28.
3. Abele JS, Miller TR, King EB, Lowhagen T. Smearing techniques for the concentration of particles from fine needle aspiration biopsy. Diagn Cytopathol. 1985;1(1):59–65.
4. Cibas ES, Ali SZ. The 2017 Bethesda system for reporting thyroid cytopathology. Thyroid. 2017;27(11):1341–6.
5. Rossi ED, Faquin WC. The Milan system for reporting salivary gland cytopathology (MSRSGC): an international effort toward improved patient care-when the roots might be inspired by Leonardo da Vinci. Cancer Cytopathol. 2018;126(9):756–66.
6. Nayar R, Wilbur DC. The pap test and Bethesda 2014. Cancer Cytopathol. 2015;123(5):271–81.
7. Zare S, Mirsadraei L, Reisian N, Liao X, Roma A, Shabaik A, Hasteh F. A single institutional experience with the Paris system for reporting urinary cytology: correlation of cytology and histology in 194 cases. Am J Clin Pathol. 2018;150(2):162–7.
8. Guidelines of the Papanicolaou Society of Cytopathology for the examination of cytologic specimens obtained from the respiratory tract. Papanicolaou society of cytopathology task force on standards of practice. Diagn Cytopathol. 1999;21(1):61–9.

9. Pinto D, Chandra A, Crothers BA, Kurtycz DFI, Schmitt F. The international system for reporting serous fluid cytopathology-diagnostic categories and clinical management. J Am Soc Cytopathol. 2020;9(6):469–77.
10. Collins BT, Chen AC, Wang JF, Bernadt CT, Sanati S. Improved laboratory resource utilization and patient care with the use of rapid on-site evaluation for endobronchial ultrasound fine needle aspiration biopsy. Cancer Cytopathol. 2013;121(10):544–51.

Chapter 2
Urinary Tract Cytology

Guoping Cai

Anatomy and histopathology of Urinary Tract

The urinary system is composed of the kidney, ureter, urinary bladder, and urethra. These organs are connected via the epithelium-lined urinary tract in the renal calyces, renal pelvis, ureter, urinary bladder, and urethra.

Urothelium:

The urothelium, lining almost the entire urinary tract except for distal urethra, is approximately three to eight cells thick, composed of superficial, intermediate, and basal cells (Fig. 2.1). The superficial cells, termed umbrella cells, have abundant eosinophilic cytology and large nuclei with frequent binucleation and multinucleation. The intermediate or pyramidal cells are relatively uniform and have a fair amount of eosinophilic cytoplasm, well-defined cell borders, and oval nuclei. The basal cells are small and have low cytoplasmic to nuclear ratios and round to oval nuclei.

Squamous epithelium:

The distal urethra is lined by squamous epithelium (Fig. 2.2), morphologically like the squamous mucosa lining in other organ systems. Squamous epithelium, likely metaplastic in nature, is commonly seen in the trigone region of the urinary bladder, especially in women.

G. Cai (✉)
Department of Pathology, Yale School of Medicine, New Haven, CT, USA
e-mail: guoping.cai@yale.edu

© The Author(s), under exclusive license to Springer Nature Switzerland AG 2023
S. M. Gilani, G. Cai (eds.), *Non-Neoplastic Cytology*,
https://doi.org/10.1007/978-3-031-44289-6_2

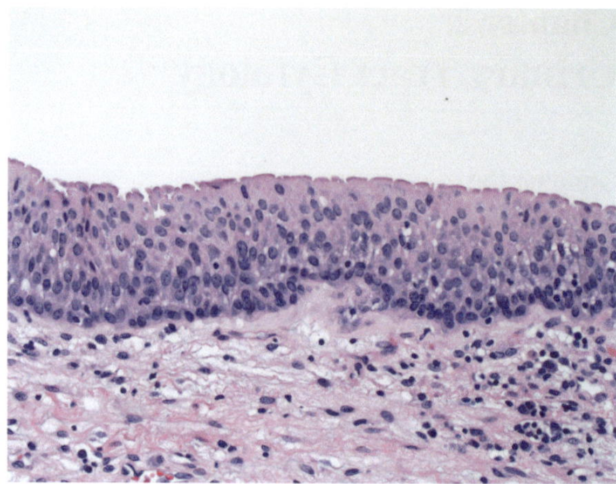

Fig. 2.1 Urothelial lining in the urinary bladder. The epithelium is composed of 5–7 layers of epithelial cells with dense cytoplasm, oval nuclei, fine granular chromatin, and small nucleoli. There are umbrella cells in the top layer of the epithelium

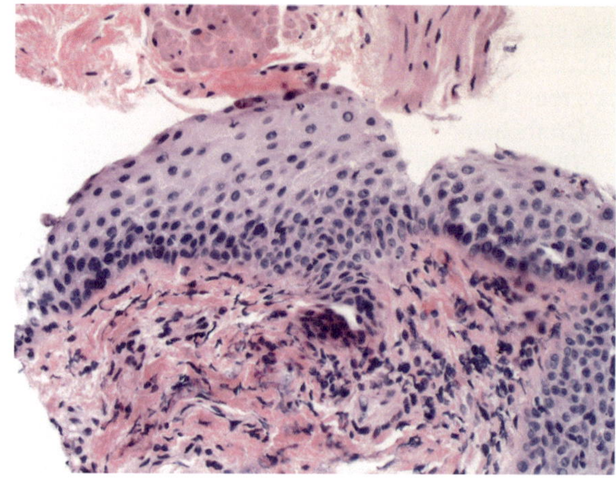

Fig. 2.2 Squamous epithelial lining in the urethra. The epithelium is composed of polygonal epithelial cells with gradual maturation from the base towards to the surface. The squamous cells have dense cytoplasm, round or oval nuclei, finely coarse chromatin, and small nucleoli. Intercellular bridges are notably seen

Sampling Methods

The cytology specimens from the urinary tract include voided urine, catheterized urine, and the samples collected by wash and brushing techniques [1]. Each of these sampling techniques has its own advantages and disadvantages (Table 2.1). Knowing the nature of sample collection methods may help avoid diagnostic pitfalls in the cytological evaluation of urine specimens.

Table 2.1 Comparison of urine sample collection methods[1]

	Utility	Advantage	Disadvantage	Diagnostic Pitfall
Voided urine	Screening test for hematuria Follow-up for patients with urothelial malignancy	Easy and inexpensive sample collection Representative of entire urinary tract	Low cellularity Degenerative changes Contaminants commonly seen	Difficult to differentiate low-grade tumors from reactive changes
Catheterized urine	Urinary tract evaluation when urinary catheter in place	Easy and inexpensive sample collection Contamination less likely Less degenerative changes	Catheterization induced reactive changes Clusters of urothelial cells commonly seen	Over-interpretation of cytological and architectural atypia related to instrumentation
Wash specimen	Evaluation of upper urinary tract lesions Evaluation of urinary bladder when no gross lesions identified during cystoscopy	Less degenerative changes Contamination less likely Evaluation of specific location	Complicated procedure Instrumentation artifacts	Over-interpretation of architectural atypia related to instrumentation Correlation with clinical and imaging findings
Brush specimen	Evaluation of upper urinary tract lesions Evaluation of urinary bladder when no gross lesions identified during cystoscopy	Less degenerative changes Contamination less likely Evaluation of specific location	Complicated procedure Instrumentation artifacts	Over-interpretation of architectural atypia related to instrumentation Correlation with clinical and imaging findings
Ileal conduit urine	Follow-up for patients with cystectomy	Easy and inexpensive sample collection	Marked degenerative changes Obscuring bacteria and/or inflammatory cells	Over-interpretation of degenerative changes as tumor diathesis

Voided Urine

The most common cytology specimen from urinary tract is voided urine, which is collected by far the easiest and least expensive method. The cells in voided urine samples may be sourced from the entire urinary tract, including upper urinary tract (renal pelvis and ureter) and lower urinary tract (urinary bladder and urethra), although most cells are likely of urinary bladder origin. The cells in voided urine samples are mostly dispersed single cells (Fig. 2.3); however, clusters of epithelial cells can be seen in neoplastic as well as nonneoplastic conditions such as inflammation, infection, and urolithiasis (Fig. 2.4). It is important in urine cytology to avoid making the diagnosis of a papillary tumor solely based on the presence of urothelial cell clusters [1] [2].

Ileal conduit urine is a special form of voided urine samples. The samples are collected from patients who have undergone cystectomy. The cells in the ileal conduit urine samples often show marked degenerative changes, mostly of intestinal epithelial origin (Fig. 2.5) [3].

Catheterized Urine

The sample is collected via a catheter. The cells in catheterized urine sample are primarily from the urinary bladder where the catheter is placed. Compared to voided urine, catheterized urine specimen more likely has clusters of urothelial cells and shows more reactive changes (Fig. 2.6).

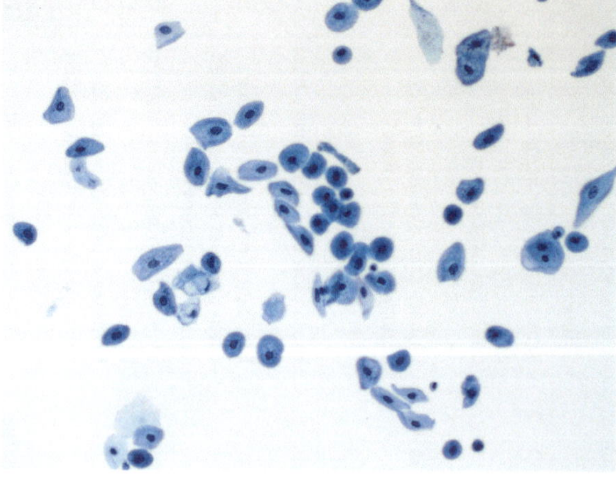

Fig. 2.3 Voided urine. Dispersed single urothelial cells composed of predominantly intermediate urothelial cells with scattered umbrella cells and rare basal cells

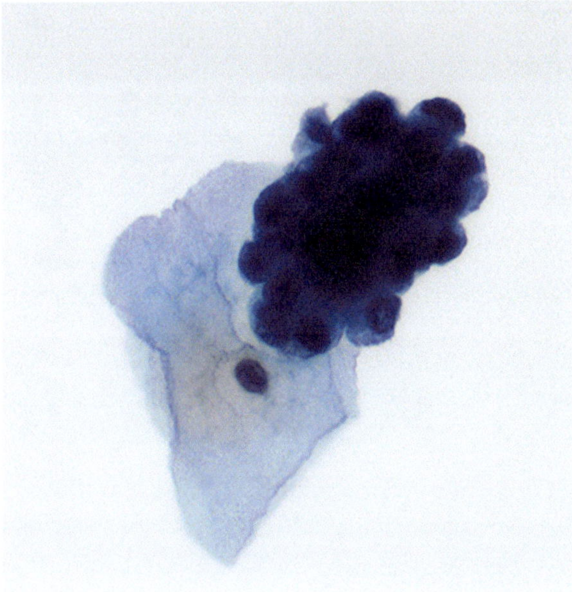

Fig. 2.4 Voided urine. A three-dimensional luster of urothelial cells. Urothelial cells are small with slightly hyperchromatic nuclei

Fig. 2.5 Ileal conduit urine. Markedly degenerated epithelial cells with apoptotic bodies and scattered inflammatory cells

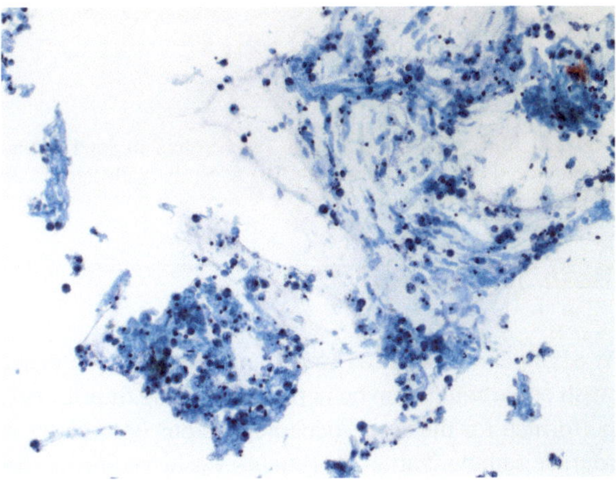

Fig. 2.6 Catheterized urine with reactive changes. Loosely cohesive group of urothelial cells with enlarged nuclei and conspicuous nucleoli. An umbrella cell with binucleation is seen

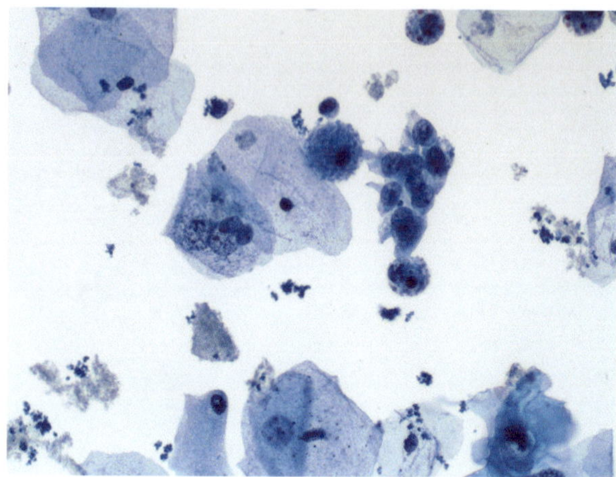

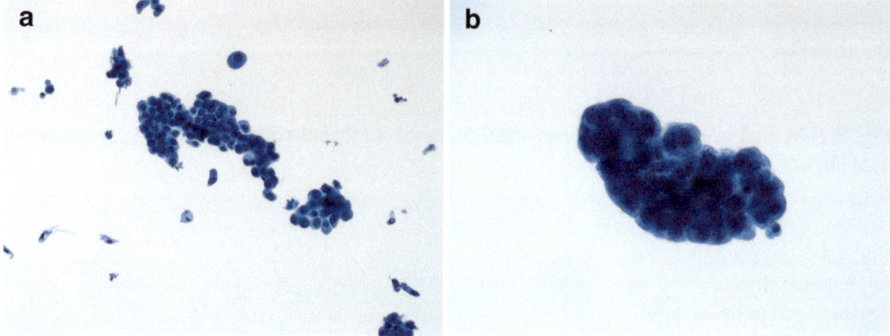

Fig. 2.7 Bladder wash specimen. (**a**) Clusters of intermediate urothelial cells with scattered umbrella cells and rare basal cells. (**b**) A papillary cluster of urothelial cells with enlarged nuclei and conspicuous nucleoli

Wash Specimen

Washing can be applied to a specific part of the urinary tract. In urinary bladder, wash or barbotage can be performed during or prior to cystoscopy. Wash can also be performed for the space-occupied lesions or stricture in upper urinary tract via retrograde catheterization. In general, wash specimens show less degenerative changes but more instrumentation artifacts (Fig. 2.7). For the upper urinary lesions, correlation with clinical and imaging findings is always recommended.

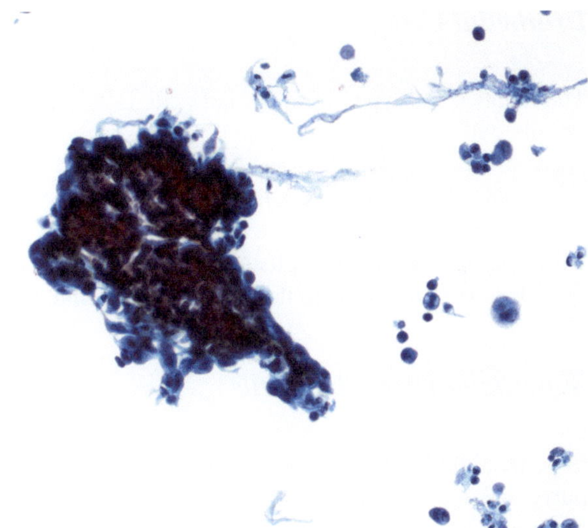

Fig. 2.8 Ureteral brush specimen. A cluster of intermediate urothelial cells with scattered umbrella cells and rare basal cells

Brush Specimen

For the space-occupied lesions or structure in the upper urinary tract, direct sampling of the lesions can be performed by brushing technique via retrograde catheterization. Like wash specimens, brush specimens also show less degenerative changes but more instrumentation artifacts (Fig. 2.8). Again, for the upper urinary lesions, correlation with clinical and imaging findings is always recommended.

Normal Urine Cytology

Adequacy

Currently, there is no well-established criteria for a specific number of cells for adequacy assessment, but a minimal volume of 30 ml for cytological evaluation of voided urine sample has been recommended [4]. Identification of any abnormal cells is considered adequate even when urine sample is less than 30 ml. For instrumented urine specimens, specific volume or cellularity requirement has not been well established. There is one study suggesting a threshold of at least 20 well-preserved, well-visualized urothelial cells per 10 high-power fields [5].

Urothelial Cells

The number and types of urothelial cells in a specimen are largely dependent on sample collection methods. Voided urine specimens are almost exclusively composed of single cells with considerable variations in cellularity. Instrumented samples often cellular with urothelial cell clusters as a common finding. Superficial and intermediate urothelial cells are the common cell types in voided urine specimens while the basal urothelial cells are more frequently seen in instrumented samples, often forming clusters with intermediate urothelial cells. (Table 2.2).

Superficial Urothelial Cells

Superficial umbrella cells are the largest urothelial cells (Fig. 2.9). These cells are polygonal and have abundant homogenous cytoplasm, occasionally with cytoplasmic vacuolation. The nuclei are round or oval with smooth nuclear contours, coarsely granular chromatin, and occasional conspicuous nucleoli. Binucleation and multinucleation are frequently seen. Although the nuclei of superficial urothelial cells, even in the single nucleated form, are larger those in the intermediate or basal cells, the superficial urothelial cells have low nuclear to cytoplasmic ratios due to abundant cytoplasm.

Intermediate Urothelial Cells

Intermediate urothelial cells are smaller than superficial urothelial cells (Fig. 2.10). These cells have fair amount of dense cytoplasm, resulting in well-defined cell borders. The nuclei are predominantly oval in shape with slightly irregular nuclear contours, fine granular chromatin, and inconspicuous nucleoli. Nuclear membrane irregularity such as nuclear grooves may become more obvious in urothelial cell clusters in instrumented samples.

Table 2.2 Cytomorphologic features of urothelial cells

	Superficial Cells	Intermediate Cells	Basal Cells
Size	Large	Intermediate	Small
Cytoplasm	Abundant, vacuolated	Modest, dense	Scant, dense
Nuclei	Larger, round	Medium, oval	Smaller, round to oval
Nuclear to cytoplasmic ratio	Low	Medium	High
Binucleation or multinucleation	Frequent	Absent	Absent
Nuclear contour	Smooth	Slightly irregular	Smooth
Chromatin	Coarsely granular	Fine granular	Fine granular
Nucleoli	Occasional conspicuous	Inconspicuous	Inconspicuous

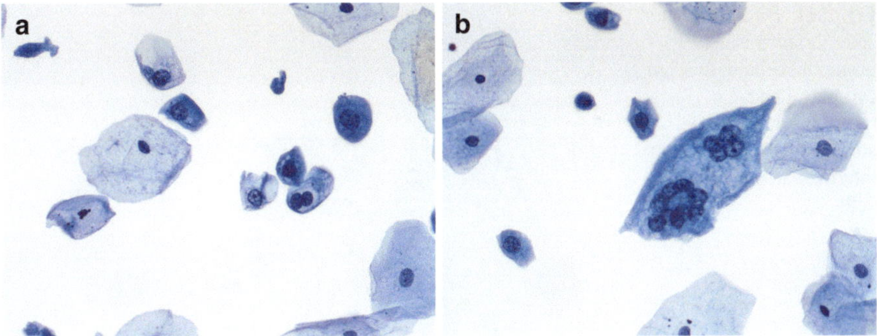

Fig. 2.9 Umbrella cells. (**a**) Umbrella cells with abundant cytoplasm, large round nuclei, and occasional binucleation. (**b**) Multinucleated umbrella cells

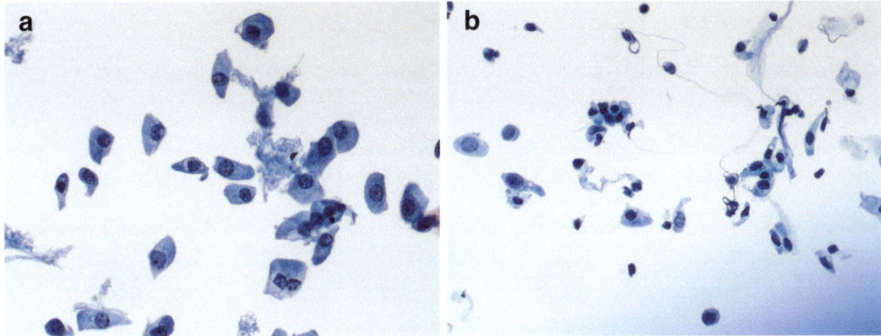

Fig. 2.10 Intermediate urothelial cells. (**a**) Dispersed polygonal urothelial cells with moderate amount of cytoplasm and round to oval nuclei. (**b**) Predominant intermediate urothelial cells with rare umbrella and basal cells

Basal Urothelial Cells

Basal cells are the smallest urothelial cells (Fig. 2.11). The cells are round in shape and have scant dense cytoplasm. The nuclei are round to oval with smooth nuclear contours, fine granular chromatin, and inconspicuous nucleoli. Although the nuclei of basal urothelial cells are small, scanty cytoplasm results in relatively high nuclear to cytoplasmic ratios.

Squamous Cells

Since distal urethra and urinary bladder trigone are lined by squamous epithelial epithelium, squamous cells are considered as a normal cellular component of urine specimens. The types of squamous cells may include polygonal superficial cells with abundant cyanophilic or orangeophilic cytoplasm and small pyknotic nuclei, intermediate cells with larger vesicular nuclei and occasionally, small parabasal

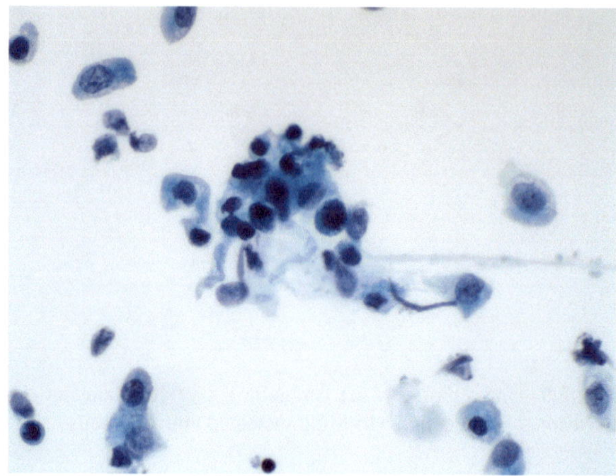

Fig. 2.11 Basal urothelial cells. A few basal urothelial cells with scant cytoplasm and hyperchromatic nuclei admixed with intermediated urothelial cells

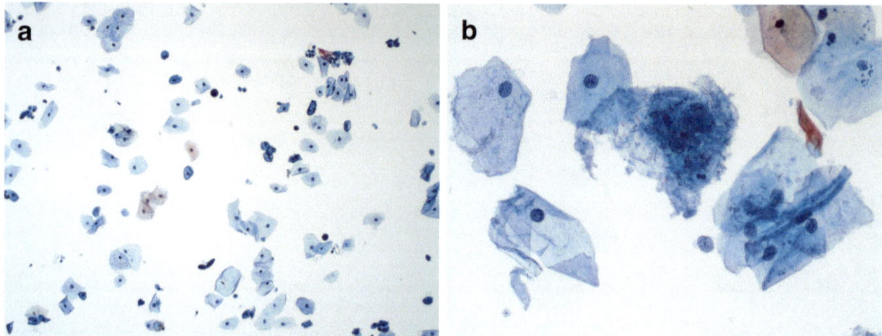

Fig. 2.12 Squamous cell contaminants. (**a**) Many superficial squamous cells admixed with scattered urothelial cells. (**b**) Superficial and intermediate squamous cells with thin bacilli, likely of vaginal contaminant

cells. When appeared in a high number and in women, squamous cells are more likely to be originated from vaginal contamination. In this setting, squamous cells may exceed the number of urothelial cells and are often accompanied by abundant bacteria (Fig. 2.12). To alleviate potential squamous cell contamination, midstream clean catch urine is highly recommended.

Other Cells

Renal tubular cells may, although infrequently, be present in urine specimens. The renal tubular cells have granular cytoplasm and round nuclei, present singly, or associated with renal casts, which might be under reported in urine specimens [6, 7]. Spermatozoa may also be identified in urine samples, sometimes associated with seminal vesicle epithelial cells (Fig. 2.13).

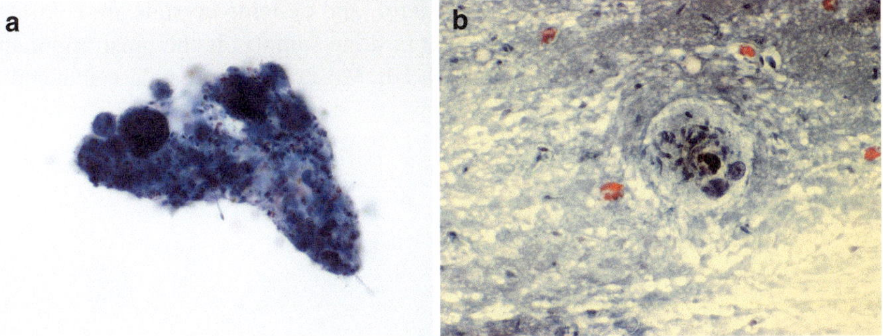

Fig. 2.13 Spermatozoa and seminal vesicle epithelial cells. (**a**) A ball of spermatozoa with rare large, degenerated cells. (**b**) Large seminal vesicle cells with intracytoplasmic lipofusion pigment

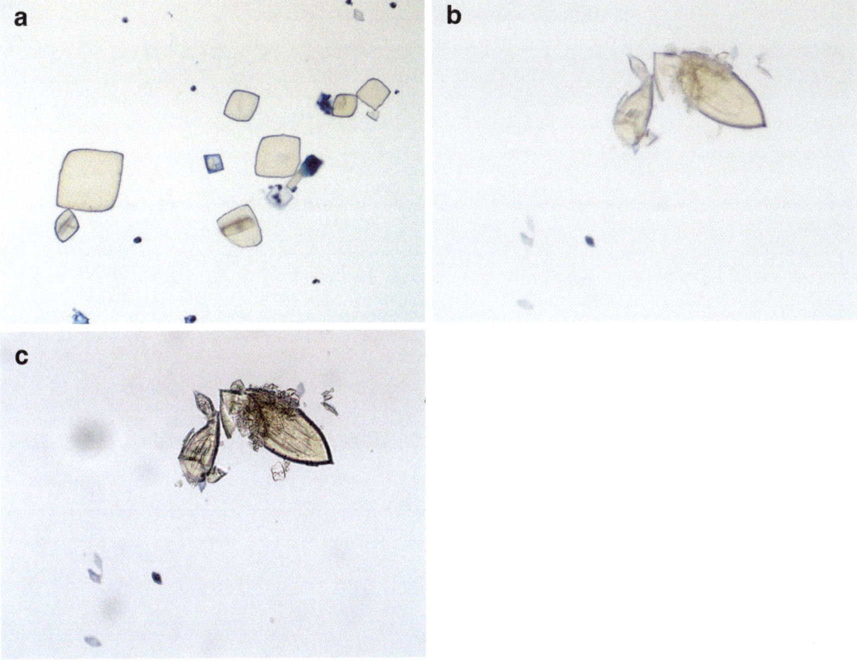

Fig. 2.14 Colored crystals. (**a, b**) Multi-shaped crystals with light brown color. (**c**) Crystals are polarizable and show reflectile feature

Crystals

The presence of crystals in urine specimens is a common finding. The crystals are composed of variable chemicals, varying in color and shape (Table 2.3) [8]. The colored crystals include uric acid, ammonium biurate, bilirubin, leucine, and sulfa crystals (Fig. 2.14). Calcium oxalate, calcium phosphate, calcium carbonate, triple phosphate, hippuric acid, tyrosine, cholesterol, and cysteine crystals are colorless and translucent (Fig. 2.15). The pH value in urine samples is the most important factor which helps formation of crystals [9, 10]. Most crystals are polarizable under

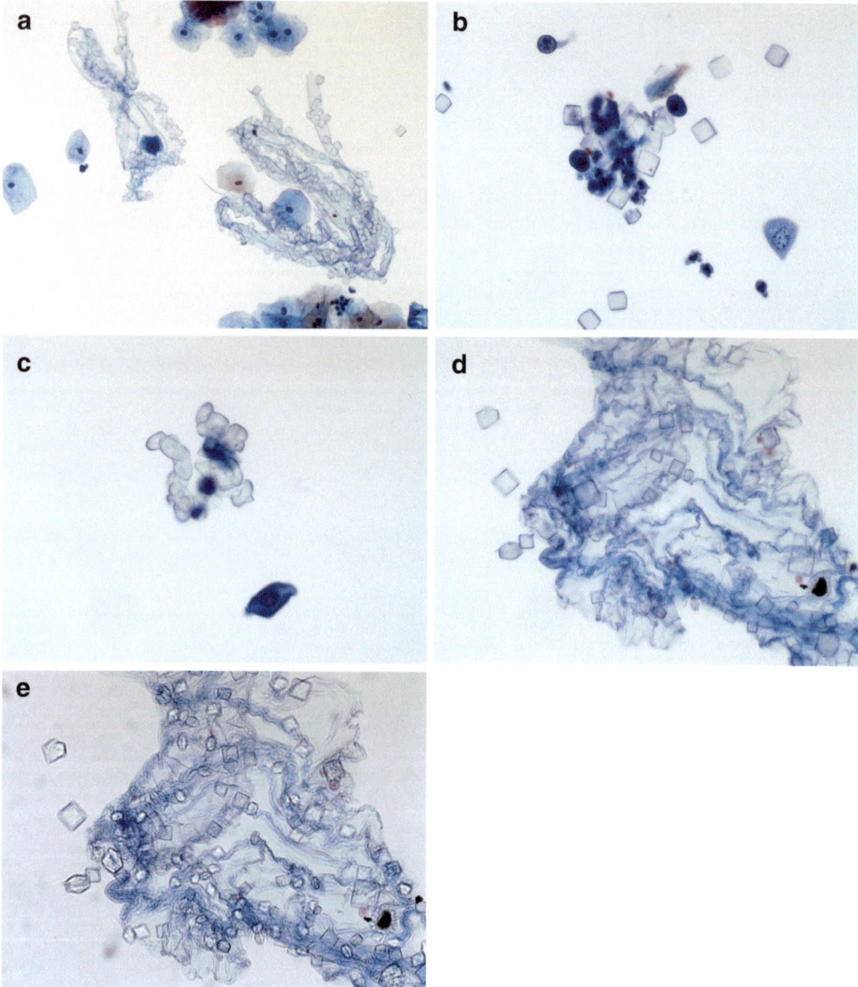

Fig. 2.15 Colorless crystals. (**a–d**) Translucent crystals in a variety shapes. (**e**) Crystals are polarizable and show refractive feature

Table 2.3 Crystals in urine specimens

Crystals	Composition	pH	Shape	Color	Significance
Uric acid	–	Acidic	Rhomboid, four-sided plates	Yellow-light brown	Possibly urate nephrolithiasis, tumor lysis syndrome
Calcium oxalate	Monohydrate or dihydrate calcium oxalate	Acidic or alkaline	Monohydrate: Dumbbells Dihydrate: Octahedral, envelope	Colorless	Possibly ethylene glycol ingestion (monohydrate)
Triple phosphate	Magnesium, ammonium, phosphate	Alkaline	Prism-shaped like a coffin lid	Colorless	Possibly infection by urease-producing bacteria
Calcium phosphate	–	Neutral or alkaline	Blunt ended needles	Colorless	
Calcium carbonate	–	Alkaline	Large dumbbells, spheres with radial striations	Colorless	
Hippuric acid	–	Acidic or neutral	Needle-like	Colorless	
Ammonium biurate	–	Alkaline	Spherical bodies with irregular protrusions	Brown or yellow brown	Possibly predisposed to urate urolithiasis
Bilirubin	Conjugated bilirubin	Acidic	Clumped needles	Yellow	Severe hepatic disorders
Cholesterol	–	Acidic	Rectangular, notched plates	Colorless	Nephritic syndrome
Sulfa	Sulfonamide	Acidic or neutral	Rosettes or sheaves of small needles	Brown	Likely administration of the drug
Leucine	–	Acidic or neutral	Spheres with concentric circles or radial striations	Yellowish brown	Possibly liver disorders
Cysteine	–	Acidic	Hexagonal	Colorless	Diagnostic of cystinuria
Tyrosine	–	Acidic or neutral	Fine needles forming clumps or rosettes	Colorless or yellow	Possibly tyrosinemia or liver disorders

polarized lens. The presence of crystals in urine specimens is usually of no diagnostic significance [11]. However, certain types of crystals may be associated with disease conditions or drug administration [12]. There is a possible but not definite linkage between the presence of crystals in urine specimens and occurrence of urolithiasis [11, 13].

Contaminants

Urine samples may be contaminated during specimen collection or processing at lab. Instrumentation is the primary source of urine contaminants. Surgical powder and lubricant gel are commonly seen in instrumented, catheterized or wash/brush, urine samples. Lubricant gel may form structures that mimic the eggs of parasites (Fig. 2.16). Alternaria, the brown and septated fungal organism, may occasionally be seen in urine specimens, which is the contaminant from lab water supply. In addition, bacterial and fungal overgrowth can occur when urine samples are left too long in room temperature, a pitfall for bacterial or fungal infection in the urinary tract (Fig. 2.17). Absence of a significant inflammatory component is a clue for the overgrowth rather than actual infection.

Reactive Changes

Reactive changes are the common findings in urine samples, which may be associated with degeneration, inflammation, infection, or therapies. Urolithiasis, stent placement, instrumentation, and surgical interventions may also cause significant cellular changes (Table 2.4). Benign-appearing glandular cells may be present in urine samples, likely because of cystitis glandularis.

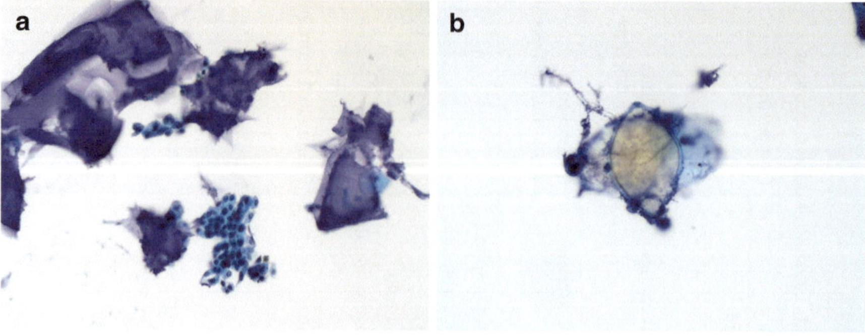

Fig. 2.16 Lubricant gel material. (**a**) Blue colored gel material with a few groups of urothelial cells. (**b**) Gel material shows a shape like parasite egg

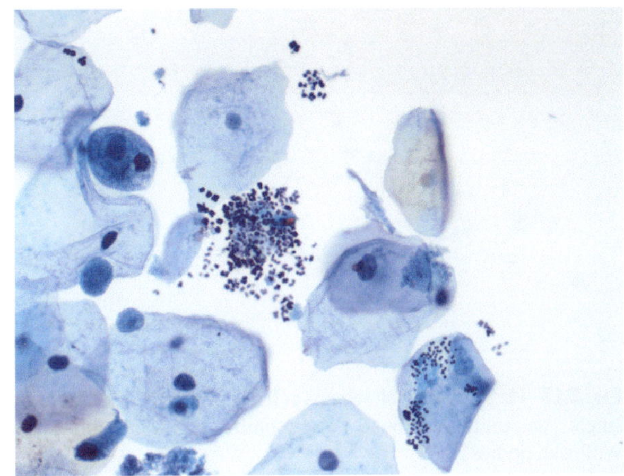

Fig. 2.17 Bacterial overgrowth. Colonies of cocci bacteria with absence of inflammation in the background

Table 2.4 Cytomorphologic features of urothelial cell degeneration, polyomavirus infection, and high-grade urothelial carcinoma

	Degeneration	Polyomavirus Infection	Urolithiasis	High-grade Urothelial Carcinoma
Architecture	Almost exclusively single cells	Almost exclusively single cells	Single cells and occasional clusters	Single cells and occasional clusters
Cell size	Small	Small to intermediate	Small to intermediate	Large
Nuclei	Small, hyperchromatic	Enlarged, ground glass appearance	Enlarged, prominent nucleoli	Large, variable in size, coarse chromatin, prominent nucleoli
Cytoplasm	Modest, vacuolated, Melamed-Wolinska bodies	Scant, dense, or vacuolated	Modest, dense, or vacuolated	Scant, dense
Background	Inflammation absent or present	Inflammation	Inflammation	Inflammation, necrosis

Degenerative Changes

Cellular degeneration is frequently encountered when evaluating urine specimens, especially those voided urine samples collected first in the morning. Degenerated urothelial cells showed loss of cellular details including enlarged pyknotic nuclei with hyperchromasia and smudged chromatin. Intracytoplasmic eosinophilic inclusions, as known as Melamed-Wolinska bodies, are frequently identified (Fig. 2.18) [14, 15]. These cytoplasmic inclusions can be found in both degenerating benign and malignant urothelial cells which have no significant diagnostic value but may suggest a urothelial origin [14, 16].

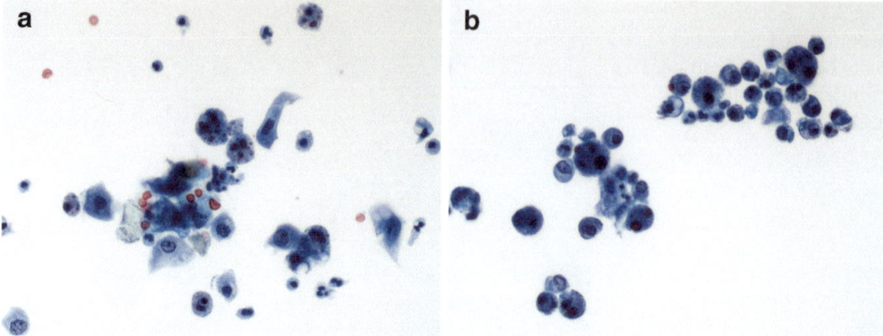

Fig. 2.18 Degenerative changes. (**a, b**) Degenerated urothelial cells show smudged chromatin and single or multiple round eosinophilic or blue intracytoplasmic inclusions (Melamed-Wolinska bodies)

Another example of degenerative changes is seen in ileal conduct samples where the glandular epithelium lined small bowel undergoes marked degenerative changes due to urine toxic environment. Therefore, the cellular element of ileal conduit urine specimen is mostly of small bowel origin. These epithelial cells are present single and in cluster. Due to degeneration, the cells are poorly preserved and do not show their usual columnar morphology. Instead, the epithelial cells are round or oval with degenerative granular cytoplasm, resembling histiocytes (Fig. 2.19). These cellular changes must be differentiated from urothelial carcinoma that might represent tumor reoccurrence in ileal conduit or derive from upper urinary tract [17, 18]. Abundant bacteria may be seen in the background. The cellular degeneration and bacteria may be alleviated or ceased long after radical surgical procedure.

Reactive Changes

Reactive changes can be caused by inflammation, infection, urolithiasis, treatments, or instrumentation. The common cellular features of reactive changes may include cytomegaly, nuclear enlargement, and prominent nucleoli although the cellular details may differ under specific conditions. In addition to urothelial cells, there may be an increase in the number of squamous cells, some in metaplastic in nature.

Acute and chronic inflammation is often caused by urinary tract infection or other nonspecific disorders, manifested by reactive epithelial changes and abundant inflammatory cells seen in the background (Fig. 2.20). In acute inflammation, neutrophils are the predominant inflammatory cells while the immune cells in chronic inflammation are dominated by lymphocytes. Granulomatous inflammation is a special form of chronic inflammation that is characterized by the presence of epithelioid histocytes with or without multinucleated giant cells. Although granulomatous

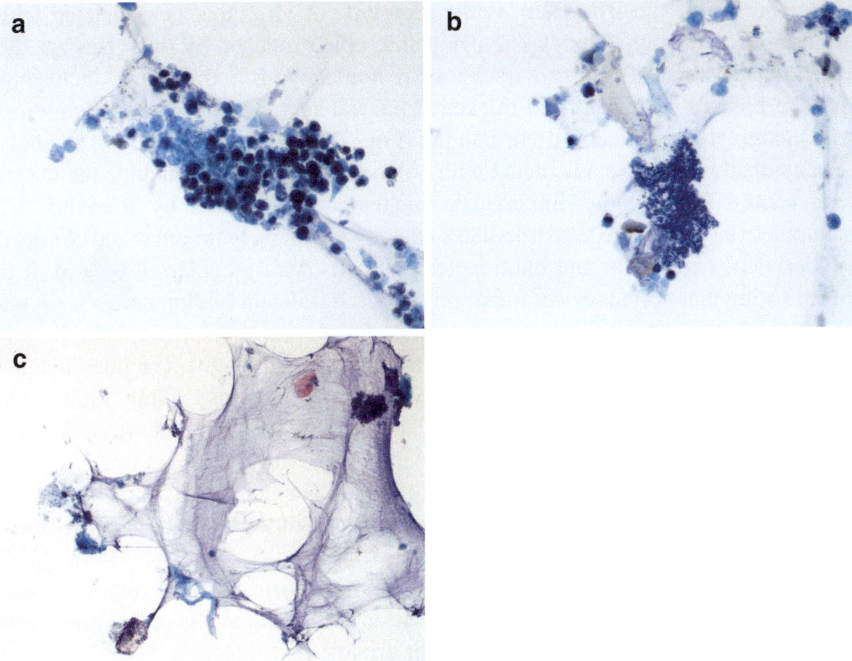

Fig. 2.19 Degenerated cells in ileal conduit specimen. (**a**) A loose group of epithelial cells with marked degenerative changes and cellular debris. (**b**) Bacterial colonies with degenerated urothelial cells. (**c**) Mucin-like material with degenerated urothelial cells

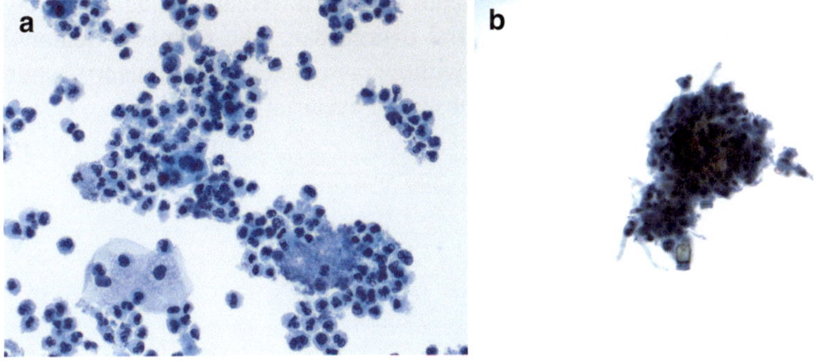

Fig. 2.20 Acute and chronic inflammation. (**a**) Abundant neutrophils. (**b**) Granuloma - a cluster of epithelioid histiocytes

inflammation is a quite common finding in patients with urothelial carcinoma following BCG treatment or transurethral tumor resection, granulomas are rarely identified in voided urine specimens. The presence of numerous eosinophils may suggest eosinophilic cystitis which is most seen in patients who receive cautery treatment.

Polyomavirus, the BK strain, is the prototype of virus that is associated with urinary tract infection. The classic cytopathic effect induced by this virus are the eccentrically located enlarged nuclei with homogenous intranuclear inclusions (packed by viral particles) and thickened nuclear membrane (nuclear membrane with marginalized/condensed chromatin) (Fig. 2.21) [19]. Other less commonly seen cytopathic changes associated with polyomavirus infection include the nuclei with central homogenous intranuclear inclusions surrounded by irregular and incomplete halo (cytomegalovirus-like), nuclei with coarsely granular and clumped (spider web) chromatin, and multinucleated nuclei with granular chromatin. It is worth noting that polyomavirus infection is not a significant finding unless it occurs in immunocompromised patients including those with renal transplant, human immunodeficiency virus infection or post-chemotherapy [20–23]. The potential pitfall is that the cells with polyomavirus cytopathic effects may mimic high-grade urothelial carcinoma, known as decoy cells [24]. Besides polyomavirus, adenovirus, cytomegalovirus, and herpes virus are the other viruses that can infect urinary tract. The koilocytic changes in squamous cells may be due to polyomavirus infection in squamous epithelium of the urethra but may more likely be resulted from vaginal/vulvar squamous cell contamination.

Bacterial infection is more likely seen in women, primarily involving lower urinary tract. Urinary tract stricture, catheterization, and malignant neoplasms are contributing factors that predispose patients for urinary tract infection. When infection persists, bacteria can reach retrogradely the upper urinary tract resulting in pyelonephritis. Bacterial infection is almost always associated with significant inflammatory responses, mostly in the form of acute inflammation but may also be chronic inflammation. Bacterial organisms, either cocci or rods, could be identified in urine specimens (Fig. 2.22). The presence of bacteria in urine specimens is not always resulted from urinary tract bacterial infection. The differential diagnosis may include vaginal contamination and bacterial overgrowth. The former is featured with abundant squamous cells with or without associated inflammatory while inflammatory cell component is virtually absent in bacterial overgrowth.

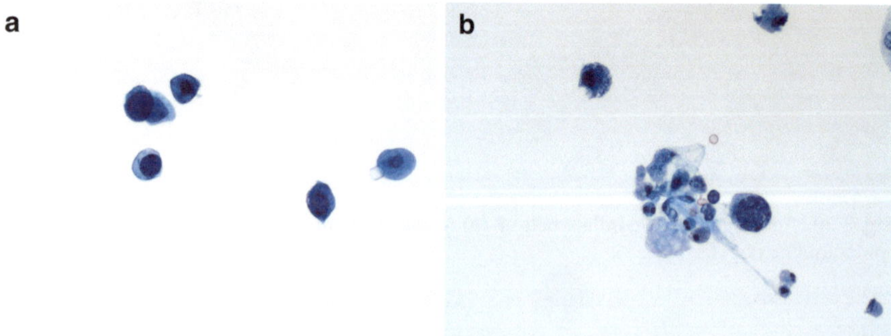

Fig. 2.21 Polyomavirus cytopathic effects. (**a**) Scattered urothelial cells with intranuclear homogenized nuclei and marginalized chromatin. (**b**) A urothelial cell with intranuclear spider-web nucleus and marginalized chromatin

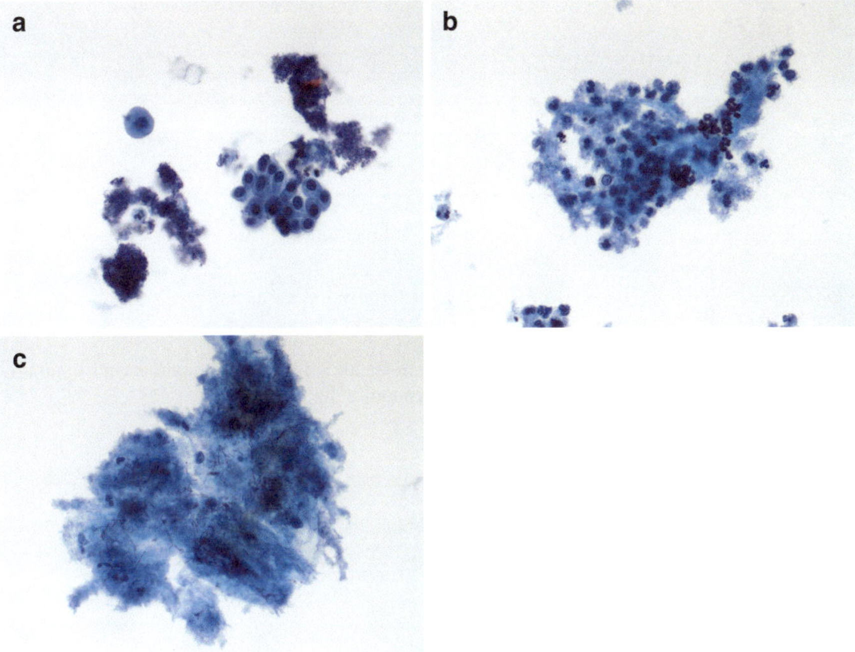

Fig. 2.22 Bacteria in urine samples. (**a**) Bacterial colonies and urothelial cells. (**b**) Coccus bacteria and inflammatory cells. (**c**) Thin bacterial rods with squamous cells, likely vaginal contaminants

Compared to bacterial infection, fungal infection is much less common in urinary tract. Candida is the most common fungal organism found in urine specimen. Candida includes yeast and pseudo-hyphae form organisms which can recognized on routine Papanicolaou-stained preparation with no need for special stain (Fig. 2.23). Other fungal infections such as aspergillosis, histoplasmosis, cryptococcosis, and blastomycosis are rarely seen. Fungal infection is often accompanied by variable cellular changes and inflammatory infiltration. Alternaria, a brown septated fungal organism, is a common lab contaminant.

Schistosoma haematobium is the most described parasite infection in urine specimens although the infection is limited to certain geographic location or to the individuals who have travel history. This organism is often identified by revelation of its ova which is characterized by a terminal spine. The most significant factor in identifying *S. haematobium* is association of its infection with squamous cell carcinoma of the urinary bladder although it is rare. A far more common finding is the presence of reactive metaplastic squamous cells. Trichomonas vaginalis is another parasite which can be seen in urine specimens usually due to vaginal contamination in female patients.

Bacillus Calmette-Guerin (BCG) treatment is a commonly used therapy for patients with urothelial carcinoma. Intra-vesicular administration of BCG induces

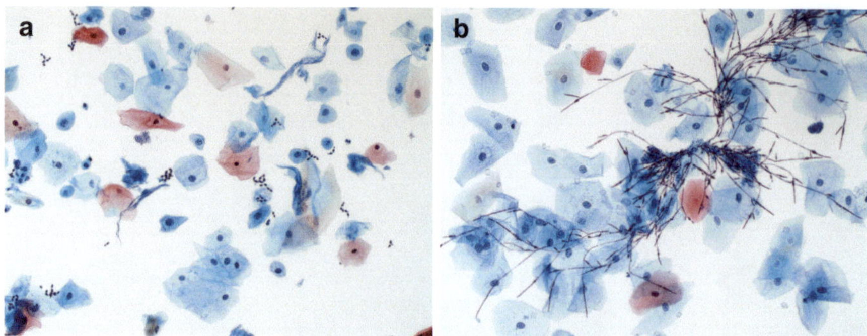

Fig. 2.23 Candida in urine samples. (**a**) Yeast-form Candida fungi with squamous cells and urothelial cells. (**b**) Candida pseudo-hyphae with squamous cells

Fig. 2.24 Therapy-related reactive changes. Scattered urothelial cells with enlarged nuclei, prominent nucleoli, and cytoplasmic vacuoles. Background inflammation

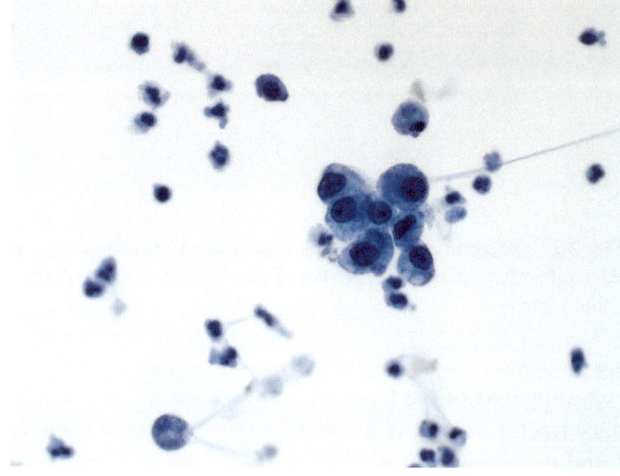

granulomatous inflammation in the wall of urinary bladder, like those of tuberculosis. The urine specimens from patients who receive BCG treatment show reactive urothelial cells and mixed inflammatory cells, it is however unusual to see granulomas, especially in voided urine samples [25].

Chemotherapy and radiation can cause similar reactive changes in urothelial cells. The reactive changes include cytomegaly, marked cytoplasmic vacuolization, nuclear enlargement, and prominent nucleoli (Fig. 2.24). Pyknotic nuclei and apoptotic bodies may also be present. It is advised to cautiously interpret the cytological atypia in the setting of post-chemotherapy or radiation to avoid diagnostic pitfall for urothelial carcinoma [26].

Urolithiasis may cause significant changes in urothelial cells, even atypical. The possible changes include nuclear enlargement, hyperchromasia, coarse chromatin, and prominent nucleoli (Fig. 2.25). The presence of urolithiasis-associated cytological atypia may pose diagnostic challenge for the differential diagnosis of

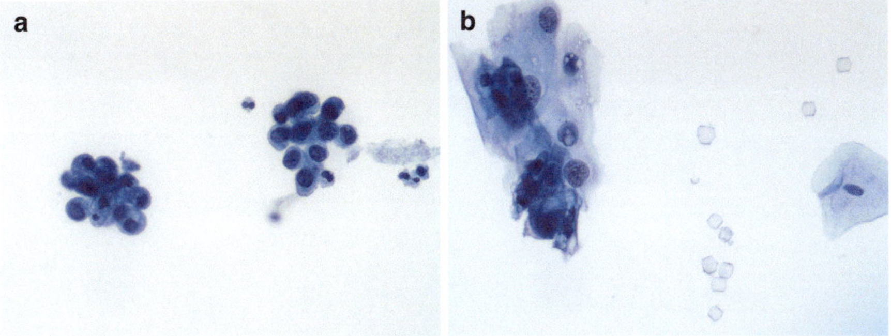

Fig. 2.25 Reactive changes related to urolithiasis. (**a**) Urothelial cells with increased nuclear to cytoplasmic ratios and nuclear hyperchromasia. (**b**) Urothelial cells with abundant cytoplasm, enlarged nuclei, and prominent nucleoli. Crystals present

urothelial carcinoma [27, 28]. It should be kept in mind that urothelial carcinoma and urolithiasis may coexist [27].

Clusters of Urothelial Cells

A urothelial cell cluster is referred as a three-dimensional group of urothelial cells in cytological specimens (Fig. 2.26). The presence of urothelial cell clusters in voided urine specimens may be considered as an abnormal finding but it alone is rarely indicative of urothelial carcinoma [29, 30]. Urothelial cell clusters are more often seen in the specimens related to urolithiasis, and instrumentation and should be differentiated from urothelial tumors, especially low-grade papillary urothelial neoplasm (Table 2.5) [31, 32].

Instrumentation procedures such as catheterization, wash and brush can artificially introduce clusters of urothelial cells in collected specimens. The urothelial cells in clusters often consist of superficial, intermediate, and basal cells and show no significant cytological changes. No real fibrovascular cores are identified within the urothelial cell clusters.

Urolithiasis-associated changes include architectural and cytological atypia [28]. The presence of clustered urothelial cell groups in voided urine samples is a common finding in patients with urolithiasis. The clustered urothelial cells can demonstrate an architecture of three-dimensional groups or papillary clusters. In addition to the architectural changes, the cells may also show nuclear changes including nuclear enlargement, hyperchromasia, and nucleoli but smooth nuclear membranes.

Low-grade urothelial neoplasm is the tumor with papillary proliferation of urothelium and mild cytological atypia [32]. Clustered urothelial groups with true fibrovascular core are commonly seen in instrumented urine samples but rarely

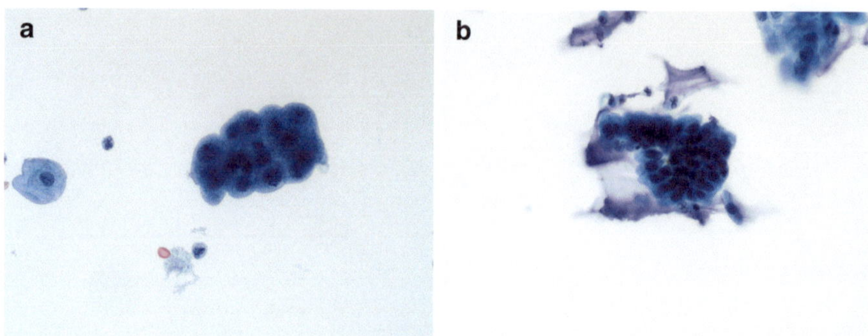

Fig. 2.26 Urothelial cell clusters. (**a**) Voided urine showing a urothelial cell cluster with enlarged nuclei and conspicuous nucleoli. (**b**) Instrumented urine showing gel material and a papillary cluster of urothelial cells with enlarged nuclei

Table 2.5 Possible causes of urothelial cell clusters in urine specimens

	Instrumentation	Urolithiasis	Low-grade Papillary Urothelial Neoplasm
Architecture	Three-dimensional cluster	Three-dimensional cluster	Three-dimensional cluster, papillary clusters
Cell composition	Superficial, intermediate, and basal cells	Predominant intermediate cells	Homogenous urothelial cells with or without superficial cells
Fibrovascular core	Absent	Absent	Likely present
Cellular changes	None or minimal	Nuclear enlargement, smooth nuclear contours, hyperchromasia, prominent nucleoli	Nuclear enlargement, irregular nuclear contours, increased nuclear to cytoplasmic ratios, hyperchromasia
Background	Clean	Inflammatory	Clean or inflammatory

identified voided urine specimens, which make a diagnosis of low-grade urothelial neoplasm in voided samples quite challenging. The tumor cells of low-grade papillary neoplasm show increased nuclear to cytoplasmic ratios, irregular nuclear contours, and hyperchromasia [33–35].

Acknowledgments None.

Conflict of Interest None.

References

1. Koss LGMM. Koss' diagnostic cytology and its histopathologic bases. 5th ed. Philadelphoa: Lippincott, Williams & Wilkins; 2006.
2. Wojcik EM. What should not be reported as atypia in urine cytology. J Am Soc Cytopathol. 2015;4(1):30–6.
3. Ajit D, Dighe SB, Desai SB. Cytology of Ileal conduit urine in bladder cancer patients: diagnostic utility and pitfalls. Acta Cytol. 2006;50(1):70–3.
4. VandenBussche CJ, Rosenthal DL, Olson MT. Adequacy in voided urine cytology specimens: the role of volume and a repeat void upon predictive values for high-grade urothelial carcinoma. Cancer Cytopathol. 2016;124(3):174–80.
5. Prather J, Arville B, Chatt G, et al. Evidence-based adequacy criteria for urinary bladder barbotage cytology. J Am Soc Cytopathol. 2015;4(2):57–62.
6. Chawla LS, Dommu A, Berger A, Shih S, Patel SS. Urinary sediment cast scoring index for acute kidney injury: a pilot study. Nephron Clin Pract. 2008;110(3):c145–50.
7. Poloni JAT, de Oliveira VA, Dos Santos CRM, Simundic AM, Rotta LN. Survey on reporting of epithelial cells in urine sediment as part of external quality assessment programs in Brazilian laboratories. Biochem Med (Zagreb). 2021;31(2):020711.
8. Lee AJ, Yoo EH, Bae YC, Jung SB, Jeon CH. Differential identification of urine crystals with morphologic characteristics and solubility test. J Clin Lab Anal. 2022;36(11):e24707.
9. Grases F, Costa-Bauzá A, Gomila I, Ramis M, García-Raja A, Prieto RM. Urinary pH and renal lithiasis. Urol Res. 2012;40(1):41–6.
10. Højgaard I, Fornander AM, Nilsson MA, Tiselius HG. The effect of pH changes on the crystallization of calcium salts in solutions with an ion composition corresponding to that in the distal tubule. Urol Res. 1999;27(6):409–16.
11. Torous VF, Dodd LG, McIntire PJ, Jiang XS. Crystals and crystalloids in cytopathology: incidence and importance. Cancer Cytopathol. 2022;130(10):759–70.
12. Frochot V, Daudon M. Clinical value of crystalluria and quantitative morphoconstitutional analysis of urinary calculi. Int J Surg. 2016;36(Pt D):624–32.
13. Hoffman A, Braun MM, Khayat M. Kidney Disease: Kidney Stones. FP Essent. 2021;509: 33–8.
14. Rashidi B, Tongson-Ignacio JE. Melamed-Wolinska bodies in urine cytology an interesting aggregate in a degenerated urothelial cell. Diagn Cytopathol. 2011;39(2):117.
15. Ayra P, Khalbuss WE, Monaco SE, Pantanowitz L. Melamed-Wolinska bodies. Diagn Cytopathol. 2012;40(2):150–1.
16. Renshaw AA, Madge R, Granter SR. Intracytoplasmic eosinophilic inclusions (Melamed-Wolinska bodies). Association with metastatic transitional cell carcinoma in pleural fluid. Acta Cytol. 1997;41(4):995–8.
17. Chen H, Liu L, Pambuccian SE, Barkan GA, Quek ML, Wojcik EM. Urine cytology in monitoring recurrence in urothelial carcinoma after radical cystectomy and urinary diversion. Cancer Cytopathol. 2016;124(4):273–8.
18. Xing J, Roy S, Monaco SE, Pantanowitz L. Cytohistologic correlation of recurrent urothelial carcinoma detected in urinary diversion specimens. Cancer Cytopathol. 2017;125(2):120–7.
19. Singh HK, Bubendorf L, Mihatsch MJ, Drachenberg CB, Nickeleit V. Urine cytology findings of polyomavirus infections. Adv Exp Med Biol. 2006;577:201–12.
20. Ramos E, Drachenberg CB, Wali R, Hirsch HH. The decade of polyomavirus BK-associated nephropathy: state of affairs. Transplantation. 2009;87(5):621–30.
21. Batal I, Franco ZM, Shapiro R, et al. Clinicopathologic analysis of patients with BK viruria and rejection-like graft dysfunction. Hum Pathol. 2009;40(9):1312–9.
22. Xing J, Procop GW, Reynolds JP, Chiesa-Vottero A, Zhang Y. Diagnostic utility of urine cytology in early detection of polyomavirus in transplant patients. J Am Soc Cytopathol. 2017;6(1):28–32.

23. Chantziantoniou N, Joudeh AA, Hamed RMA, Al-Abbadi MA. Significance, cytomorphology of decoy cells in polyomavirus-associated nephropathy: review of clinical, histopathological, and virological correlates with commentary. J Am Soc Cytopathol. 2016;5(2):71–85.
24. Allison DB, Olson MT, Lilo M, Zhang ML, Rosenthal DL, VandenBussche CJ. Should the BK polyomavirus cytopathic effect be best classified as atypical or benign in urine cytology specimens? Cancer Cytopathol. 2016;124(6):436–42.
25. Takashi M, Schenck U, Koshikawa T, Nakashima N, Ohshima S. Cytological changes induced by intravesical bacillus Calmette-Guérin therapy for superficial bladder cancer. Urol Int. 2000;64(2):74–81.
26. Nguyen L, Nilforoushan N, Krane JF, Bose S, Bakkar R. Should "suspicious for high-grade urothelial carcinoma" and "positive for high-grade urothelial carcinoma" remain separate categories? Cancer Cytopathol 2021;129(2):156–163.
27. Beyer-Boon ME, Cuypers LH, de Voogt HJ, Brussee JA. Cytological changes due to urinary calculi: a consideration of the relationship between calculi and the development of urothelial carcinoma. Br J Urol. 1978;50(2):81–9.
28. Kannan V, Gupta D, Calculus artifact. A challenge in urinary cytology. Acta Cytol. 1999;43(5):794–800.
29. Onur I, Rosenthal DL, VandenBussche CJ. Benign-appearing urothelial tissue fragments in noninstrumented voided urine specimens are associated with low rates of urothelial neoplasia. Cancer Cytopathol. 2015;123(3):180–5.
30. Wojcik EM, Kurtycz DFI, Rosenthal DL. We'll always have Paris the Paris system for reporting urinary cytology 2022. J Am Soc Cytopathol. 2022;11(2):62–6.
31. Kannan V, Bose S. Low grade transitional cell carcinoma and instrument artifact. A challenge in urinary cytology. Acta Cytol. 1993;37(6):899–902.
32. Raab SS, Lenel JC, Cohen MB. Low grade transitional cell carcinoma of the bladder. Cytologic diagnosis by key features as identified by logistic regression analysis. Cancer. 1994;74(5):1621–6.
33. Zhang ML, Rosenthal DL, VandenBussche CJ. The cytomorphological features of low-grade urothelial neoplasms vary by specimen type. Cancer Cytopathol. 2016;124(8):552–64.
34. Bansal S, Pathuthara S, Joseph S, Dighe S, Menon S, Desai SB. Is diagnosis of low-grade urothelial carcinoma possible in urine cytology? J Cytol. 2021;38(2):64–8.
35. Chandler JB, Colunga M, Celli R, Lithgow MY, Baldassarri RJ. Applicability of the Paris system for veterans: high rates of undiagnosed low-grade urothelial neoplasia. J Am Soc Cytopathol. 2021;10(4):357–65.

Chapter 3
Cervical and Vaginal Cytology

Tong Sun and Syed M. Gilani

The Bethesda system provides a uniform reporting system for cervical cytology specimens. Recommended adequacy for liquid-based preparation is at least 5000 squamous cells, and for conventional smears is between 8000 and 12,000 squamous cells [1] (Fig. 3.1).

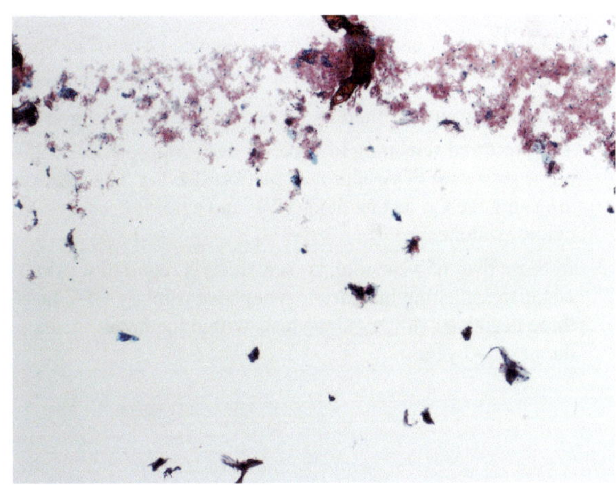

Fig. 3.1 Unsatisfactory for evaluation due to lack of sufficient squamous component (ThinPrep × 40)

T. Sun (✉)
Department of Pathology, Yale School of Medicine, New Haven, CT, USA
e-mail: tong.sun@yale.edu

S. M. Gilani
Department of Pathology, Albany Medical Center, Albany Medical College,
Albany, NY, USA

S. M. Gilani, G. Cai (eds.), *Non-Neoplastic Cytology*,
https://doi.org/10.1007/978-3-031-44289-6_3

Different Preparations and Screening Procedures [2] (Table 3.1)

Two commonly used techniques for collecting Pap smears are liquid-based and conventional.

- Conventional Smear
  Often obtained using the combination of a spatula and brush.
- Liquid-Based Cytology
  It can provide the opportunity to prepare duplicate slides and cell blocks and the option of additional testing, including HPV, *chlamydia*, and gonorrhea. It is also a substrate for automated screening devices.

  - *ThinPrep* uses a methanol-based preservative solution (PreservCyt Solution). The preparation method involves dispersion, and cell collection, followed by cell transfer to slides.
  - *SurePath* uses an ethanol-based preservative solution. The preparation method involves vortexing, disaggregation, and transfer to a sedimentation tube, and a pallet is obtained, sedimentation by gravity, followed by cell deposition and Papanicolaou staining.

Table 3.1 Cervical cancer screening guidance (American Society for Colposcopy and Cervical Pathology 2021) [3]

1.	In an age group less than 25 years, no screening is suggested
2.	The preferred screening method for age groups between 25 and 65 years is HPV testing alone (using an FDA-approved platform) every 5 years. However, other acceptable options are using the Co-test method (HPV and cytology) every 5 years or every 3 years with cytology alone
3.	In those over 65 years old, no screening is required if prior screening is negative. This negative screening includes two negative primary HPV tests, or two negative co-tests, or three negative cytology alone tests within the last 10 years (with the most recent test within the past 3–5 years)

Normal Elements (Superficial, Intermediate, Parabasal, and Navicular) [1, 4]

- Squamous cells include basal cells, parabasal cells, and intermediate cells.

    Basal cells are usually small cells along the basement membrane and resemble small histocytes, as seen in the atrophic specimen primarily as syncytial aggregates.

    Parabasal cells are the first to acquire squamous features, dense cytoplasm, and distinct cell boundaries. In addition, they have moderately abundant cytoplasm and round to oval nuclei. Parabasal cell predominates in atrophic specimens and can also be seen in postpartum conditions or related to the intake of oral contraception (progesterone).

    Intermediate cells provide essential nuclear size reference (average 35mm^2, the size of a red blood cell). Intermediate cells have abundant and transparent cytoplasm. Any squamous nucleus significantly larger and more hyperchromatic than an intermediate cell is likely a dysplastic cell.

    Superficial cells have pyknotic nuclei and delicate transparent cytoplasm.
- Endocervical cells are cohesive fat sheets or strips of uniform cells, appearing "honeycomb" pattern (opposing view) or "picket fence" pattern (side view). The cell shape (nuclei and cytoplasm) can be tall columnar and may have abundant mucinous cytoplasm.

    Reactive endocervical cells can have significant nuclear enlargement, hyperchromasia, and prominent nucleoli but maintain smooth nuclear membranes and fine chromatin, abundant cytoplasm with distinct cell borders, low nuclear/cytoplasmic ratios, and without crowding or overlapping [5]. In addition, they can show binucleation or multinucleation and should not be confused with herpes virus changes.
- Endometrial cells.

    Exfoliated endometrial cells can be seen if a Pap sample is taken during the first 12 days of the menstrual cycle. Morphologically, they appear as a spherical cluster, small cells with a dark nucleus and scant cytoplasm. They are associated with menstrual cycle changes, endometrial pathology (such as endometritis, endometrial polyps, or neoplasia), and exogenous changes (intrauterine devices, IUDs, and others). Exodus represents a group of endometrial cells with endometrial stroma (darker area) in the center surrounded by endometrial glandular cells (Fig. 3.2). Directly sampled endometrial cells present large and small tissue fragments with a combination of glands and stroma.

    Endometrial cells are needed to be reported in women 45 years of age or older. The differential diagnoses of exfoliated endometrial cells include high-grade intraepithelial lesion (HSIL), squamous cell carcinoma, adenocarcinoma in situ (AIS), endometrial carcinoma and rarely a small cell carcinoma.

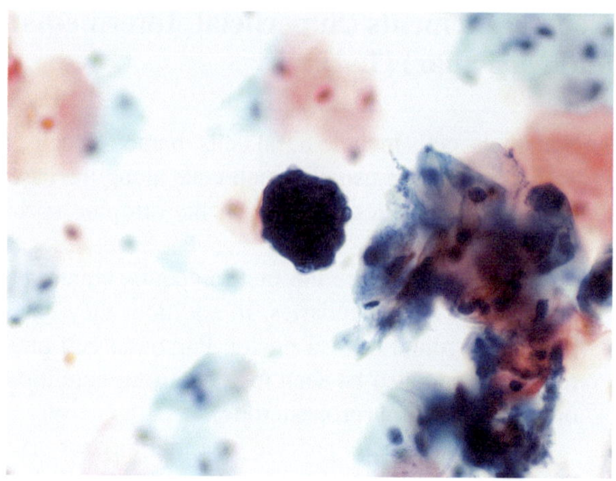

Fig. 3.2 Cluster of endometrial cells with dark central area and lighter periphery (SurePath × 400)

Benign Findings [1, 4] (Table 3.2)

- Parakeratosis is a benign reactive change caused by chronic irritation. It usually shows keratinized squamous cells with dense organophilic cytoplasm and small pyknotic nuclei. However, if nuclear atypia is present, then the term "atypical parakeratosis" is used and categorized as "epithelial cell abnormality" such as ASCUS (atypical squamous intraepithelial lesion) or SIL (squamous intraepithelial lesion), depending on the extent of the abnormality.
- Hyperkeratosis is a benign response of stratified squamous epithelium due to chronic mucosal irritation, as in uterine prolapse. Squamous cells manifested as anucleate, mature, polygonal isolated cells or plaques of tightly adherent isolated cells. Differential diagnosis includes contaminated cells of the skin.
- Atrophic changes happen in late post-menopause (Fig. 3.3), postpartum (Fig. 3.4), lactation, and childhood (except newborn). Atrophic changes can show nuclear enlargement with mild hyperchromasia. However, the nuclear membrane is still uniform, and the chromatin is evenly distributed but often smudgy. There are usually syncytial groups of parabasal cells and may show background inflammation and cell degeneration. A granular basophilic background may be present, and mummified parabasal cells, "blue blobs," can be evident. The differential diagnosis includes endometrial cells, HSIL, or malignancy.
- Pregnancy-related changes include a predominance of intermediate cells and an increase in navicular cells (glycogenated intermediate cells). Other changes and cell types seen in pregnancy are as follows: Syncytiotrophoblastic cells, decidual cells, arias-stella reaction, and cockleburs.

Table 3.2 Differential diagnosis of benign findings in Pap smears

	Differential diagnosis
Atrophy	HSIL Endometrial cells
IUD-related changes	Atypical glandular cells or adenocarcinoma, ASC-H, or HSIL
Pregnancy-related changes	Arias-Stella reaction: Clear cell carcinoma Decidual cells: Squamous intraepithelial lesion (ASCUS or LSIL) Syncytiotrophoblasts: Herpes infection (Fig. 3.11)
Hormone-related changes	Atrophy, HSIL
Repair	Squamous cell carcinoma
Radiation changes	LSIL, malignancy
Endometrial cells	HSIL, atypical glandular cells, or AIS
Lower uterine segment	Atypical glandular cells
Metaplastic cells	ASC-H or HSIL
Glandular cells post hysterectomy	Atypical glandular cells or well-differentiated adenocarcinoma
Follicular cervicitis	Endometrial cells, ASC-H or HSIL, lymphoma

HSIL high-grade squamous intraepithelial lesion, *ASC-H* atypical squamous cells cannot exclude high grade squamous intraepithelial lesion, *IUD* intrauterine device, *LSIL* low-grade squamous intraepithelial lesion

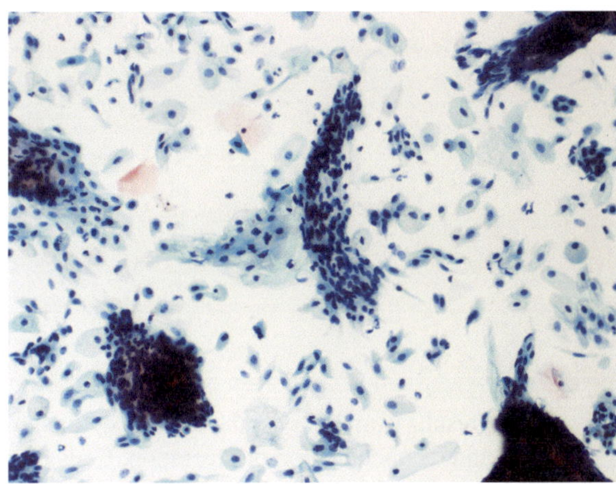

Fig. 3.3 Syncytial groups of parabasal cells suggesting atrophy (SurePath × 200)

- Syncytiotrophoblastic cells are rare findings on Pap smears and may be associated with history of pregnancy. They are large cells with abundant cytoplasm and multiple nuclei.
- Decidual cells are isolated cells with abundant granular cytoplasm, a large vesicular nucleus, and a prominent nucleolus.
- Arias-Stella reaction shows nuclear enlargement, pleomorphism, and hyperchromasia. They have abundant vacuolated cytoplasm without any increase in mitosis and can mimic clear cell carcinoma. It is usually due to hormonal stimulation from pregnancies or trophoblastic disease.

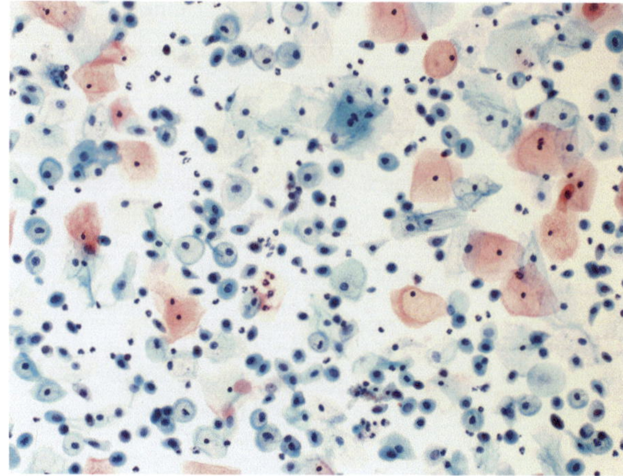

Fig. 3.4 Postpartum changes includes more parabasal cells and less superficial cells (SurePath × 400)

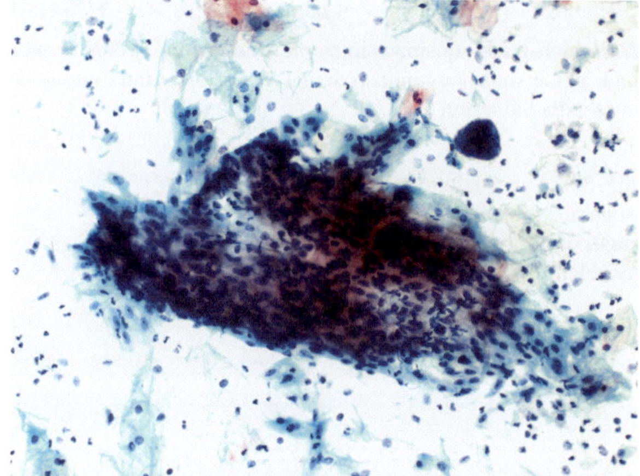

Fig. 3.5 Reactive cellular changes with streaming sheet of cells (ThinPrep × 200)

- Repair

  - Repair results from injury to the cervical epithelium, the proliferation of reserve cells, and reepithelization of ulceration. Cells maintain a uniform polarity that gives the sheets the appearance of streaming or being pulled out, with large nuclei with marked size variation and prominent nucleolus, sometimes irregular in shape (Fig. 3.5). Often, background inflammation can be seen.

- IUD-related changes

  - The characteristic of IUD effect includes the combination of two types of cells a vacuolated cell (Fig. 3.6) and a small dark cell with scant cytoplasm. Sometimes reparative changes are also present, and the background is inflamed. IUD changes may also include reactive changes and inflammation, bacterial vaginosis, and actinomyces [6] (Fig. 3.7). Reactive changes are more prominent in glandular cells and may stimulate an "atypical glandular cells" diagnosis [6].

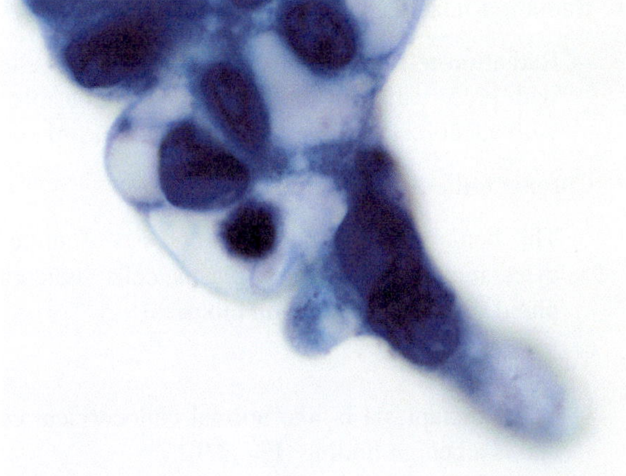

Fig. 3.6 IUD changes include vacuolated cells with large nuclei (ThinPrep × 600)

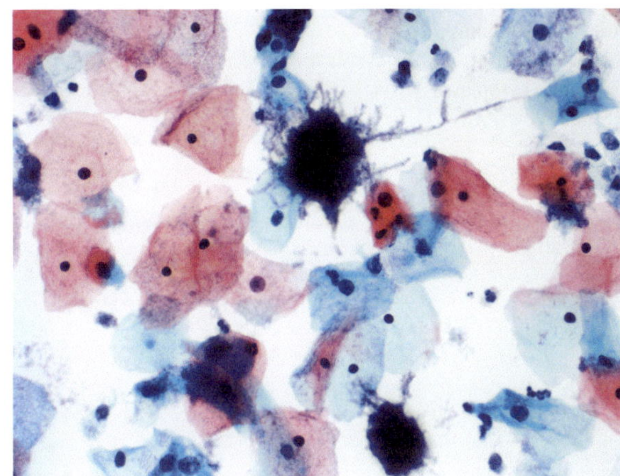

Fig. 3.7 Actinomyces forming a ball-like structure with peripheral filamentous protrusions (SurePath × 400)

- Hormone-related changes

  - The squamous epithelium of the cervix and vagina responds to various stimuli, especially hormones. Estrogen stimulation results in the predominance of a superficial layer. The progesterone effect shows a predominance of intermediate cells. Lack of estrogen effect may result in atrophic pattern smears, which can show a predominance of parabasal cells [7].

- Maturation index: It measures the relationship between the three layers of squamous epithelium (parabasal layer, intermediate cell layer, and superficial layer). The maturation index ratio with the right shift shows an estrogen effect (0/5/95), while the left shift is usually seen in atrophic pattern smears (95/5/0). The mid-zone increase suggests a progesterone effect with an increase in the intermediate cell layer (0/95/5).

- Radiation-related changes

  - Radiation-related changes can show marked cellular and nuclear enlargement with preservation of the nuclear-to-cytoplasmic ratio, abundant cytoplasmic with vacuolization (Fig. 3.8), and cytoplasmic polychromasia.

- Chronic follicular cervicitis

  - This benign reactive condition consists of numerous polymorphous lympho-cytes, including occasional plasma cells, indicating follicular cervicitis (lymphoid follicle formation on biopsies).

- Tubal metaplasia

  - Tubal metaplasia is like normal endocervical cells, except for having cilia, and is a benign finding (Fig. 3.9).

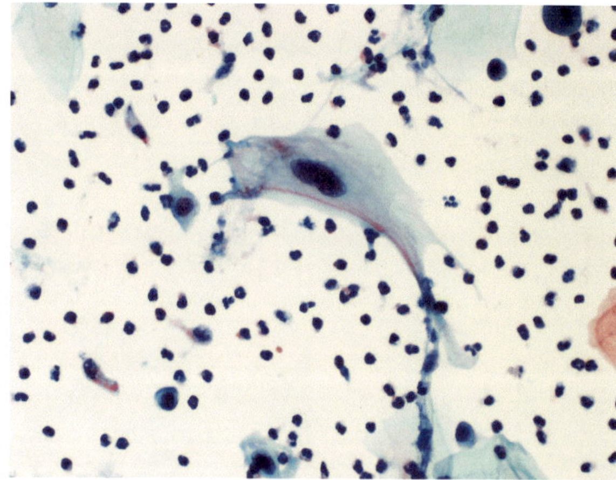

Fig. 3.8 Radiation changes with abundant cytoplasm (SurePath × 400)

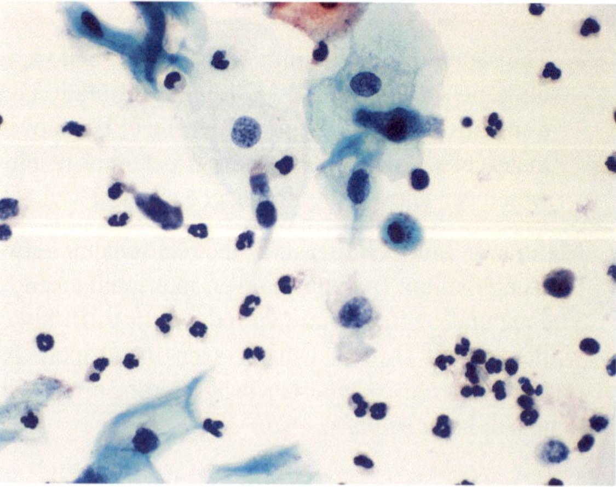

Fig. 3.9 Tubal metaplasia with ciliated epithelial cells (SurePath × 600)

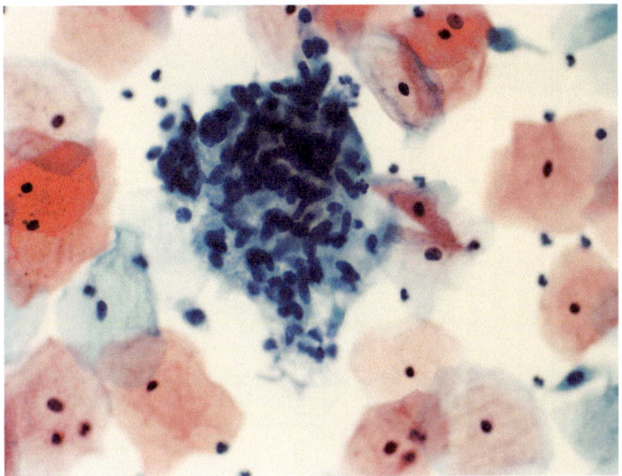

Fig. 3.10 Collection of histiocytes, forming a vaguely formed granuloma (SurePath × 400)

- Glandular cells post-hysterectomy
- Glandular cells post hysterectomy present in a very low subset of vaginal Paps from women who had a total hysterectomy and are benign and usually metaplastic. They resemble normal endocervical cells.
- Other reactive changes:

  - Other reactive changes such as histiocytic collection or granulomatous-type inflammation can be seen (Fig. 3.10).

Organisms and the Pap Test [8]

- Normal Flora and Cytolysis.

  - The vagina epithelium is colonized by Gram-positive, rod-shaped bacteria (*Lactobacillus*), which produce lactic acid, reduce the ambient pH, and may cause cytolysis. *Lactobacillus* can form long rods and mimic fungi or other bacteria.

- Other Organisms and Specific Infections.

  - The common causative viral, bacterial, fungal, and parasite were summarized in Table 3.3.

Table 3.3 Cytomorphologic features, cytomorphologic mimics and molecular studies of common organisms seen on cervical Pap specimens

Microorganisms	Cytomorphology	Differential diagnosis	Ancillary tests
Viruses			
HPV	LSIL: Koilocytosis with perinuclear clearing, nuclear enlargement, nuclear membrane irregularity, hyperchromasia, and binucleation. HSIL: Nuclear membrane irregularity scant cytoplasm, hyperchromasia, nuclear membrane irregularity	Reactive changes or glycogenated cells can mimic LSIL. Parabasal/basal cells may mimic HSIL	Molecular studies: Hybrid capture II assay, Cervista HPV tests, APTIMA HPV assay, Cobas HPV tests DNA and RNA in situ hybridization studies P16 immunostain
HSV	Triad of multinucleation, margination, and molding (Fig. 3.11); background with inflammation and ulceration	Reactive epithelial changes, multinucleated endocervical cells, and radiation changes	PCR on fluids Immunostains for HSV-1 and HSV-2
CMV	Nuclear enlargement, margination, large intranuclear inclusion with a surrounding halo, and small cytoplasmic inclusions	Reactive epithelial changes from ulceration, herpes infection	PCR on fluids; immunostain
Bacteria			
Actinomyces	Gram-positive; thin long filamentous, bacterial forms a ball-like structure with peripheral protrusion of filaments; sulfur granules may be seen	More commonly seen in patients with IUDs *Nocardia* spp., other bacteria or fungi	Not routinely performed
Neisseria gonorrhea [12]	Gram-negative diplococci	Other bacteria	PCR on fluids
Gardnerella vaginalis	A shift in flora: Short bacilli (coccobacilli), curved bacilli, or mixed bacteria; "clue cells" (Fig. 3.12)	Actinomyces	Vaginal pH The amine-odor "whiff" test after addition of potassium hydroxide [KOH]
Leptothrix	Long filamentous bacteria (Fig. 3.13) can be associated with *trichomonas*	Candida	Not routinely performed
Fungal			
Candida	Budding yeast form; may contain true or Pseudohyphae (Fig. 3.14)	Other yeast form fungi	Not routinely performed
Parasite			
Trichomonas vaginalis (Fig. 3.15)	Extracellular flagellated protozoa, pear-shaped; 15–30 µm, red cytoplasmic granules, eccentric nucleus, reactive changes that can mimic koilocytosis	LSIL	*Wet-mount microscopy, rapid antigen-testing* PCR on fluids

Fig. 3.11 Herpes viral changes with multinucleation, margination, and molding (SurePath × 600)

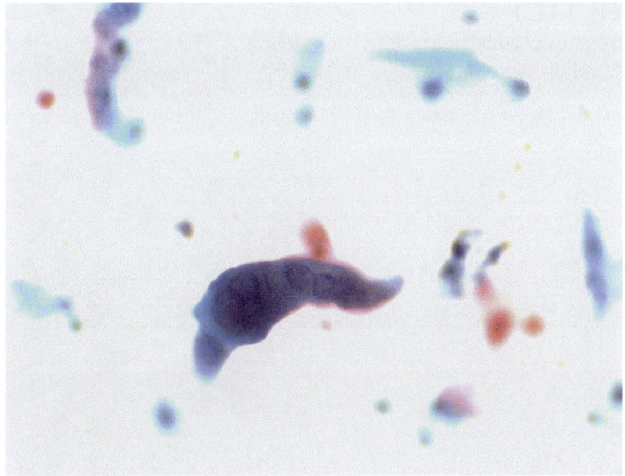

Fig. 3.12 Bacterial colonies on squamous cells "clue cell" (SurePath × 400)

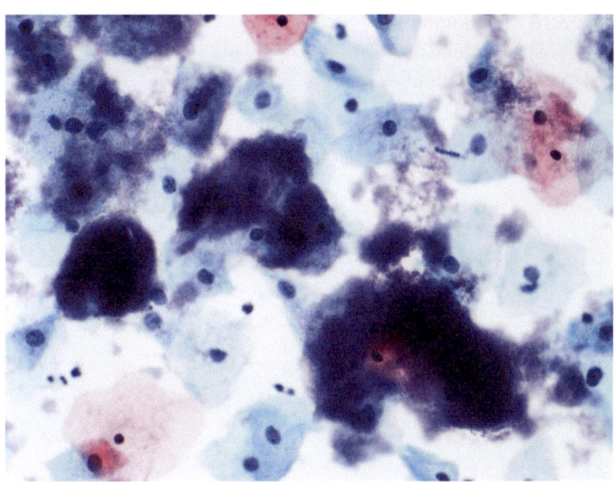

Fig. 3.13 Leptothrix. Long filamentous bacteria (ThinPrep × 200)

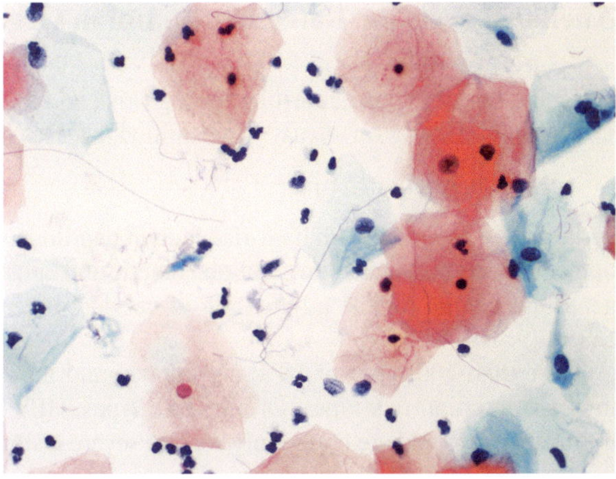

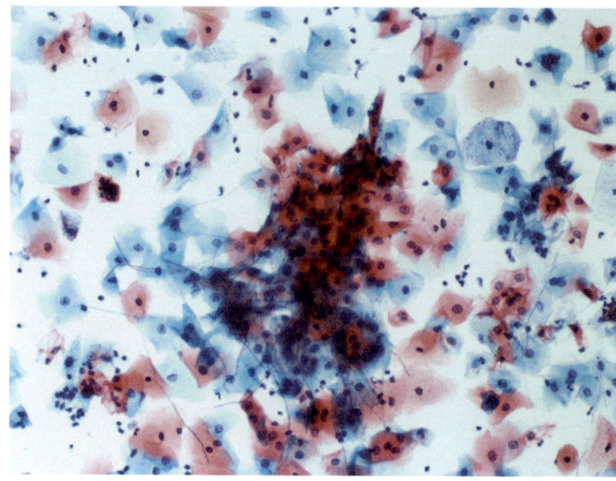

Fig. 3.14 Fungal organisms consistent with Candida (SurePath × 200)

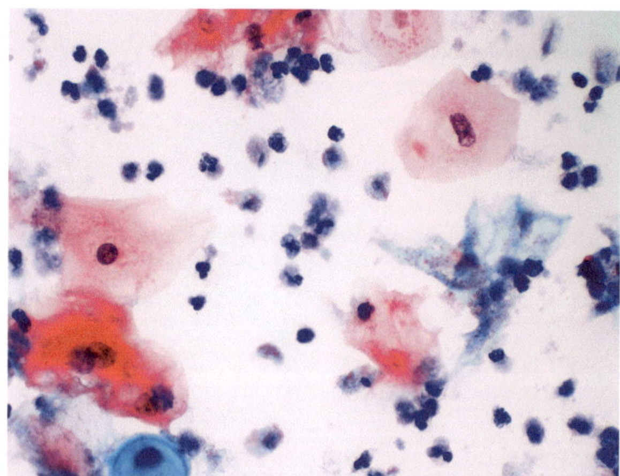

Fig. 3.15 Trichomonas. Pear-shaped organism with red cytoplasmic granules (SurePath × 600)

Ancillary Tests for Detecting Common Organisms in Cervix

- Liquid-based molecular testing for high-risk and low-risk HPV genotype.
- Molecular testing for sexually transmitted diseases (Table 3.3).

  - Human Papilloma virus:

Persistent infection with high-risk human papillomavirus can result in the development of cervical cancer. In addition, genetic and epigenetic alterations in host cell genes are crucial for the progression of cervical precancerous lesions to invasive cancer [9, 10].

More than 100 types of HPV are known, and they are further subdivided into low-risk and high-risk types. Of high-risk types, HPV16 and HPV18 are the most important types and are commonly seen in severe lesions.

According to protein expression during the viral cycle, two functional genome regions have been identified: (1) an early genes region, encoding E1, E2, E4, E5, E6, and E7, and (2) a two late genes region, encoding the major (L1) and minor (L2) capsid proteins [11].

The viral proteins E6 and E7 are overexpressed and block apoptosis and uncouple cell growth arrest by inactivating p53 and pRb, respectively. The inactivation of pRb by E7 forces infected cells to remain proliferative, stimulates the S-phase gene, and fails to stop the cell cycle. This accumulation of DNA damage, centrosome abnormalities, and chromosomal segregation defects eventually leads to genomic instability and carcinogenesis.

Table 3.4 Artifacts, contaminates, and miscellaneous findings features in Pap smears

Findings	Causes/Subcategories	Features
Artifact		
Cornflaking [13]	Air trapped on superficial squamous cells (Fig. 3.16)	Refractile brown or black artifact which obscures nuclear details
Cockleburs [14]	Can be seen in pregnancy but also without pregnancy such as in women with IUDs	Refractile crystalline structures surrounded by inflammatory cells/histocytes (Fig. 3.17)
Contaminates		
Airborne fungal spores [15]		
	Alternaria	Brown pigmented structure
	Aspergillus	Characteristic "fruiting body," septate hyphae with acute angle branching
Pollen grains [16]	Microscopic masculine cells that come from flower-bearing plants	Mono or multilayer cell wall May be mistaken for protozoa cysts or SIL
Vegetable cells [16] (Fig. 3.18)		May be mistaken for abnormal cells or certain microorganisms
Miscellaneous findings		
Psammoma bodies [17]	Associate with a benign condition in more than half of cases. Clinical and imaging correlation to search for a neoplastic process (such as *Mullerian tumors*)	Concentrically laminated calcifications (Fig. 3.19)
Collagen balls	Commonly seen in serous body cavity fluid but rarely reported in Pap [18]	Translucent blue-green, spheroid hyalinized collagen bodies
Hematoidin crystals [19]	Can be seen in pregnancy or postpartum conditions	Needle shaped brown crystalline material forming rosette-like structure
Blue blobs [20]	Condensed mucus-like material or degenerated nuclei (cyanophilic bodies), seen in some atrophic smears. Should not be interpreted as significant abnormality	Calcifications, HSIL

Fig. 3.16 Cornflaking. Brown refractile artifact due to air trapping (ThinPrep × 200)

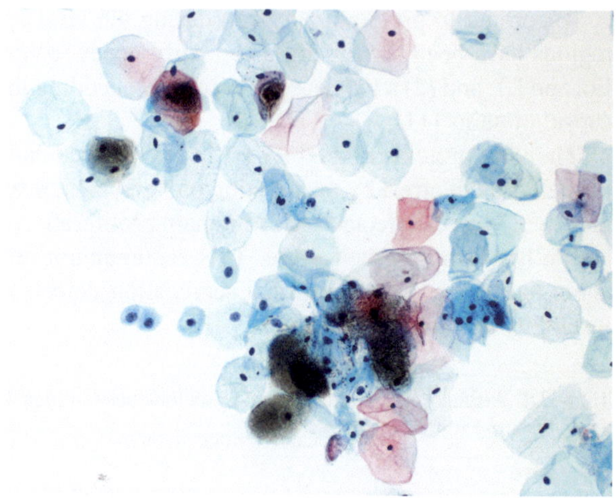

Fig. 3.17 Cockleburs. Refractile crystalline structures surrounded by histocytes (SurePath × 400)

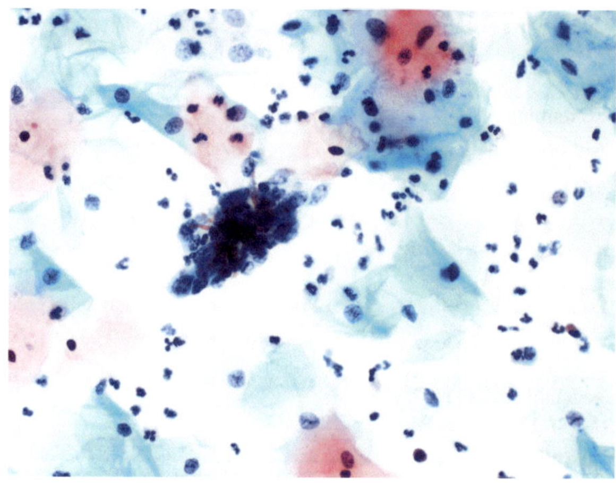

Fig. 3.18 Vegetable material (SurePath × 400)

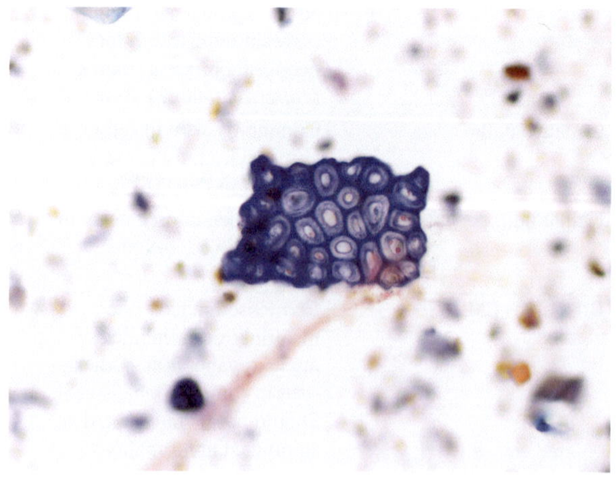

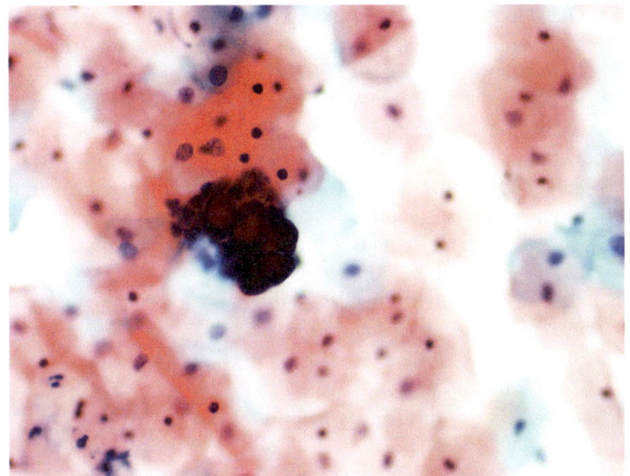

Fig. 3.19 Psammoma calcifications (SurePath × 400)

Acknowledgments None.

Conflict of Interest None.

References

1. Nayar R, Wilbur DC. The pap test and Bethesda 2014. Cancer Cytopathol. 2015;123(5):271–81.
2. Makde MM, Sathawane P. Liquid-based cytology: technical aspects. Cytojournal. 2022;14(19):41.
3. Marcus JZ, Cason P, Downs LS Jr, Einstein MH, Flowers L. The ASCCP cervical cancer screening task force endorsement and opinion on the American Cancer Society updated cervical cancer screening guidelines. J Low Genit Tract Dis. 2021;25(3):187–91.
4. Kamal M, Topiwala F. Nonneoplastic Cervical Cytology. Cytojournal. 2022;29(19):25.
5. Pulkkinen J, Huhtala H, Krogerus LA, Hollmén S, Laurila M, Kholová I. Endocervical cytology: inter- and intra-observer variability in conventional pap smears. Acta Cytol. 2022;66(3):206–15.
6. Bariş İİ, Keleş AN. Mardin Bölgesinden Verilerle Servikal Sitolojide RIA Etkisine Bir Bakış [A review on the impact of IUD in cervical cytology: Mardin region data]. Turk Patoloji Derg. 2013;29(1):51–7.
7. Demay RM. The pap test: exfoliative gynecologic cytology. 1st ed. American Society for Clinical Pathology; 2005.
8. Fitzhugh VA, Heller DS. Significance of a diagnosis of microorganisms on pap smear. J Low Genit Tract Dis. 2008;12(1):40–51.
9. Crosbie EJ, Einstein MH, Franceschi S, Kitchener HC. Human papillomavirus and cervical cancer. Lancet. 2013;382(9895):889–99.
10. Schiffman M, Castle PE, Jeronimo J, Rodriguez AC, Wacholder S. Human papillomavirus and cervical cancer. Lancet. 2007;370(9590):890–907.
11. McBride AA. Mechanisms and strategies of papillomavirus replication. Biol Chem. 2017;398:919–27.
12. Chernesky M, Freund GG, Hook E 3rd, Leone P, D'Ascoli P, Martens M. Detection of chlamydia trachomatis and Neisseria gonorrhoeae infections in north American women by testing SurePath liquid-based pap specimens in APTIMA assays. J Clin Microbiol. 2007;45(8):2434–8.

13. Okayama K, Ishii Y, Fujii M, Oda M, Okodo M. Causation of cornflake artifacts: possible association of poor dehydration with drying before mounting in Papanicolaou stain. Diagn Cytopathol. 2022;50(10):E301–5.
14. Kapila K, Al-Juwaiser A, Haji BE. Crystalline bodies in pap smear: a forgotten entity. Diagn Cytopathol. 2007;35(7):423.
15. Martínez-Girón R, Ribas-Barceló A, García-Miralles MT, López-Cabanilles D, Tamargo-Peláez ML, Torre-Bayón C, Fernández-Alvarez L. Airborne fungal spores, pollen grains, and vegetable cells in routine Papanicolaou smears. Diagn Cytopathol. 2004;30(6):381–5.
16. Rivasi F, Tosi G, Ruozi B, Curatola C. Vegetable cells in Papanicolaou-stained cervical smears. Diagn Cytopathol. 2006;34(1):45–9.
17. Zreik TG, Rutherford TJ. Psammoma bodies in cervicovaginal smears. Obstet Gynecol. 2001;97(5 Pt 1):693–5.
18. Szporn A, Chen X, Wu M, Burnstein DE. Collagen balls in cervica-vaginal smears. Acta Cytol. 2005;49(3):262–4.
19. Thakur A, Sarin H. Hematoidin crystals in pap smear: a revisit. Diagn Cytopathol. 2020;48(1):92.
20. Abdulla M, Hombal S, Kanbour A, Becich M, Stankovich D, Ries A, Kanbour-Shakir A. Characterizing "blue blobs". Immunohistochemical staining and ultrastructural study. Acta Cytol. 2000;44(4):547–50.

Chapter 4
Peritoneal Washings and Ovary

Tong Sun and Syed M. Gilani

Peritoneal Washings

- Benign findings and immunohistochemical study [1, 2].

  - Mesothelial cells are arranged in flat sheets (Fig. 4.1) with some space ("windows") between each cell. They have round or oval nuclei and a moderate amount of cytoplasm. Immunochemistry study shows positive mesothelial markers such as calretinin (+), WT1(+), and cytokeratin 5/6 (+).
  - Collagen balls are spheres of collages surrounded by flattened mesothelial cells (Fig. 4.2), which are seen in up to 50% peritoneal washing. They have no known significance.
  - Histocytes usually are present as aggregates or as isolated cells. They have granular or vacuolated cytoplasm, oval or folded nuclei, and show immunoactivity for CD68 and CD163.
  - Skeletal and adipose tissue can occasionally be found in peritoneal washings. Detached ciliary tufts (Fig. 4.3), presumed from endosalpingiosis, can also be seen.

- Benign/reactive findings and their mimickers [3, 4].

  - Endometriosis is a potential diagnostic pitfall and is rarely diagnosed solely by peritoneal washing. All essential diagnostic elements should be present for definitive diagnosis, including hemosiderin-laden macrophages (Fig. 4.4)

T. Sun (✉)
Department of Pathology, Yale School of Medicine, New Haven, CT, USA
e-mail: tong.sun@yale.edu

S. M. Gilani
Department of Pathology, Albany Medical Center, Albany Medical College,
Albany, NY, USA

S. M. Gilani, G. Cai (eds.), *Non-Neoplastic Cytology*,
https://doi.org/10.1007/978-3-031-44289-6_4

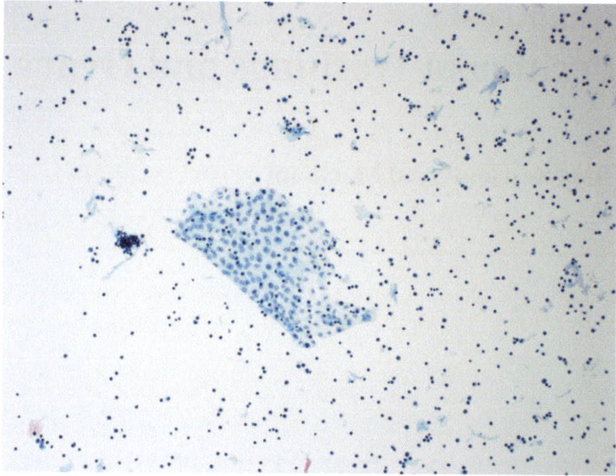

Fig. 4.1 Flat sheets of mesothelial cells are present (ThinPrep × 100)

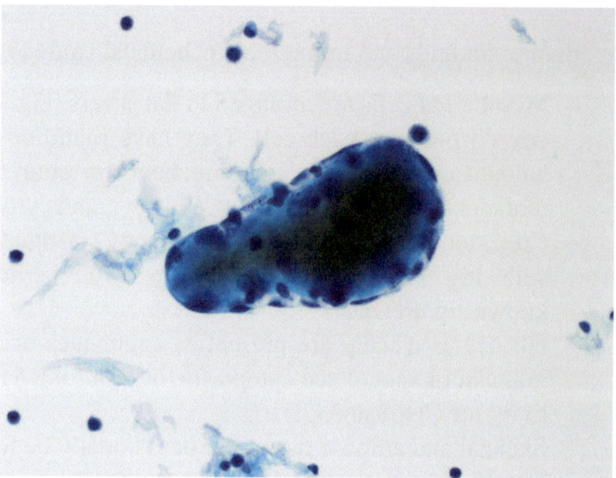

Fig. 4.2 Collagen ball (ThinPrep × 400)

or hemolyzed blood, endometrial epithelial cells, and endometrial stromal cells [5]. Additionally, the presence of glandular cells (endometrial cells) within the peritoneal washing may raise a differential diagnosis of malignancy, especially adenocarcinoma, which also stains positive for epithelial markers (Ber-Ep4 and Moc-31). In such cases, a cautious approach is advisable to avoid overinterpretation.

- Endosalpingiosis (Fig. 4.5) is present as benign ciliated epithelial cells with small nuclei and vacuolated cytoplasm in peritoneal washing. Association with psammoma bodies is common (Fig. 4.6). The differential diagnosis includes endometriosis and malignancy (Table 4.1).
- Peritoneal washing usually shows flat sheets of mesothelial cells, but frequently reactive mesothelial proliferations and hyperplasia can be seen, which can be diagnostically challenging. Reactive mesothelial proliferation can morphologically present as clusters, including papillary groups with promi-

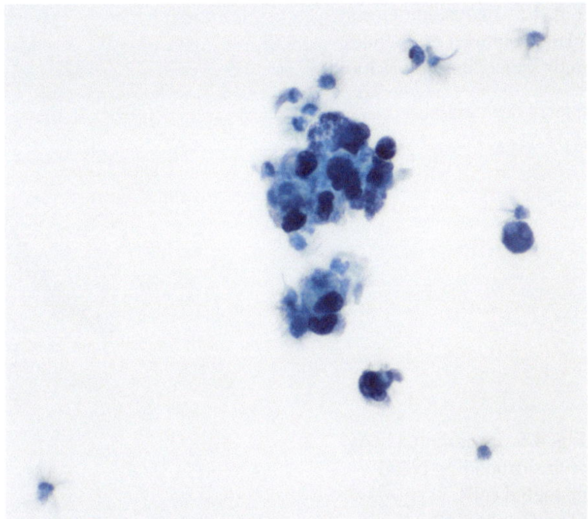

Fig. 4.3 Scattered detached ciliary tufts can be seen (ThinPrep × 600)

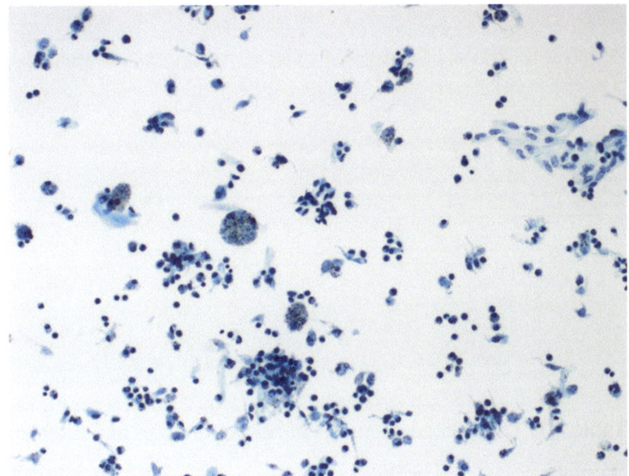

Fig. 4.4 Hemosiderin-laden histiocytes, few inflammatory cells and mesothelial cells are present (ThinPrep × 200)

nent nucleoli, and may show some atypia, multinucleation, cytoplasmic vacuoles, and occasionally psammoma bodies. Psammoma bodies are concentric lamination of calcification. The presence of psammoma bodies is not a sign of malignancy [6, 7]. However, it includes a list of differential diagnoses such as serous carcinoma, borderline serous tumors, serous cystadenoma, serous adenofibroma, benign mesothelial proliferation, endometriosis, and other Mullerian inclusion cysts.

- Artifacts

  - Mucoid-like material produced in surgical suction liner bags, made from thick opaque material, can mimic mucin. Diagnostically, it will pose more challenges if there is a prior history of the mucinous tumor.
  - Adhesion artifacts bring fibrin and histocytes in peritoneal washings.

Fig. 4.5 Endosalpingiosis: bland columnar epithelial cells seen (ThinPrep × 400)

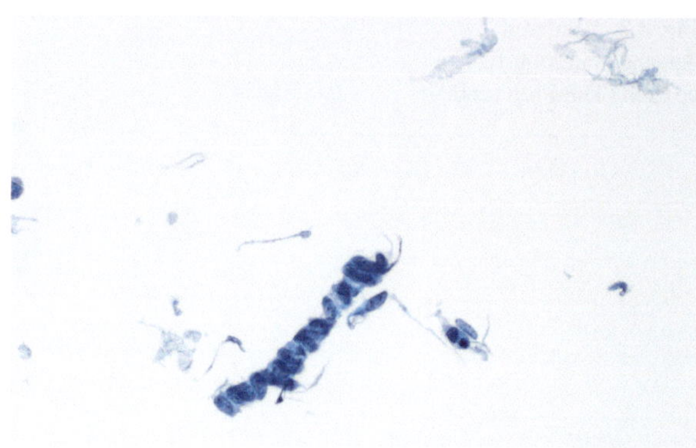

Fig. 4.6 Psammoma body with surrounding bland epithelial cells (ThinPrep × 400)

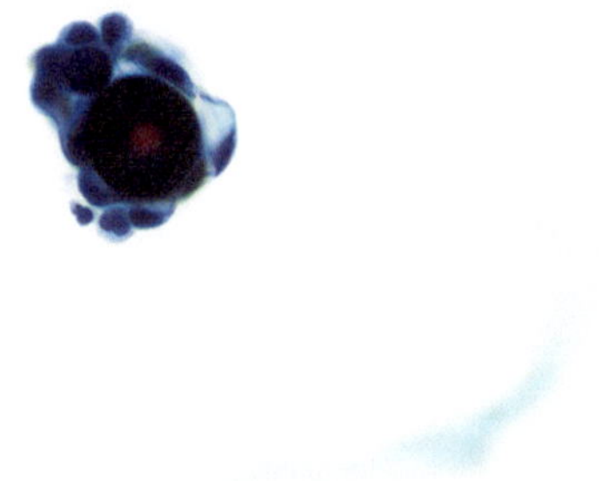

Table 4.1 Differential diagnosis of benign findings in peritoneal washings

Entities	Features	Differential diagnosis
Endometriosis	Presence of endometrial epithelial cells and/or stromal cells, histiocytes	Endosalpingiosis, Endometroid adenocarcinoma
Endosalpingiosis	Ciliated glandular epithelial cells	Endometriosis, reactive mesothelial hyperplasia, serous neoplasms, adenocarcinoma
Psammoma bodies	Concentric lamination of calcification	Endosalpingiosis, benign mesothelial proliferation, serous borderline tumor, and serous carcinoma
Reactive mesothelial cells	Cluster of cells with variable cytologic atypia	Mesothelioma Adenocarcinoma

Ovary

- Normal cytology [8, 9].

  - Ultrasound-guided fine needle aspiration (FNA) of cystic ovarian lesions occasionally is performed. This procedure is usually used to evaluate small, incidental cystic masses that appear benign on ultrasound or laparoscopic examination, tubo-ovarian abscesses, or rarely to confirm malignancy.
  - Ovarian cystic lesion FNA has variable sensitivity and false-negative rates, especially for borderline tumors [10].

- Non-neoplastic cysts [8–10].

  Follicle cyst, corpus luteum cyst, endometrioma, and paratubal cyst are non-neoplastic cystic lesions and cytomorphology features, and differential diagnosis are summarized in Table 4.2.

Table 4.2 Ovarian benign non-neoplastic cysts and differential diagnosis

Ovarian non-neoplastic cysts	Cytomorphological features	Differential diagnosis
Cystic follicle and follicle cyst	• Variable cellularity • Isolated cells and clusters of granulosa cells	Granulosa cell tumor
Corpus luteum cyst	• Variably cellular, cohesive aggregates of luteinized cells which have small dark nuclei and abundant foamy or granular cytoplasm with background hemosiderin laden macrophages	Granulosa cell tumor Endometriotic cyst
Endometriotic cyst	• Thick, chocolate-colored fluid (degenerative blood) is often only finding • Diagnostic triad: endometrial epithelial cells and stroma cells, hemosiderin laden macrophages	Endometroid adenocarcinoma
Simple ovarian and paratubal cyst	Sparsely cellular, mostly of macrophages and a few degenerated epithelial cells in sheets with round to oval nuclei, fine chromatin, and inconspicuous nucleoli	Follicle cyst Hydrosalpinx

Acknowledgments None.

Conflict of Interest None.

References

1. Zuna RE. Diagnostic cytopathology of peritoneal washings. Cytojournal. 2022;19:9.
2. Schulte JJ, Lastra RR. Abdominopelvic washings in gynecologic pathology: A comprehensive review. Diagn Cytopathol. 2016;44:1039–57.
3. Selvaggi SM. Diagnostic pitfalls of peritoneal washing cytology and the role of cell blocks in their diagnosis. Diagn Cytopathol. 2003;28:335–41.
4. Yu GH, Song SJ. Cytology of benign peritoneal fluids and pelvic washing specimens: diagnostic cytomorphologic features and pitfalls. Acta Cytol. 2023;10:1–9.
5. Cantley RL, Yoxtheimer L, Molnar S. The role of peritoneal washings in the diagnosis of endometriosis. Diagn Cytopathol. 2018;46:447–51.
6. Sun T, Pitman MB, Torous VF. Determining the significance of psammoma bodies in pelvic washings: a 10-year retrospective review. Cancer Cytopathol. 2021;129:83–9.
7. Parwani AV, Chan TY, Ali SZ. Significance of psammoma bodies in serous cavity fluid: a cytopathologic analysis. Cancer. 2004;102:87–91.
8. Zhou AG, Levinson KL, Rosenthal DL, VandenBussche CJ. Performance of ovarian cyst fluid fine-needle aspiration cytology. Cancer Cytopathol. 2018;126:112–21.
9. Gupta N, Rajwanshi A, Dhaliwal LK, Khandelwal N, Dey P, Srinivasan R, Nijhawan R. Fine needle aspiration cytology in ovarian lesions: an institutional experience of 584 cases. Cytopathology. 2012;23:300–7.
10. Papathanasiou K, Giannoulis C, Dovas D, Tolikas A, Tantanasis T, Tzafettas JM. Fine needle aspiration cytology of the ovary: is it reliable? Clin Exp Obstet Gynecol. 2004;31:191–3.

Chapter 5
Body Cavity Fluid Cytology

Minhua Wang

Serous effusion is excessive fluid accumulation in the pleural, pericardial, and peritoneal cavities. All serous effusions are pathological processes resulting from a variety of causes, which can be either malignant or benign [1]. Needle aspiration of fluid from the thorax (thoracocentesis), peritoneal cavity (abdominal paracentesis), or pericardial cavity (pericardiocentesis) is a minimally invasive procedure, and serous effusions can be analyzed cytologically to offer clinical information with minimal risk to patients.

Clinically, effusions are classified as transudative or exudative, and the distinction between these two categories has therapeutic implications. Transudative effusions are caused by an imbalance between hydrostatic and oncotic pressures, while an exudative effusion is defined when one or more of the following conditions are met: [1] Fluid protein/serum protein level is greater than 0.5; [2] Fluid lactate dehydrogenase (LDH)/serum LDH level is greater than 0.6; or [3] Fluid LDH concentration is higher than 200 IU/L (or greater than 67% of the upper normal limit for serum LDH) [2]. Table 5.1 summarizes the distinction between transudates and exudates.

Most effusions are benign. The most common causes of pleural effusion are infection, congestive heart failure, hemodynamic disturbances, pneumonia, pulmonary embolism, and cancer [1, 3, 4]. Most peritoneal effusions, i.e., ascites, are transudates. Liver cirrhosis is the most prevalent cause, accounting for 75% of ascites, followed by malignancy (10%), heart failure (3%), tuberculosis (2%), and pancreatitis (1%) [5]. Most pericardial effusions, on the other hand, are exudates, usually resulting from damage to the pericardial membrane, such as through infection, autoimmune disease, or malignancy. Lastly, pericardial transudates are caused by congestive heart failure, renal insufficiency, and hypoalbuminemia [6].

M. Wang (✉)
Department of Pathology, Yale School of Medicine, New Haven, CT, USA
e-mail: minhua.wang@yale.edu

S. M. Gilani, G. Cai (eds.), *Non-Neoplastic Cytology*,
https://doi.org/10.1007/978-3-031-44289-6_5

Table 5.1 Differential diagnosis of transudates vs. exudates [2]

	Transudates	Exudates
Mechanism	Watery ultrafiltrate of the plasma	Damage of the serous membrane and mesothelium, usually due to inflammation or cancer
Gross appearance	Clear, pale, yellow, cloudy fluid	Cloudy, yellow, or bloody
Lactate dehydrogenase (LDH)	Fluid LDH/serum LDH < =0.6 Fluid LDH < =200 IU/L (or fluid LDH /serum LDH < =67% (2/3) of the upper normal limit for serum LDH)	Fluid LDH/serum LDH >0.6 Fluid LDH >200 IU/L (or fluid LDH /serum LDH >67% (2/3) of the upper normal limit for serum LDH)
Protein	Protein content <3 g/L (<2 in ascites) Fluid protein/serum protein level < =0.5	Protein content >3 g/L Fluid protein/serum protein level > 0.5
Lower specific gravity	<1.015	>1.015
Causes	Usually benign, only 5% of malignant effusions	Malignant effusions are usually exudates

Benign Elements

In all serous effusions, mesothelial cells, lymphocytes, and histiocytes are typical benign cellular components.

Mesothelial Cells

Mesothelial cells are either dispersed or form small clusters in effusions (Figs. 5.1 and 5.2). The border of a cluster is typically lobulated, or "knobby" like a flower Fig. 5.2a, as opposed to smooth borders as seen in carcinoma clusters. Mesothelial cells feature a two-tone cytoplasm with a dense perinuclear zone and a clear outer rim (a lacy "skirt") composed of microvilli. The nuclei are round to oval with a smooth nuclear contour, vesicular chromatin, and a low N:C ratio. A mesothelial cell usually has one small nucleus, but binucleation and rarely multinucleation can be seen. Microvilli form intercellular spaces ("windows") in cell clusters (Fig. 5.2b). Cytoplasmic arms embracing an adjacent ("hugging") can be seen in mesothelial cells (Fig. 5.2c). Differential diagnoses of reactive mesothelial cells include metastatic carcinoma and malignant mesothelioma.

Reactive mesothelial cells can have marked nuclear atypia. However, the atypia represents a spectrum of changes. Although their nuclei are enlarged, mesothelial cells still contain a smooth nuclear contour, vesicular chromatin, and a normal N:C ratio (Table 5.2). Features favoring mesothelioma include high cellularity, presence of complex papillary structures or tissue fragments, variation in size and shape and marked cytologic atypia. Desmin immunostaining shows strong cytoplasmic

Fig. 5.1 Normal elements in pleural fluid (ThinPrep). The reactive mesothelial cells show two-tone cytoplasmic staining, denser cytoplasm around the nucleus, and a clear outer rim (lacy skirt) formed by microvilli. The nuclei are round with vesicular chromatin and small nucleoli. Histiocytes show bean-shaped nuclei and vacuolated cytoplasm. Lymphocytes are small with scant cytoplasm. 600×

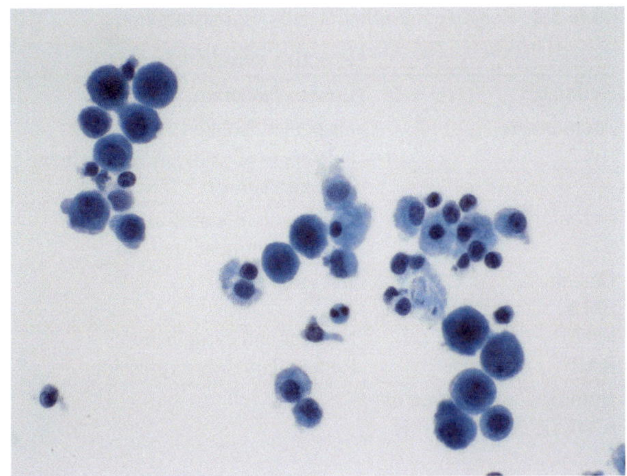

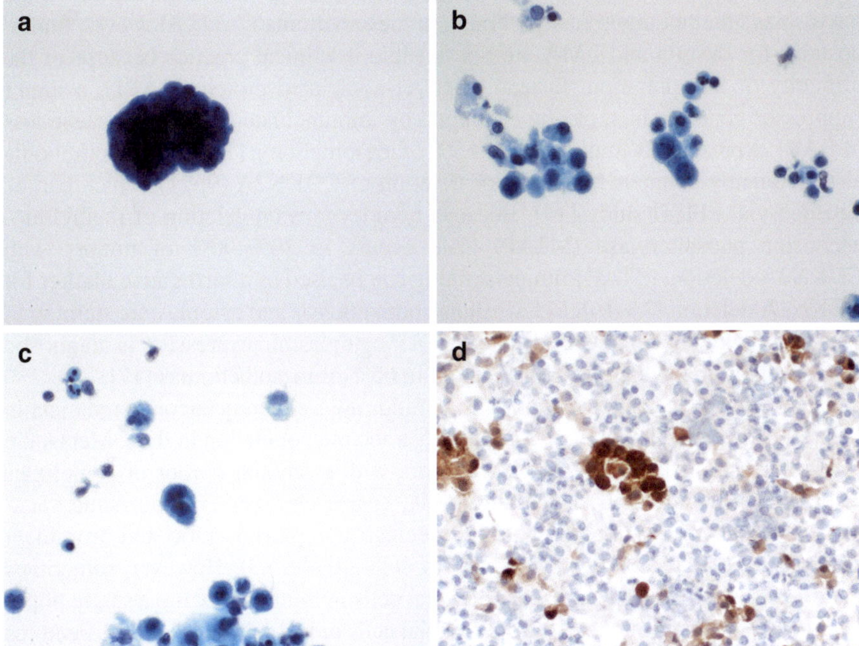

Fig. 5.2 Reactive mesothelial cells. (**a**) A small cluster of reactive mesothelial cells shows a scalloped border. (**b**) There is a "slit-like" separation between mesothelial cells, referred to as a "window." (**c**) One mesothelial cell seems to be enveloped by an adjacent mesothelial cell, referred to as "hugging." (**d**) Calretinin highlights mesothelial cells. (**a, b**) 600×; (**d**) 400×

Table 5.2 Reactive mesothelial cells vs. mesothelioma

	Reactive mesothelial cells	Mesothelioma
Cellularity	Low to moderate	High
Architecture	Dispersed isolated cells, small clusters (<12 cells), and flat sheet, 2D aggregates	Large clusters (>12 cells), complex, papillae 3D aggregates
Cytomorphology	Comparatively uniform Small prominent nucleoli	Pleomorphic Macronucleoli
Desmin	+ (cytoplasmic)	–
EMA	–	+ (membranous)
MTAP	Nuclear and cytoplasm	Loss of cytoplasmic staining
BAP1	Retained nuclear expression	Loss of nuclear expression
Homozygous deletion of p16/CDKN2A by FISH	–	+

staining patterns in benign mesothelium but are negative in malignant mesothelioma [7, 8]. EMA, on the other hand, shows no expression in benign mesothelium, but displays membranous bushy staining in mesothelioma [7–11]. However, immunostains for desmin and EMA are not feasible in clinical practice because of the difficulty of interpretation. Instead, BRCA1-associated protein (BAP1), a tumor suppressor gene product, can be examined by immunohistochemistry because loss of BAP1 expression is found in up to 65% of mesothelioma [12, 13]. Mesothelioma also frequently contains homozygous deletion of CDKN2A (9p21), which can be detected via a FISH study [14]. Because homozygous co-deletion of methylthioadenosine phosphorylase (MTAP) gene occurs in 80%–90% of tumors with CDKN2A deletion, MTAP immunostaining can be used as a surrogative marker for CDKN2A deletion [14–16]. MTAP shows both nuclear and cytoplasmic staining in benign mesothelial cells. Only loss of MTAP cytoplasmic expression is diagnostic for mesothelioma, which is reported in up to 65% of mesotheliomas [17].

Distinction of metastatic carcinomas in fluids are frequently encountered in daily practice. The general approach is to identify a second population in fluid. Metastatic carcinoma can form tightly packed clusters with a smooth border or sometimes dispersed individual cells. Hyperchromasia, coarse chromatin, cytoplasmic vacuoles, irregular nuclear membrane, high nuclear: cytoplasmic ratio and prominent nucleoli are typical features of carcinoma cells (Table 5.3). However, sometimes tumor cells may exhibit dispersed individual cells in fluid, producing a single population of cells that mimic reactive mesothelial cells or histiocytes (Fig. 5.3). Features favor reactive mesothelial cells include a smooth nuclear contour, vesicular chromatin, and small nucleoli (Table 5.3).

In daily practice, a panel of two mesothelial markers and two epithelial markers is commonly used for distinguishing reactive mesothelial cells from metastatic carcinoma. Mesothelial markers include calretinin, CK5/6, D2–40, and WT1 (Fig. 5.2d) [1]. A new antibody, HEG1, has been reported to be highly sensitive for mesothelial cells but negative for carcinoma, making it a potentially good marker for mesothelial differentiation [15]. Epithelial markers include claudin-4, MOC31,

Table 5.3 Reactive mesothelial cells vs. adenocarcinoma

	Reactive mesothelium	Adenocarcinoma
	Native cells	Foreign cells
Architecture	Individual, small berry-like clusters Clear spaces between cells ("window") and cytoplasmic arms embracing an adjacent ("hugging")	Glandular formation, solid aggregates, clusters with a smooth border, intracytoplasmic lumen
Cytology	Two-tone cytoplasm (dense center, pale edge)	Delicate cytoplasm
	Lacy cell border ("skirt")	Sharp cell border
	Low N/C ratio	High N/C ratio
	Smooth nuclear contour	Irregular nuclear membrane
	Vesicular chromatin	Hyperchromasia
	Small nucleoli	Large conspicuous nucleoli Intracytoplasmic mucin
Epithelial markers	–	(+) for MOC31, Ber-Ep4, and claudin 4
Mesothelial markers	(+) for Calretinin, CK5/6, D2–40, WT1, HEG1	–

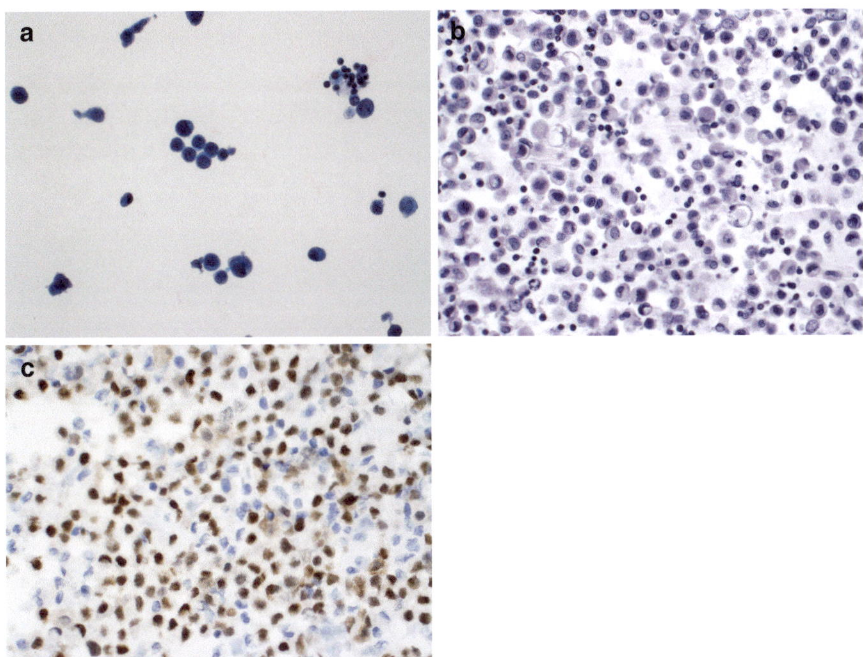

Fig. 5.3 Metastatic lobular carcinoma from breast primary. (**a**) Tumor cells are dispersed in pleural fluid. (**b**) Intracytoplasmic lumina is present (**c**) GATA3 labels the tumor cells. (**a–c**) 400×

Ber-Ep4, BG-8, B72.3, CD15 (LeuM1), and CEA [7, 18, 19]. It needs to be pointed out that focal reactivity of epithelial markers, such as MOC31 and Ber-Ep4, can also be found in reactive mesothelial cells (Fig. 5.4) [20]. Claudin-4 is highly sensitive for epithelial cells and completely negative for mesothelioma and reactive mesothelial cells, making it a good epithelial marker [20–23]. It has been reported that a combination of claudin 4 and Ber-Ep4 likely yields the highest combined sensitivity and specificity [21].

Histiocytes

Histiocytes appear as either single cells or in loosely cohesive groups (Figs. 5.1 and 5.5). They can exhibit great variability in size and morphology. The cells usually feature small, folded nuclei (bean-shaped), open chromatin and small or indistinct nucleoli. Binucleation and multinucleation are also commonly seen. Cytoplasm can be granular or dense but is typically foamy or vacuolated. Histiocytes with cytoplasmic hemosiderin are commonly seen as well. Histiocytes express CD68 and CD163. Differential diagnosis includes metastatic carcinoma.

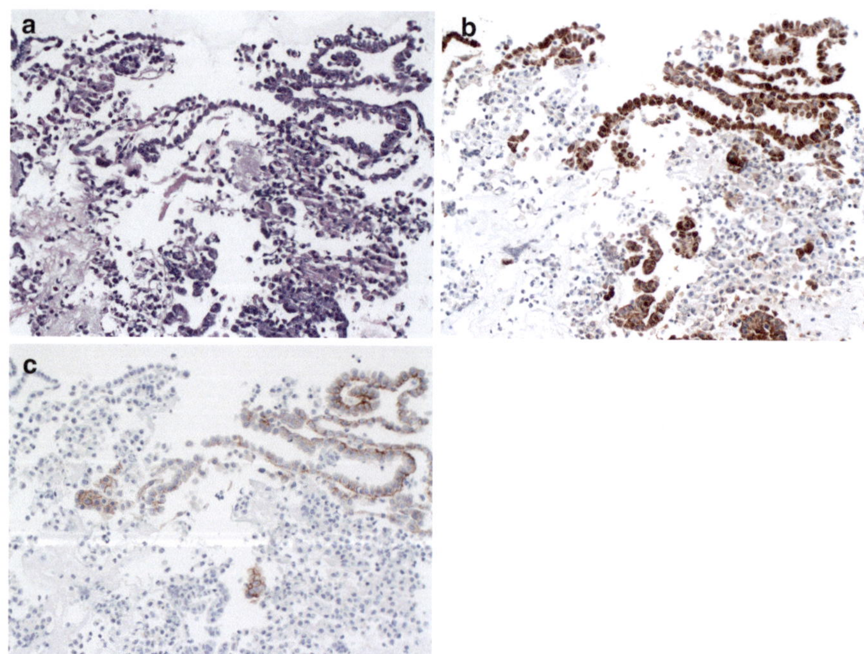

Fig. 5.4 Focal positivity of epithelial markers can be seen in mesothelial cells. (**a**) Reactive mesothelial cells and histiocytes. (**b**) Calretinin highlights reactive mesothelial cells. (**c**) Focal MOC-31 positivity is seen in reactive mesothelial cells. (**a–c**) 200×

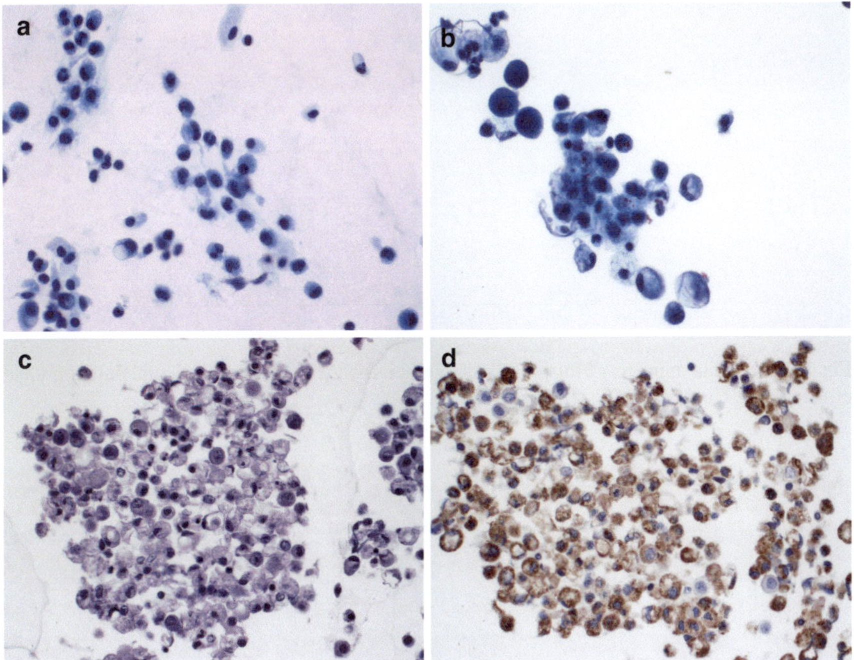

Fig. 5.5 Histiocytes. (**a–c**) Histiocytes are dispersed or form loosely cohesive groups with foamy or vacuolated cytoplasm. (**d**) CD68 highlights histiocytes. (**a–c**) 600×; (**d**), 400×

Acute Inflammatory effusion

Numerous neutrophils indicate acute inflammatory processes (purulent effusion) (Fig. 5.6). Empyema is caused by bacterial infection of the pleura in the setting of pneumonia. Acute inflammation in peritoneal fluid is frequently caused by inflammation of or injury to the bowel. Bacteria, fungi, or microorganisms can be detected using special stains, such as GMS and PAS.

Lymphocytic effusion

Lymphocytic effusion contains predominantly small to intermediate-sized lymphocytes. Scattered large lymphoid cells may also be seen (Fig. 5.7).

Polymorphous lymphocytes with a spectrum of maturation are characteristic in a reactive process in effusion, which is a common finding in daily practice. Abundant lymphocytes can also be seen in chylous effusions, while an abundance of lymphocytes without mesothelial cells are characteristic of tuberculous effusions. CD45, CD20, and CD3 are lymphocytic markers commonly used in clinical practice. A reactive process is characterized by predominantly CD3-positive T-lymphocytes with scattered CD20-positive B-lymphocytes (Fig. 5.7) [24].

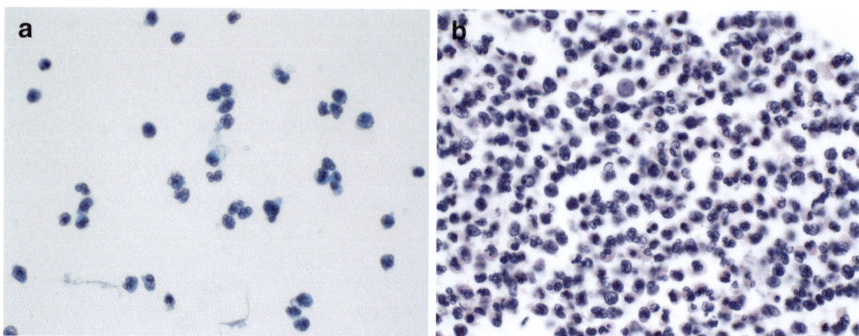

Fig. 5.6 Acute inflammatory effusion. Numerous neutrophils are present in pleural fluid (purulent effusion). (**a**) ThinPrep, 600×; (**b**) H&E, 600×

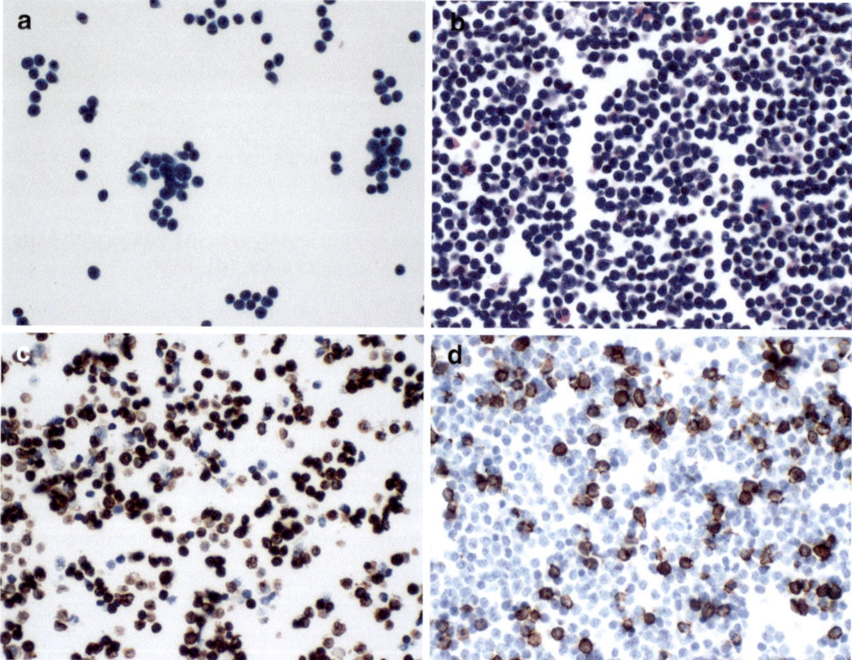

Fig. 5.7 Lymphocytic effusion. (**a, b**) Predominantly small to intermediate-sized lymphocytes with scattered large lymphocytes. (**c**) CD3 labels T-lymphocytes. (**d**) CD20 highlights scattered B-lymphocytes. (**a**) ThinPrep, 600×; (**b**) H&E, 600×; (**c, d**) 60×

The presence of monomorphic small lymphocytes or atypical lymphoid cells suggests a lymphoproliferative disorder. The differential diagnosis includes small lymphocytic lymphoma/chronic lymphocytic leukemia (SLL/CLL), small cell carcinoma and poorly differentiated adenocarcinoma. In SLL/CLL, neoplastic lymphocytes are monomorphic with scant cytoplasm, irregular nuclear membrane, and coarsely clumped chromatin, resulting in the so-called lumpy cells [25, 26]. However, it is almost impossible to distinguish a reactive process from low-grade lymphoma by morphology alone. The combined application of flow cytometry, immunohistochemical study, polymerase chain reaction (PCR), and fluorescence in situ hybridization (FISH) can be helpful in most lymphomatous effusion cases. It should be noted that lymphoma is rarely present in effusions as the initial manifestation [27, 28].

Differential diagnosis also includes metastatic small cell carcinoma and poorly differentiated carcinoma. In small cell carcinoma, tumor cells have scant cytoplasm and salt and pepper chromatin. Tumor clusters with nuclear molding are characteristic for small cell carcinoma and express neuroendocrine markers, such as INSM1, synaptophysin, and chromogranin (Fig. 5.8). Tumor cells in metastatic poorly differentiated carcinoma contain scant to moderate cytoplasm with prominent nucleoli.

Plasma Cells

Plasma cell can occur in chronic inflammation, rheumatoid effusions, tuberculosis, cancer, lymphocytosis/lymphoma, and myeloma.

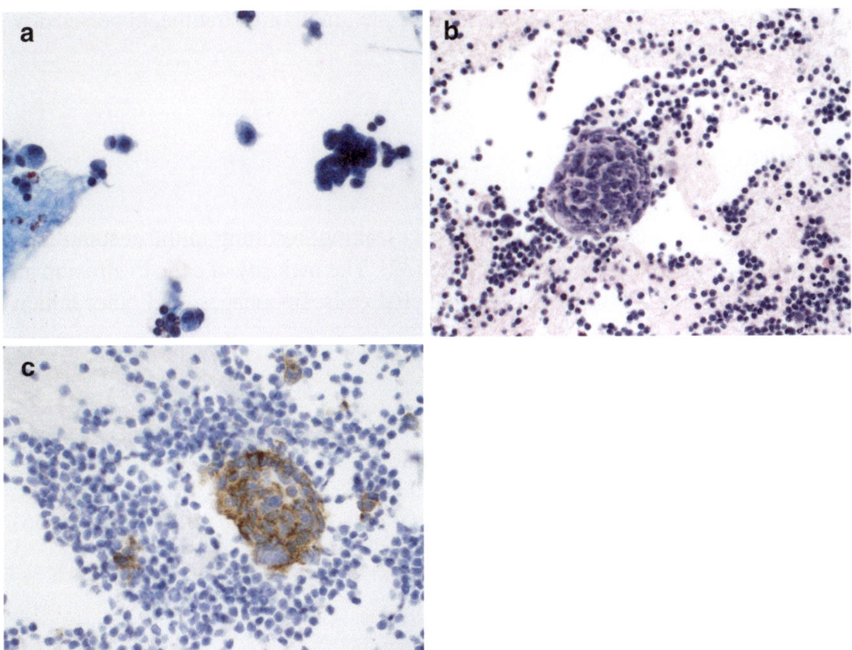

Fig. 5.8 Metastatic small cell carcinoma in pleural fluid. (**a, b**) Tumor clusters show nuclear molding. (**c**) GATA3 highlights tumor cells. (**a**) ThinPrep, 60×; (**b**) H&E, 40×; (**c**) 40×

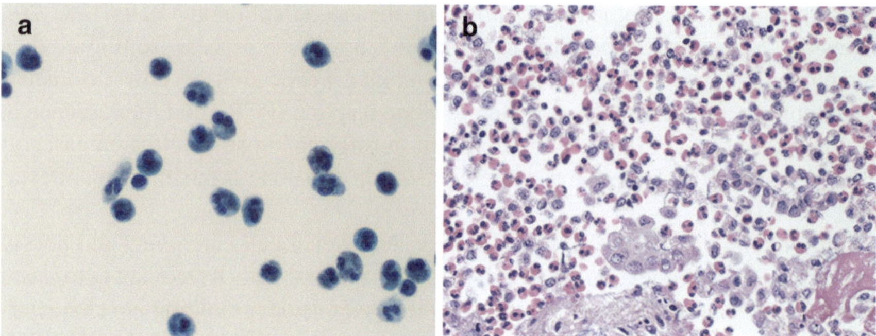

Fig. 5.9 Eosinophilic effusion. Eosinophils comprise more than 10% of the nucleated cells. (**a**) ThinPrep, 800×; (**b**) H&E, 400×

Eosinophilic effusion

Eosinophils have characteristic cytoplasmic granules that appear red in Romanowsky and hematoxylin and eosin (H&E) staining (Fig. 5.9). Eosinophilic effusion is defined as eosinophils comprising more than 10% of the nucleated cells [29, 30]. The most common cause of eosinophilic effusion is air or blood in the body cavities [30, 31]. Other associated conditions include pneumothorax, trauma, hypersensitivity, parasites, and infection [30, 31].

Chylous effusion

Chylous effusion is caused by thoracic duct leaking, resulting in the accumulation of lymphatic fluid (chyle) in pleural space [32]. The majority of cells in effusion are small lymphocytes, admixed with mesothelial cells, lipophages, and other inflammatory cells that are present.

Parapneumonic and Empyema

A parapneumonic effusion is a pleural effusion associated with pneumonia [33–35]. Empyema refers to the presence of pus in a body cavity.

Infectious Effusions

An effusion caused by organisms, such as bacteria, viruses, mycoplasma, chlamydia, fungi, bacteria, and parasites.

Tuberculous effusion

Abundant lymphocytes and absent/sparse mesothelial cells are characteristic of tuberculous effusions [36]. Clumps formed by fibrin exudation and trapped cells are another common feature. Differential diagnosis includes low-grade lymphoma, and flow cytometry or immunohistochemical study on cell blocks can help with the distinction. Most lymphocytes in tuberculous effusion are mature T-cells, while most low-grade lymphomas are of B-cell origin [37].

Rheumatoid effusion

Rheumatoid effusion is usually associated with rheumatoid arthritis. Triads of rheumatoid effusions include multinucleated giant cells, elongated histiocytes, and granular and necrotic debris, which is diagnostic of rheumatoid effusion [38]. Multinucleated cells are present in most cases. Granular debris is a fluffy and amorphous material, which can stain green, pink, red, or orange with Papanicolaou staining [39]. Histiocytes are usually round or spindled and elongated. In rare cases, spindled histiocytes resemble fibroblasts or tadpole cells of squamous cell carcinoma. They can degenerate and may show orangeophilic due to staining artifact, which is not true keratinization. Mesothelial cells are scant or absent; mixed population of inflammatory cells are present.

Systemic Lupus Erythematous (SLE)

Systemic lupus erythematous (SLE) is an autoimmune disease. Effusion manifestation occurs in approximately 30% to 40% of SLE patients [1]. The LE cell, the characteristic cell, is a neutrophil or macrophage with a glassy, homogeneous cytoplasmic inclusion (hematoxylin body) [40]. LE cells are highly suggestive of but not specific for SLE effusions. LE cells can be found in effusions associated with infection, rheumatoid arthritis, hepatitis, and medication [40–42]. LE cells must be distinguished from nonspecific tart cells, which are macrophages phagocytosing a nucleus of another cell, showing ingested non-homogeneous nuclei with visible chromatin structures [40, 42].

Contaminants

Occasionally, miscellaneous cell types can be seen in fluid specimens. These include ciliated bronchial cells, squamous cells from the skin, hepatocytes, and skeletal muscle (Fig. 5.10). The cells may be "picked-up" when the needle goes through

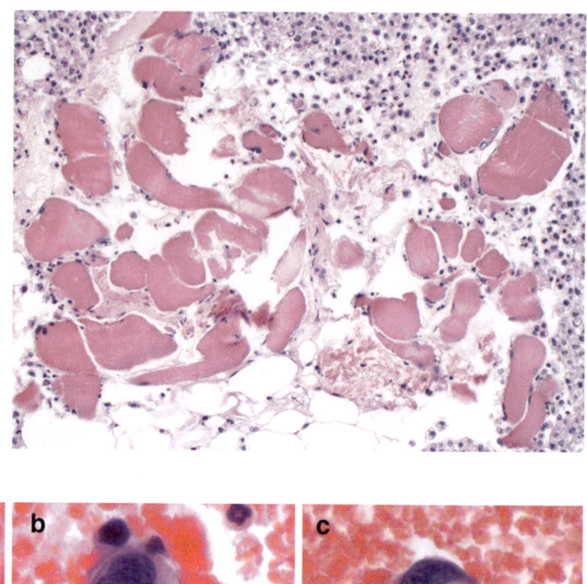

Fig. 5.10 Skeletal muscle in pleural fluid. 200×

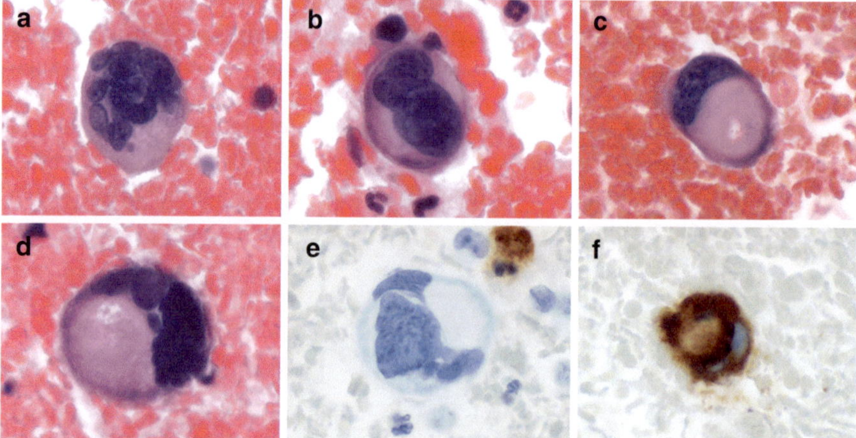

Fig. 5.11 Megakaryocytes in pleural fluid. (**a–d**) Megakaryocytes. (**e**) Pan cytokeratin is negative in megakaryocytes. (**f**) CK61 labels megakaryocytes. (**a–f**) 600×

tracheobronchial tree, skin and liver during the procedure. Blood elements, such as red blood cells and white blood cells, are therefore common contaminants. For hematopoietic diseases, contaminant hematopoietic cells can be misdiagnosed as atypical/neoplastic cells (Fig. 5.11).

Declarations of Interest The author declares no conflicts of interest.

References

1. Lepus CM, Vivero M. Updates in effusion cytology. Surg Pathol Clin. 2018;11(3):523–44. https://doi.org/10.1016/j.path.2018.05.003.
2. Feller-Kopman D, Light R. Pleural Disease. N Engl J Med. 2018;378(8):740–51. https://doi.org/10.1056/NEJMra1403503.
3. Skok K, Hladnik G, Grm A, Crnjac A. Malignant pleural effusion and its current management: a review. Medicina (Kaunas). 2019;55(8):490. https://doi.org/10.3390/medicina55080490.
4. Light RW. Pleural effusions. Med Clin North Am. 2011;95(6):1055–70. https://doi.org/10.1016/j.mcna.2011.08.005.
5. Oey RC, van Buuren HR, de Man RA. The diagnostic work-up in patients with ascites: current guidelines and future prospects. Neth J Med. 2016;74(8):330–5.
6. Azarbal A, LeWinter MM. Pericardial Effusion. Cardiol Clin. 2017;35(4):515–24. https://doi.org/10.1016/j.ccl.2017.07.005.
7. Mneimneh WS, Jiang Y, Harbhajanka A, Michael CW. Immunochemistry in the work-up of mesothelioma and its differential diagnosis and mimickers. Diagn Cytopathol. 2021;49(5):582–95. https://doi.org/10.1002/dc.24720.
8. Attanoos RL, Griffin A, Gibbs AR. The use of immunohistochemistry in distinguishing reactive from neoplastic mesothelium. A novel use for desmin and comparative evaluation with epithelial membrane antigen, p53, platelet-derived growth factor-receptor, P-glycoprotein and Bcl-2. Histopathology. 2003;43(3):231–8. https://doi.org/10.1046/j.1365-2559.2003.01686.x.
9. Saad RS, Cho P, Liu YL, Silverman JF. The value of epithelial membrane antigen expression in separating benign mesothelial proliferation from malignant mesothelioma: a comparative study. Diagn Cytopathol. 2005;32(3):156–9. https://doi.org/10.1002/dc.20208.
10. Ikeda K, Tate G, Suzuki T, Kitamura T, Mitsuya T. Diagnostic usefulness of EMA, IMP3, and GLUT-1 for the immunocytochemical distinction of malignant cells from reactive mesothelial cells in effusion cytology using cytospin preparations. Diagn Cytopathol. 2011;39(6):395–401. https://doi.org/10.1002/dc.21398.
11. Shen J, Pinkus GS, Deshpande V, Cibas ES. Usefulness of EMA, GLUT-1, and XIAP for the cytologic diagnosis of malignant mesothelioma in body cavity fluids. Am J Clin Pathol. 2009;131(4):516–23. https://doi.org/10.1309/ajcpwfw7o1fvflkt.
12. Cigognetti M, Lonardi S, Fisogni S, et al. BAP1 (BRCA1-associated protein 1) is a highly specific marker for differentiating mesothelioma from reactive mesothelial proliferations. Mod Pathol. 2015;28(8):1043–57. https://doi.org/10.1038/modpathol.2015.65.
13. Andrici J, Sheen A, Sioson L, et al. Loss of expression of BAP1 is a useful adjunct, which strongly supports the diagnosis of mesothelioma in effusion cytology. Mod Pathol. 2015;28(10):1360–8. https://doi.org/10.1038/modpathol.2015.87.
14. Marjon K, Cameron MJ, Quang P, et al. MTAP Deletions in Cancer Create Vulnerability to Targeting of the MAT2A/PRMT5/RIOK1 Axis. Cell Rep. 2016;15(3):574–87. https://doi.org/10.1016/j.celrep.2016.03.043.
15. Hiroshima K, Wu D, Hamakawa S, et al. HEG1, BAP1, and MTAP are useful in cytologic diagnosis of malignant mesothelioma with effusion. Diagn Cytopathol. 2021;49(5):622–32. https://doi.org/10.1002/dc.24475.
16. Churg A, Naso JR. The separation of benign and malignant mesothelial proliferations: new markers and how to use them. Am J Surg Pathol. 2020;44(11):e100–12. https://doi.org/10.1097/pas.0000000000001565.
17. Michael CW. The cytologic diagnosis of mesothelioma: are we there yet? J Am Soc Cytopathol. 2023;12(2):89–104. https://doi.org/10.1016/j.jasc.2022.12.001.
18. Husain AN, Colby T, Ordonez N, et al. Guidelines for pathologic diagnosis of malignant mesothelioma: 2012 update of the consensus statement from the international mesothelioma interest group. Arch Pathol Lab Med. 2013;137(5):647–67. https://doi.org/10.5858/arpa.2012-0214-OA.

19. Lyons-Boudreaux V, Mody DR, Zhai J, Coffey D. Cytologic malignancy versus benignancy: how useful are the "newer" markers in body fluid cytology? Arch Pathol Lab Med. 2008;132(1):23–8. https://doi.org/10.5858/2008-132-23-cmvbhu.

20. Bernardi L, Bizzarro T, Pironi F, et al. The "Brescia panel" (Claudin-4 and BRCA-associated protein 1) in the differential diagnosis of mesotheliomas with epithelioid features versus metastatic carcinomas. Cancer Cytopathol. 2021;129(4):275–82. https://doi.org/10.1002/cncy.22368.

21. Najjar S, Gan Q, Stewart J, Sneige N. The utility of claudin-4 versus MOC-31 and Ber-EP4 in the diagnosis of metastatic carcinoma in cytology specimens. Cancer Cytopathol. 2022;131:245. https://doi.org/10.1002/cncy.22672.

22. Patel A, Borczuk AC, Siddiqui MT. Utility of Claudin-4 versus BerEP4 and B72.3 in pleural fluids with metastatic lung adenocarcinoma. J Am Soc Cytopathol. 2020;9(3):146–51. https://doi.org/10.1016/j.jasc.2019.12.003.

23. Oda T, Ogata S, Kawaguchi S, et al. Immunocytochemical utility of claudin-4 versus those of Ber-EP4 and MOC-31 in effusion cytology. Diagn Cytopathol. 2016;44(6):499–504. https://doi.org/10.1002/dc.23476.

24. Ghosh AK, Spriggs AI, Mason DY. Immunocytochemical staining of T and B lymphocytes in serous effusions. J Clin Pathol. 1985;38(6):608–12. https://doi.org/10.1136/jcp.38.6.608.

25. Molina M, Ortega G, Martínez F, Sola J. B-lymphocytes in the pleural effusion of chronic lymphocytic leukemia. Med Clin (Barc). 1995;105(12):478. Linfocitos B en el derrame pleural de la leucemia linfática crónica.

26. Seidel TA, Garbes AD. Cellules grumelées: old terminology revisited. Regarding the cytologic diagnosis of chronic lymphocytic leukemia and well-differentiated lymphocytic lymphoma in pleural effusions. Acta Cytol. 1985;29(5):775–80.

27. Das DK, Al-Juwaiser A, George SS, et al. Cytomorphological and immunocytochemical study of non-Hodgkin's lymphoma in pleural effusion and ascitic fluid. Cytopathology. 2007;18(3):157–67. https://doi.org/10.1111/j.1365-2303.2007.00448.x.

28. Patel T, Patel P, Mehta S, Shah M, Jetly D, Khanna N. The value of cytology in diagnosis of serous effusions in malignant lymphomas: an experience of a tertiary care center. Diagn Cytopathol. 2019;47(8):776–82. https://doi.org/10.1002/dc.24197.

29. Bower G, Eosinophilic pleural effusion. A condition with multiple causes. Am Rev Respir Dis. 1967;95(5):746–51. https://doi.org/10.1164/arrd.1967.95.5.746.

30. Matthai SM, Kini U. Diagnostic value of eosinophils in pleural effusion: a prospective study of 26 cases. Diagn Cytopathol. 2003;28(2):96–9. https://doi.org/10.1002/dc.10227.

31. Heidecker J, Kaplan A, Sahn SA. Pleural fluid and peripheral eosinophilia from hemothorax: hypothesis of the pathogenesis of EPE in hemothorax and pneumothorax. Am J Med Sci. 2006;332(3):148–52. https://doi.org/10.1097/00000441-200609000-00011.

32. Jhala N, Jhala D, Shidham VB. Serous fluid: Reactive conditions. Cytojournal. 2022;19:14. https://doi.org/10.25259/cmas_02_06_2021.

33. Hamm H, Light RW. Parapneumonic effusion and empyema. Eur Respir J. 1997;10(5):1150–6. https://doi.org/10.1183/09031936.97.10051150.

34. Light RW. Parapneumonic effusions and empyema. Proc Am Thorac Soc. 2006;3(1):75–80. https://doi.org/10.1513/pats.200510-113JH.

35. Taryle DA, Potts DE, Sahn SA. The incidence and clinical correlates of parapneumonic effusions in pneumococcal pneumonia. Chest. 1978;74(2):170–3. https://doi.org/10.1378/chest.74.2.170.

36. Light RW. Update on tuberculous pleural effusion. Respirology. 2010;15(3):451–8. https://doi.org/10.1111/j.1440-1843.2010.01723.x.

37. Pettersson T, Klockars M, Hellström PE, Riska H, Wangel A. T and B lymphocytes in pleural effusions. Chest. 1978;73(1):49–51. https://doi.org/10.1378/chest.73.1.49.

38. Montes S, Guarda LA. Cytology of pleural effusions in rheumatoid arthritis. Diagn Cytopathol. 1988;4(1):71–3. https://doi.org/10.1002/dc.2840040117.

39. Boddington MM, Spriggs AI, Morton JA, Mowat AG. Cytodiagnosis of rheumatoid pleural effusions. J Clin Pathol. 1971;24(2):95–106. https://doi.org/10.1136/jcp.24.2.95.
40. Naylor B. Cytological aspects of pleural, peritoneal and pericardial fluids from patients with systemic lupus erythematosus. Cytopathology. 1992;3(1):1–8. https://doi.org/10.1111/j.1365-2303.1992.tb00014.x.
41. Good JT Jr, King TE, Antony VB, Sahn SA. Lupus pleuritis. Clinical features and pleural fluid characteristics with special reference to pleural fluid antinuclear antibodies. Chest. 1983;84(6):714–8. https://doi.org/10.1378/chest.84.6.714.
42. Hargraves MM, Richmond H, Morton R. Presentation of two bone marrow elements; the tart cell and the L.E. cell. Proc Staff Meet Mayo Clin. 1948;23(2):25–8.

Chapter 6
Salivary Gland

Syed M. Gilani

Salivary Gland Origin, Types, and Locations

Major salivary glands are derived from primitive oral epithelium and usually seen around 6 weeks of gestation. [1] There are three major salivary glands that include parotid gland, submandibular gland, and sublingual gland.

- Parotid gland: The parotid gland is located below and in front of the external ear. It covers a portion of the mandible (ramus) and is divided into superficial and deep lobes based on its relationship to facial nerve [2]. The deep lobe is irregular in shape and extends to parapharyngeal space. The gland weighs 15–28 g, consisting of serous acini and small ducts connecting with the Stensen (main duct).
- Submandibular gland: The submandibular gland is in a submandibular triangle in the deep posterior floor of the mouth. It is relatively smaller in size (7–8 g) and consists of mixed acini (serous and mucus) and Wharton's duct (main duct).
- Sublingual gland: The sublingual gland is in the sublingual area at the anterior floor of the mouth. It is smaller than the other two major glands (close to 4 g) and mainly consists of mucous-type acini. In addition, Bartholin's duct (main duct) and numerous small ducts help in draining secretions.

1. Minor salivary gland is located throughout different locations such as the lip, oral cavity, palate, paranasal sinuses, larynx, and tracheobronchial area and may involve non-neoplastic and neoplastic etiologies. Salivary gland tissue/or heterotopia/or ectopic can be found in locations as follows [3–20]:

   (a) External auditory canal
   (b) Middle ear

S. M. Gilani (✉)
Department of Pathology, Albany Medical Center, Albany Medical College,
Albany, NY, USA
e-mail: gilanis@amc.edu

© The Author(s), under exclusive license to Springer Nature
Switzerland AG 2023
S. M. Gilani, G. Cai (eds.), *Non-Neoplastic Cytology*,
https://doi.org/10.1007/978-3-031-44289-6_6

    (c) Mandible
    (d) Pituitary gland
    (e) Rathke's cleft
    (f) Cerebellopontine angle
    (g) Neck
    (h) Thyroid gland
    (i) Parathyroid gland
    (j) Thyroid gland
    (k) Breast
    (l) Chest wall
  (m) Mediastinum
    (n) Esophagus
    (o) Gastroesophageal junction
    (p) Large intestine
    (q) Rectum
    (r) Lymph nodes (neck, mediastinum)

Morphology of Salivary Gland

1. Acini: They can be serous, mixed, and mucous type. Serous acini have dense basophilic cytoplasm. Mucous type acinic are larger in size (Fig. 6.1).
2. Ducts: There are two subtypes: intralobular ducts and interlobular ducts (excretory ducts).

    (a) Intralobular ducts: Intercalated ducts are lined by cuboidal epithelium and present within the acini. Striated ducts are lined by columnar epithelium and show parallel striation and eosinophilic cytoplasm due to increased mitochondria. Tumors arise from intercalated ducts that usually show epithelial

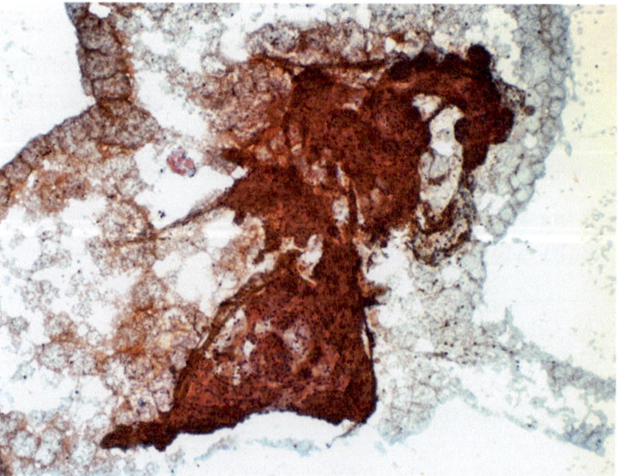

Fig. 6.1 Salivary gland acini in lobular architecture (Papanicolaou stain × 100)

and myoepithelial differentiation, while oncocytic tumors (Warthin tumor or oncocytoma) arise from striated ducts.

(b) Interlobular ducts are larger ducts, and they are in the septal tissue close to vasculature and may contain goblet cells.

3. Myoepithelial cells and basal cells: They are flat, have long cytoplasmic projections, and may share epithelial and mesenchymal structures. They are located outside the basement membrane outside the acinar cells and intercalated ductal cells. Basal cells are present outside striated ducts and excretory ducts. Myoepithelial cells and basal cells are also called abluminal cells. However, alteration in myoepithelial cells can be a manifestation of a neoplastic process. These altered myoepithelial cells can be epithelial, spindle, plasmacytoid, or stellate/chondromyxoid types.

4. Oncocytic epithelium: Oncocytic epithelium can be seen in interlobular ducts, mostly due to increased mitochondria. With advancing age, they are most frequent and can be seen in reactive and neoplastic processes.

5. Intra-parenchymal lymph node: Lymph nodes can be seen in the parotid gland and usually show a polymorphous population of lymphocytes (Fig. 6.2).

6. Sebaceous glands: The sebaceous gland can be seen in the salivary gland and are more frequent in the parotid gland. There is a suggestion that sebaceous gland or sebaceous differentiation in the salivary gland is likely due to a metaplastic process. Primary sebaceous neoplasms can arise from these glands [21].

7. Metaplastic changes: Metaplastic changes are variable and can include squamous metaplasia, mucous metaplasia, presence of goblet cells, and ciliated changes in the epithelium.

8. Adipose tissue: With advancing age, more adipose tissue is seen.

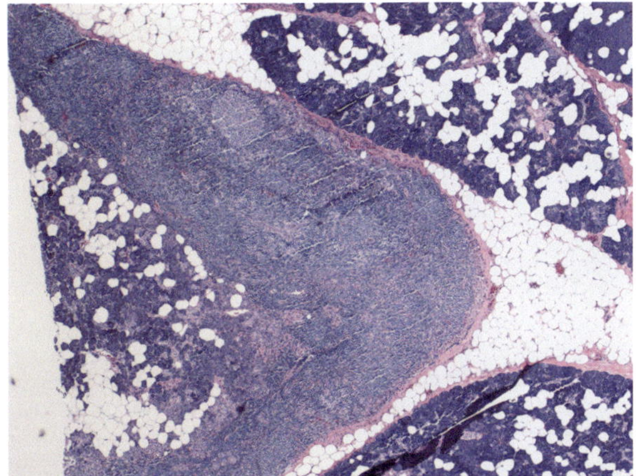

Fig. 6.2 Intraparotid lymph node (H&E × 40)

Table 6.1 Immunohistochemistry in benign salivary gland

Stains	Salivary gland component (Positive)	Negative
Keratins (cytokeratin AE/AE3 or pancytokeratin	Ductal cells, acinar cells, and myoepithelial and basal cells	–
CEA	Ductal and acinar cells	Myoepithelial and basal cells
EMA	Ductal cells, acinar and sebaceous cells	Myoepithelial and basal cells
Calponin	Myoepithelial cells	Ductal cells, acini cells, basal cells of striated and excretory ducts
S100	Myoepithelial cells (all type, variable expression) can show staining in intercalated ducts	Other ductal cells, acini cells, basal cells of striated and excretory ducts
SMA	Myoepithelial cells (but less in plasmacytoid cells)	Ductal cells and acini cells, basal cells of striated and excretory ducts
P63 and p40	Myoepithelial cells and basal cells (all types)	Ductal cells and acini cells
Muscle-specific antigen (MSA)	Myoepithelial cells (variable expression)	Ductal cells and acini cells, basal cells of striated and excretory ducts
SOX10	Intercalated ducts and mostly serous acini	Ductal cells of mucous acini, striated ducts, and interlobular ducts
DOG-1	Apical luminal membranous staining in acini (serous>mucous) and intercalated ducts	Striated ducts and excretory ducts
PAS (periodic acid-Schiff)	Acini cells (zymogen granules)	

Immunohistochemistry

Immunohistochemistry in the normal salivary gland [22–25] is discussed in Table 6.1.

Cystic Lesions

Cystic lesions in the salivary gland can be neoplastic and non-neoplastic. The non-neoplastic cystic lesion and the differential diagnosis is discussed in Table 6.2 [26–29].

Table 6.2 Benign Cystic lesion

Cystic lesions	Cytomorphologic features	Differential diagnosis	Diagnostic clues
Lymphoepithelial cyst (LEC) (Figs. 6.3 and 6.4)	• Cyst wall with lymphoid component • Cyst lining is mostly squamous but can be columnar with or without goblet cells • Mainly in parotid gland	• Other cystic lesions (HIV-associated) • Warthin tumor • Squamous cell carcinoma (SCC) • Mucoepidermoid carcinoma, low grade (MEC-LG)	• *HIV-associated cysts:* Similar morphology but usually multiple and can have multinucleated giant cells • *Warthin tumor:* Typical bi-layered oncocytic epithelium • *SCC:* Cystic SCC usually shows atypical epithelial cells and necrotic debris. P16 and HPV testing can be valuable in HPV-associated SCCs. Prior clinical history is also important • *MEC-LG:* Usually show mucous cells, intermediate and epidermoid cells. Tumor-associated lymphoid cells can be seen
Mucocele	• Mostly mucous admixed with inflammatory cells and histiocytes • Usually, no epithelial cells • Can be due to mucus extravasation reaction (more common) associated with trauma • Or due to mucous retention (less common)	• Salivary duct cyst (SDC) • MEC, LG	• *SDC:* Usually after 60 years of age and show bland cuboidal/ or columnar epithelial lining • *MEC, LG:* Should have other components such as epidermoid and intermediate cells. Oftentimes distinction is difficult in paucicellular cytology specimens
Epidermoid cyst	• Keratinizing squamous epithelium, anucleated squamous cells and keratin debris	• Dermoid cyst • LEC • SCC, well differentiated	• *Dermoid cyst:* Usually have skin appendages • *LEC:* Lymphoid component is prominent • *SCC, well-differentiated:* Cytologic atypia, keratin with atypical changes, or mitosis

(continued)

Table 6.2 (continued)

Cystic lesions	Cytomorphologic features	Differential diagnosis	Diagnostic clues
Polycystic disease	• Low cellularity specimen with histiocytes with or without red blood cells and scant epithelial cells • Bilateral enlarged gland with multi-cystic dilatation of ducts	• LEC • Cystic salivary gland neoplasms	• *LEC:* Have more lymphoid component while polycystic disease usually doesn't have overt lymphoid component • *Cystic salivary gland neoplasm:* More epithelial proliferation
Salivary duct cyst (SDC)	• Dilated excretory duct, mostly single layer epithelial undulating lining (cuboidal or columnar) • Metaplastic changes (oncocytic, ciliated, mucous, or squamous), can be seen	• Mucocele • Cystadenoma • MEC-LG	• *Mucocele*: Younger age (<40 years as compared to SDC, sixth decade), common site lip and trauma history • *Cystadenoma*: Usually have more epithelial proliferation • *MEC-LG:* Usually have mucous cells, epidermoid (squamoid, eosinophilic cytoplasm) cells, intermediate cells (small dark nuclei and pale cytoplasm), more p63 staining as compared to SDC (which show only basal cell staining)

SCC squamous cell carcinoma, *MEC-LG* mucoepidermoid carcinoma, low grade, *SDC* salivary duct cyst, *LEC* lymphoepithelial cyst

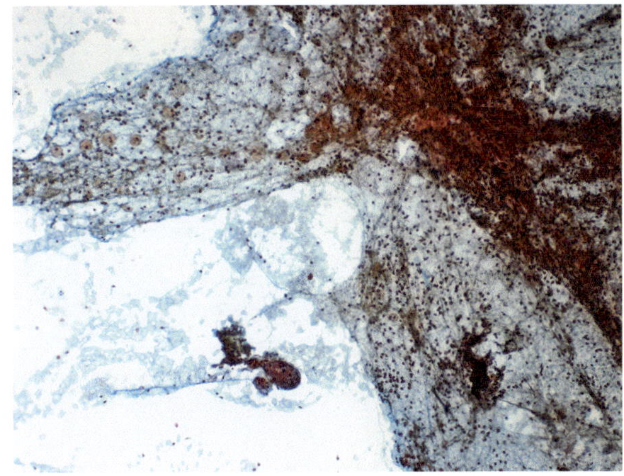

Fig. 6.3 Lymphoepithelial cyst with scattered lymphocytes, salivary gland acini and histiocytes (Papanicolaou stain × 100)

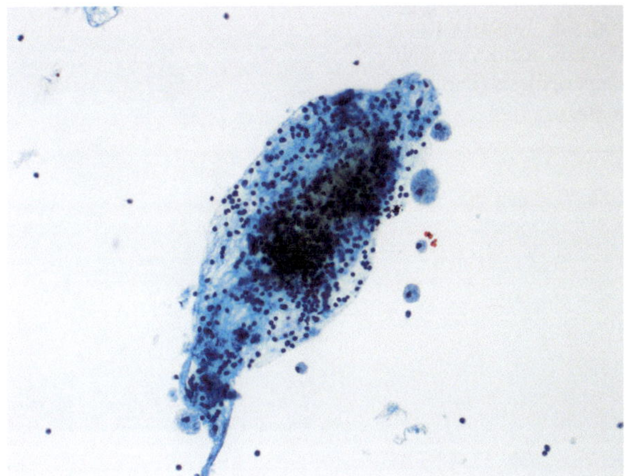

Fig. 6.4 Lymphoepithelial cyst with scattered lymphocytes, salivary gland acini and histiocytes (ThinPrep × 200)

Salivary Gland Reactive and Inflammatory Conditions

IgG4-Related Disease

IgG4-related salivary gland disease (IgG4-RSGD) is a chronic fibroinflammatory condition that may result in swelling. It appears as a mass-forming lesion of the gland and frequently involves the submandibular gland compared to others [30, 31]. Cytology specimens can be paucicellular due to fibrosis. Cytology smears can show salivary gland parenchymal cells (acini and ductal cells) with associated chronic inflammatory cells (mixed lymphocytes and plasma cells) (Fig. 6.5). Lobular architecture is usually maintained with acinar atrophy. Serum IgG4 levels are usually elevated. Immunohistochemistry for IgG4 and IgG is helpful. IgG4-positive plasma cells and IgG4/IgG ratio > 40%, along with morphologic features, are required to

                                                                    S. M. Gilani

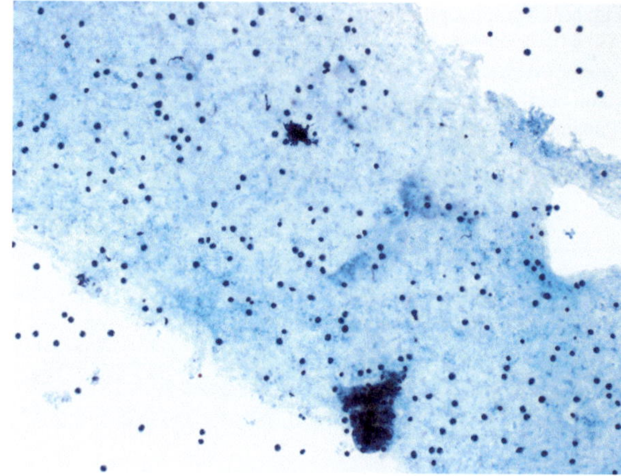

Fig. 6.5 Chronic inflammation involving salivary gland acini (ThinPrep × 200)

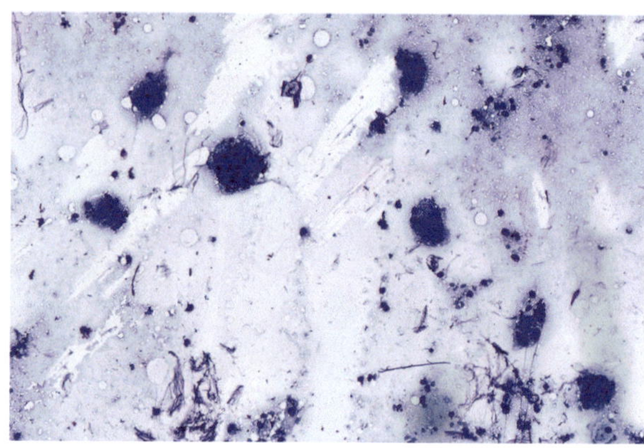

Fig. 6.6 Rosai-Dorfman disease, histiocytes with emperipolesis (Diff-Quik × 400)

diagnose IgG-RSGD [32]. The differential diagnosis includes Sjogren syndrome (SS), which usually have antiSSA antibody, lack IgG4-positive plasma cells, and can show lymphoepithelial lesion consisting of lymphocytes and epithelial cells. Marginal zone lymphoma is a B-cell lymphoma that typically shows the proliferation of monocytoid cells with abundant pale cytoplasm and variable degree of admixed plasma cells. Immunohistochemistry for B-cell markers and flow cytometry is helpful for definitive diagnosis. Extra-nodal Rosai-Dorfman disease usually shows a collection of histiocytes which typically show emperipolesis (the presence of intact hematopoietic cells within histiocytic cytoplasm) (Fig. 6.6). Histiocytes are positive for S100, OCT-2, and cyclin-D1 but negative for CD1a [33, 34].

Necrotizing Sialometaplasia

Necrotizing sialometaplasia is an inflammatory process that usually affects minor salivary glands, especially the hard palate [35]. It may present as swelling, which is followed by ulceration. Morphologically lobular architecture is maintained with areas of necrosis, inflammatory infiltrates, and squamous metaplasia. The differential diagnosis includes squamous cell carcinoma (SCC). SCC should have cytologic atypia and irregular borders. However, in paucicellular specimens, a cautious approach would be helpful to avoid overinterpretation.

Sialadenitis

Sialadenitis can represent an acute or chronic inflammatory process involving salivary gland parenchymal tissue, either due to infectious etiology or chronic conditions, or obstruction due to sialolithiasis. Infectious etiology includes viral, bacterial, mycobacterial, and fungal infections. Granulomatous-type inflammatory reactions can be seen in mycobacterial, fungal infections, sarcoidosis, and special stains can be helpful. A cytologic examination can show salivary gland parenchymal cells and acute or chronic inflammatory cells with or without granuloma formation. Crystals such as amylase crystals can be seen (Fig. 6.7).

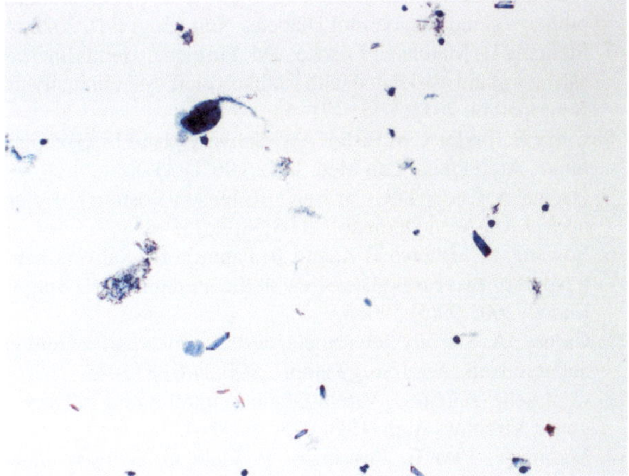

Fig. 6.7 Salivary gland acini and crystalline material (ThinPrep × 200)

Post-FNA Changes in Salivary Gland

Fine needle aspiration of the salivary gland can result in various alterations in the tissue morphology. For example, post-FNA tissue infarction/necrosis and hemorrhage can be seen [36]. Other changes, such as fibrosis, granulation tissue formation, and metaplastic changes, can rarely be seen.

Acknowledgments None.

Conflict of Interest None.

References

1. Holmberg KV, Hoffman MP. Anatomy, biogenesis and regeneration of salivary glands. Monogr Oral Sci. 2014;24:1–13.
2. Bialek EJ, Jakubowski W, Zajkowski P, Szopinski KT, Osmolski A. US of the major salivary glands: anatomy and spatial relationships, pathologic conditions, and pitfalls. Radiographics. 2006;26(3):745–63.
3. Raghavan V, Moorthy PE, Srinivasan S. Salivary gland Choristoma in external Auditory Canal: a case report. Fetal Pediatr Pathol. 2022;5:1–4.
4. Morimoto N, Ogawa K, Kanzaki J. Salivary gland choristoma in the middle ear: a case report. Am J Otolaryngol. 1999;20(4):232–5.
5. Dorman M, Pierse D. Ectopic salivary gland tissue in the anterior mandible: a case report. Br Dent J. 2002;193(10):571–2.
6. Iglesias P, Fernández-Mateos C, Tejerina E. Symptomatic salivary gland choristoma of the pituitary gland. Endocrinol Diabetes Nutr (Engl Ed). 2022;69(7):544–6.
7. Stefanits H, Matula C, Frischer JM, Furtner J, Hainfellner JA, Woehrer A. Innervated ectopic salivary gland associated with Rathke's cleft cyst clinically mimicking pituitary adenoma. Clin Neuropathol. 2013;32(3):171–5.
8. Curry B, Taylor CW, Fisher AW. Salivary gland heterotopia: a unique cerebellopontine angle tumor. Arch Pathol Lab Med. 1982;106(1):35–8.
9. Haemel A, Gnepp DR, Carlsten J, Robinson-Bostom L. Heterotopic salivary gland tissue in the neck. J Am Acad Dermatol. 2008;58(2):251–6.
10. Edwards PC, Bhuiya T, Kahn LB, Fantasia JE. Salivary heterotopia of the parathyroid gland: a report of two cases and review of the literature. Oral Surg Oral Med Oral Pathol Oral Radiol Endod. 2005;99(5):590–3.
11. Carney JA. Salivary heterotopia, cysts, and the parathyroid gland: branchial pouch derivatives and remnants. Am J Surg Pathol. 2000;24(6):837–45.
12. Cameselle-Teijeiro J, Varela-Durån J. Intrathyroid salivary gland-type tissue in multinodular goiter. Virchows Arch. 1994;425(3):331–4.
13. Maffini F, Pisa E, Possanzini P, Viale G. Salivary gland choristoma of breast. Breast J. 2012;18(2):181.
14. Shin CE, Kim SS, Chwals WJ. Salivary gland choristoma of the anterior chest wall. J Pediatr Surg. 2000;35(10):1506–7.
15. Feigin GA, Robinson B, Marchevsky A. Mixed tumor of the mediastinum. Arch Pathol Lab Med. 1986;110(1):80–1.
16. Ryu DG, Choi CW, Kim SJ. Esophageal wall thickening due to salivary gland heterotopia. Korean J Intern Med. 2022;38:139.

17. Abdul Karim L, Kwon DH, Ozdemirli M. Salivary gland heterotopia in the gastroesophageal junction: a case series and review of the literature. Case Rep Gastrointest Med. 2018;30(2018):6078581.
18. Maffini F, Vingiani A, Lepanto D, Fiori G, Viale G. Salivary gland choristoma in large bowel. Endoscopy. 2012;44(Suppl 2 UCTN):E13–4.
19. Lewis AL, Truong LD, Cagle P, Zhai QJ. Benign salivary gland tissue inclusion in a pulmonary hilar lymph node from a patient with invasive well-differentiated adenocarcinoma of the lung: a potential misinterpretation for the staging of carcinoma. Int J Surg Pathol. 2011;19(3):382–5.
20. Shinohara M, Harada T, Nakamura S, Oka M, Tashiro H. Heterotopic salivary gland tissue in lymph nodes of the cervical region. Int J Oral Maxillofac Surg. 1992;21(3):166–71.
21. Gnepp DR, Brannon R. Sebaceous neoplasms of salivary gland origin. Report of 21 cases. Cancer. 1984;53(10):2155–70.
22. Nagao T, Sato E, Inoue R, Oshiro H, Takahashi RH, Nagai T, Yoshida M, Suzuki F, Obikane H, Yamashina M, Matsubayashi J. Immunohistochemical analysis of salivary gland tumors: application for surgical pathology practice. Acta Histochem Cytochem. 2012;45(5):269–82.
23. Furuse C, Sousa SO, Nunes FD, Magalhães MH, Araújo VC. Myoepithelial cell markers in salivary gland neoplasms. Int J Surg Pathol. 2005;13(1):57–65.
24. Hsieh MS, Lee YH, Chang YL. SOX10-positive salivary gland tumors: a growing list, including mammary analogue secretory carcinoma of the salivary gland, sialoblastoma, low-grade salivary duct carcinoma, basal cell adenoma/adenocarcinoma, and a subgroup of mucoepidermoid carcinoma. Hum Pathol. 2016;56:134–42.
25. Chênevert J, Duvvuri U, Chiosea S, Dacic S, Cieply K, Kim J, Shiwarski D, Seethala RR. DOG1: a novel marker of salivary acinar and intercalated duct differentiation. Mod Pathol. 2012;25(7):919–29.
26. Stojanov IJ, Malik UA, Woo SB. Intraoral salivary duct cyst: clinical and histopathologic features of 177 cases. Head Neck Pathol. 2017;11(4):469–76.
27. Layfield LJ, Gopez EV. Cystic lesions of the salivary glands: cytologic features in fine-needle aspiration biopsies. Diagn Cytopathol. 2002;27(4):197–204.
28. Bowers EMR, Schaitkin B. Management of Mucoceles, Sialoceles, and Ranulas. Otolaryngol Clin N Am. 2021;54(3):543–51.
29. Ozcan KM, Dere H, Ozcan I, Gun T, Unal T. An epidermal cyst in the parotid gland following ear surgery: a case report. B-ENT. 2006;2(4):193–5.
30. Puxeddu I, Capecchi R, Carta F, Tavoni AG, Migliorini P, Puxeddu R. Salivary gland pathology in IgG4-related disease: a comprehensive review. J Immunol Res. 2018;2018:6936727.
31. Migliora P, Barizzi J, Torre A, Ermanni S, Fulciniti F. A hard mass of the right submandibular gland in an 83-Yr-old lady. Acta Cytol. 2021;65(2):194–6.
32. Umehara H, Okazaki K, Nakamura T, Satoh-Nakamura T, Nakajima A, Kawano M, Mimori T, Chiba T. Current approach to the diagnosis of IgG4-related disease - combination of comprehensive diagnostic and organ-specific criteria. Mod Rheumatol. 2017;27(3):381–91.
33. Ojha J, Rawal YB, Hornick JL, Magliocca K, Montgomery DR, Foss RD, Torske KR, Accurso B. Extra nodal Rosai-Dorfman disease originating in the nasal and paranasal complex and gnathic bones: a systematic analysis of seven cases and review of literature. Head Neck Pathol. 2020;14(2):442–53.
34. Ravindran A, Goyal G, Go RS, Rech KL. Mayo Clinic Histiocytosis working group. Rosai-Dorfman disease displays a unique monocyte-macrophage phenotype characterized by expression of OCT2. Am J Surg Pathol. 2021;45(1):35–44.
35. Chateaubriand SL, de Amorim Carvalho EJ, Leite AA, da Silva Leonel ACL, Prado JD, da Cruz Perez DE. Necrotizing sialometaplasia: A diagnostic challenge. Oral Oncol. 2021;118:105349.
36. Mukunyadzi P, Bardales RH, Palmer HE, Stanley MW. Tissue effects of salivary gland fine-needle aspiration. Does this procedure preclude accurate histologic diagnosis? Am J Clin Pathol. 2000;114(5):741–5.

Chapter 7
Thyroid Gland

Syed M. Gilani

Normal Cytology

The thyroid gland is an endocrine organ located anterior to the trachea and consists of two lobes connected at the midline by the isthmus. Depending on demographics and nutritional factors, the thyroid gland weighs between 14 and 18.5 g [1–3]. Pyramidal lobe, a normal component of the thyroid gland, can be seen in 15–75% [4]. Ultimobranchial bodies give rise to C cells (calcitonin-secreting cells), mostly seen in the mid-upper portion of thyroid lobes rather than peripheral areas and isthmus [4].

Fine needle aspiration (FNA) examination of the thyroid gland usually shows thyroid follicular cells that are smaller in size, arranged in a macrofollicular pattern, monolayer sheets, or often in mixed macro- and microfollicular patterns (Figs. 7.1 and 7.2). Follicular cells are small, close to the size of red blood cells, with round to oval nuclei, finely granular chromatin material, and smooth nuclear membrane. In addition, follicular cells can show pigment accumulation, such as hemosiderin. Colloid is usually present in the background, and appearance is variable in different cytology preparations and can either be watery or dense or thick. A watery colloid consists of a thin colloid layer and should be distinguished from the background serum. Color appearance is also variable and pink-orange or green in Papanicolaou and violet-blue with or without cracking artifact in Diff-Quik stain preparations. Calcium oxalate crystals can also be seen [5].

Other elements that are present include macrophages, cyst lining cells, lymphocytes, and Hurthle cells. Hurthle cells are oncocytic or oxyphilic cells with abundant granular cytoplasm and nucleoli that can be conspicuous [6]. They appear green or orange on the Papanicolaou stain and purple on Diff-Quik preparation.

S. M. Gilani (✉)
Department of Pathology, Albany Medical Center, Albany Medical College,
Albany, NY, USA
e-mail: gilanis@amc.edu

S. M. Gilani, G. Cai (eds.), *Non-Neoplastic Cytology*,
https://doi.org/10.1007/978-3-031-44289-6_7

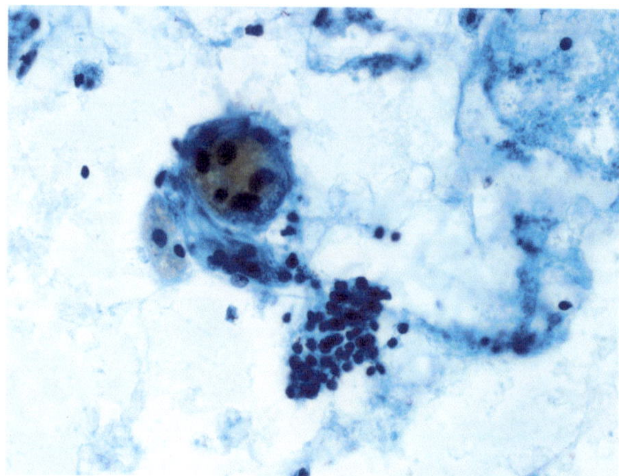

Fig. 7.1 Benign follicular cells with histiocytes (Papanicolaou stain × 400)

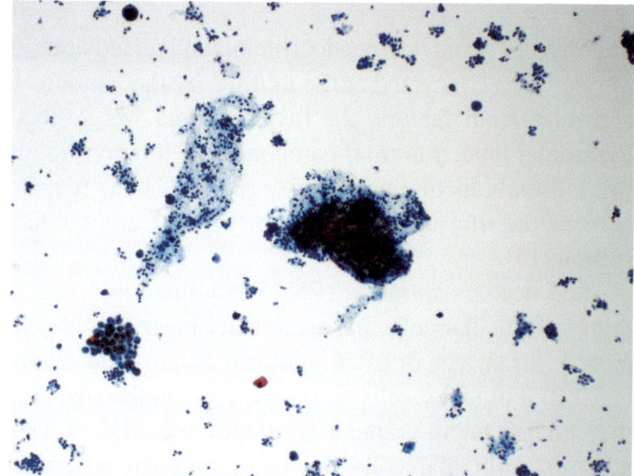

Fig. 7.2 Cellular specimen with mixed microfollicular and macrofollicular cells with histiocytes. No cytologic atypia is seen. Overall features showed mix population of cells and consistent with cellular goiter (ThinPrep × 100)

Adequacy Criteria

Thyroid FNA cytology evaluation should have at least six groups of follicular cells with at least ten cells in each group, preferably on one slide. There are a few exceptions to this adequacy criterion in certain scenarios, such as abundant colloid (Figs. 7.3 and 7.4), lymphocytic thyroiditis, or nuclear atypia in follicular cells [7]. Follicular cells should be well preserved without any obscuring artifact.

Fig. 7.3 Thin colloid with background histiocytes (Diff-Quik × 100)

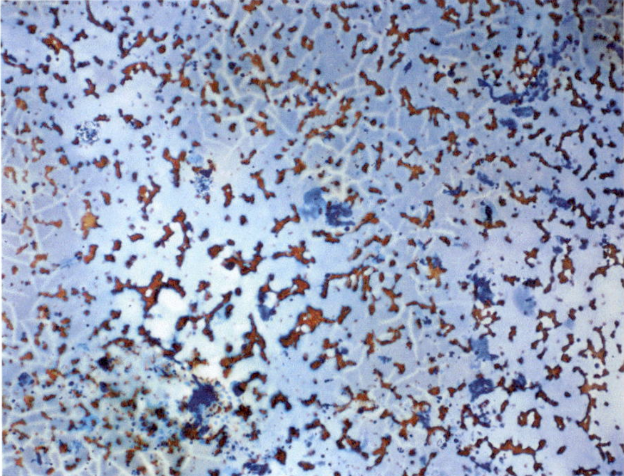

Fig. 7.4 Thick colloid and background red blood cells (Diff-Quik × 200)

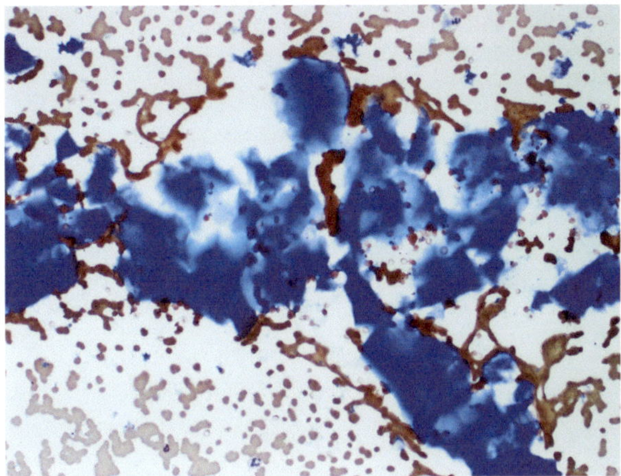

Artifacts

Certain artifacts should be in consideration while evaluating thyroid FNA cytology specimens. (Table 7.1).

Table 7.1 Artifacts and contaminants

	Differential diagnosis
Presence of cells form adjacent structures	
Ultrasound gel material (Fig. 7.5)	Colloid
Skeletal muscle (Fig. 7.6)	Colloid
Parathyroid tissue	Follicular cells
Thymic tissue [8]	Lymphocytes Lymphoma
Ciliated respiratory epithelial cells	Follicular cells
Presence of thyroid lesional cells	
Stripped follicular cells in smears (Fig. 7.7)	Lymphocytes
Macrophages (specially in ThinPrep)	Hurthle cells
Epithelioid histiocytes with elongated pale nuclei	Nuclear atypia/PTC

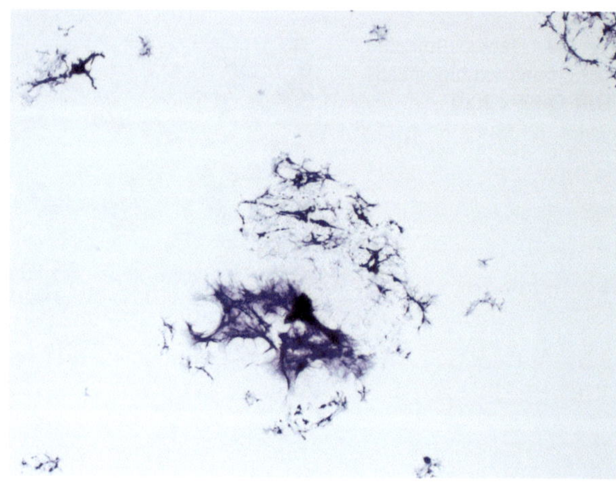

Fig. 7.5 Gel material used during the ultrasound procedure appears as amorphous material and should not be confused with colloid (ThinPrep × 400)

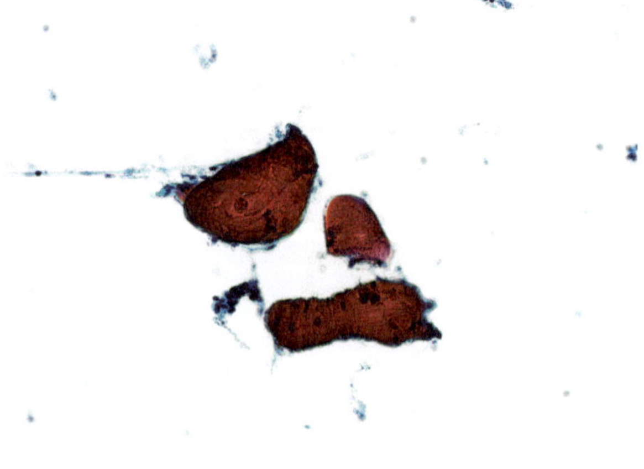

Fig. 7.6 Skeletal muscle fibers with striations can mimic colloid (Papanicolaou stain × 400)

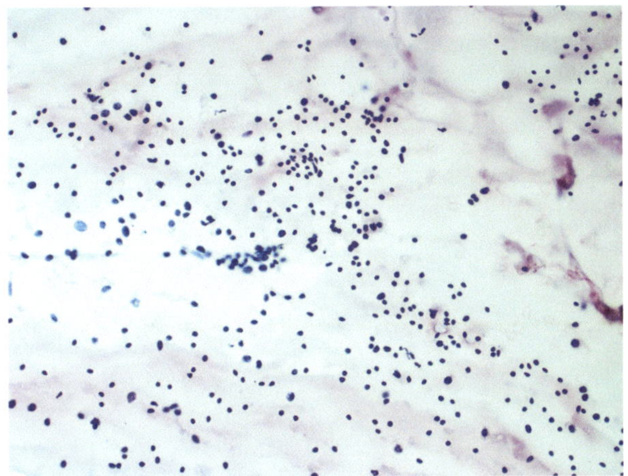

Fig. 7.7 Smearing artifact can produce a discohesive population of follicular cells which can resemble lymphocytes (Papanicolaou stain × 200)

Graves' Disease

Graves' disease is an important cause of hyperthyroidism and is an autoimmune condition caused by circulating autoantibodies [21]. On ultrasound, it may show hypervascularization with an "inferno pattern" can be seen in color-doppler studies [22, 23]. Thyroid scintigraphy can show diffusely elevated uptake within the gland [24]. Overall, there is a diffuse enlargement of the gland which can cause hyperplastic thyroid follicles and peripherally scalloped colloid. Tall columnar cells with eosinophilic cytoplasm and scattered lymphocytes can be seen. However, nuclei are usually round, but nuclear clearing and papillary hyperplasia can pose diagnostic challenges. After radioactive iodine treatment, nuclear atypia and oncocytic metaplasia can be seen. The differential diagnosis includes papillary thyroid carcinoma; identifying the clinical history of Graves' disease or RAI treatment is essential in such cases. Recognizing isolated nuclear features should be evaluated cautiously to avoid overinterpretation in the background of Graves' disease.

Hashimoto's (Chronic Lymphocytic) Thyroiditis

Hashimoto's thyroiditis (HT) is an important cause of hypothyroidism and is autoimmune thyroiditis caused by antithyroid antibodies (such as antithyroid peroxidase and anti-thyroglobulin) [25]. Radiologically, it appears as a diffusely enlarged gland with various patterns (echogenicity) and can show variable changes [26]. Morphologic evaluation of the specimen shows oncocytic cells, a mixed population of lymphocytes, and plasma cells with a variable number of colloid materials (Fig. 7.8). Isolated nuclear cytologic atypia can be seen in HT, which may result in overinterpretation (Fig. 7.9) [27]. Oncocytic cells (Hurthle cells) can also show atypia which is more recognized as an endocrine type of atypia or degenerative

Fig. 7.8 Lymphocytic
thyroiditis (Papanicolaou
stain × 200)

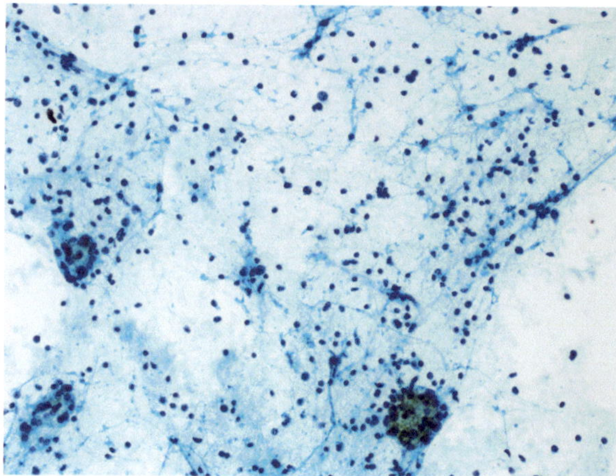

Fig. 7.9 Lymphocytic
thyroiditis with reactive
nuclear changes
(Papanicolaou stain × 400)

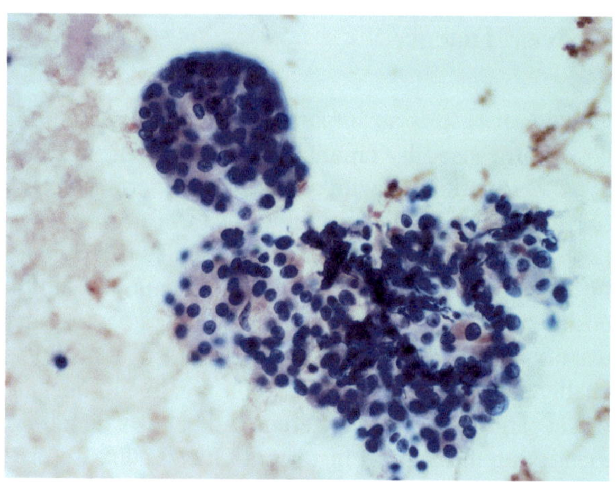

atypia. The differential diagnosis includes lymphoma or papillary thyroid carcinoma. B-cell lymphoma is the most common primary thyroid non-Hodgkin lymphoma [28]. Lymphoma shows a monomorphic population of neoplastic lymphoid cells, while in HT, lymphocytes are polymorphous. Obtaining an additional pass for flow cytometry would be helpful in suspected cases of lymphoma. Papillary thyroid carcinoma should have typical nuclear features such as nuclear crowding, clearing, grooves, enlargement, and intranuclear pseudoinclusions.

De Quervain (Sub-Acute Granulomatous) Thyroiditis

De Quervain (sub-acute granulomatous) thyroiditis is a self-limiting inflammatory condition, mostly due to viral infection, usually presents with pain in the thyroid gland and hyperthyroidism. On imaging, color doppler studies usually show

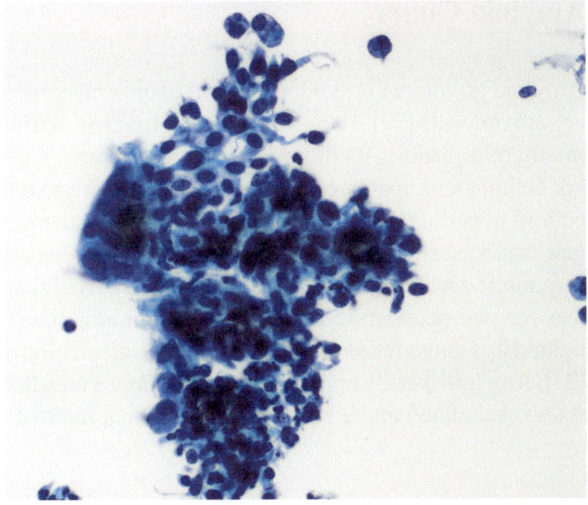

Fig. 7.10 Histiocytic aggregate with a multinucleated giant cell and background inflammatory cells (ThinPrep × 400)

decreased flow with low uptake on radionucleotide scans [29]. Morphologic evaluation shows epithelioid histiocytes, multinucleated giant cells, and inflammatory cells (neutrophils in the early stage, then lymphocyte and plasma cells) (Fig. 7.10). The differential diagnosis includes other forms of thyroiditis, such as granulomatous thyroiditis, palpation thyroiditis, and papillary thyroid carcinoma. Granulomatous thyroiditis usually shows epithelioid histiocytes, and granuloma formation and infectious etiology (fungal and mycobacteria) should be ruled out. Palpation thyroiditis can have multinucleated giant cells but usually lack inflammatory infiltrate. Papillary thyroid carcinoma can come in differential diagnosis, especially in cellular cytology specimens with many multinucleated giant cells and epithelioid histiocytes, which can show nuclear clearing and overlapping. However, the lack of atypical nuclear features of PTC and the presence of inflammatory infiltrate with multinucleated giant cells and epithelioid histiocytes help to differentiate these two entities.

Riedel Thyroiditis

It is an uncommon fibrosing process involving the thyroid gland and usually presents as a firm neck mass [30]. There is a suggestion in the literature that Riedel thyroiditis is within the spectrum of IgG4-related diseases. [31] Morphologically, it shows fibrosis and inflammatory infiltrates, mostly plasma cells. Due to fibrosis, the cytology specimen is usually paucicellular. The differential diagnosis includes a paucicellular variant of anaplastic thyroid carcinoma (ATC) [14]. However, atypia is more in ATC cases, and PAX-8 stain would be helpful for further characterization.

Amyloid Goiter

Amyloid goiter can present as thyroid gland enlargement due to primary or secondary amyloidosis [32]. However, the most frequent setting in which amyloid is seen in the thyroid gland is medullary thyroid carcinoma. Cytology specimens are usually not cellular and mainly consist of amorphous amyloid material, which can resemble colloid material (Figs. 7.11 and 7.12). However, the presence of associated vasculature can be seen in amyloid [33]. Amyloid has been reported in parathyroid, which can mimic medullary thyroid carcinoma [34]. Medullary carcinoma is usually positive for neuroendocrine markers and calcitonin stains. Amyloid material is highlighted by Congo red stain and shows apple-green birefringence under polarized light [35]. Amyloid usually appears as *bright yellow-green* fluorescence when Thioflavin-T stain is examined under an immunofluorescent microscope. See Table 7.2.

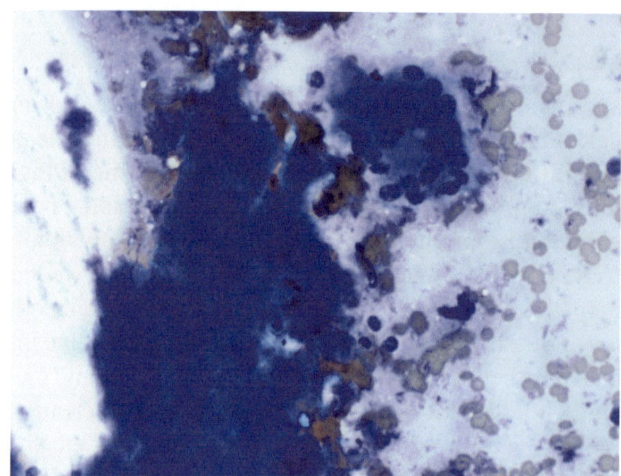

Fig. 7.11 Amyloid material with scattered spindle cells and multinucleated giant cells (Diff-Quik x 400)

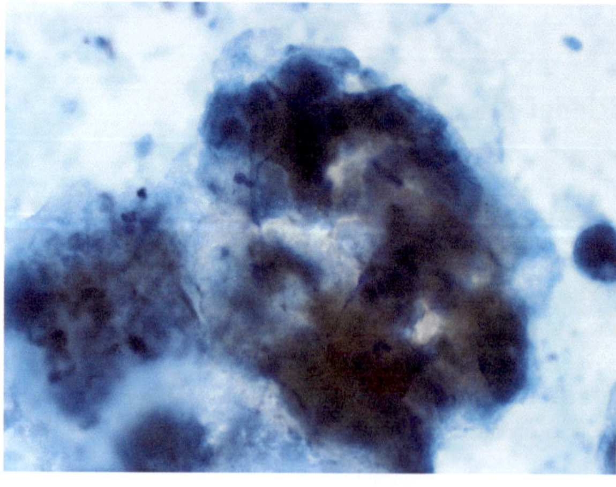

Fig. 7.12 Amyloid material with scattered spindle cells and multinucleated giant cells (Papanicolaou stain × 400)

Table 7.2 Benign and reactive conditions and differential diagnosis

Conditions	Cytomorphologic features	Differential diagnosis	Diagnostic clues
Graves' disease	Hyperplastic changes but decrease with treatment, papillary projections with scalloped colloid	Papillary thyroid carcinoma (PTC)	PTC—nuclear features of PTC are present
	RAI effects: Nuclear atypia, cytoplasmic vacuolization, lymphocytes, histocytes, Hurthle cell changes, and lack of microfollicular and papillary archetecture [9, 10]	PTC, and other higher-grade carcinomas (primary/ anaplastic, metastatic carcinoma) [11]	RAI—prior history of RAI
Chronic lymphocytic (Hashimoto's) thyroiditis	Mature mixed lymphocytes, scattered plasma cells, Hurthle cells which may show focal nuclear atypia, tingible-body macrophages, colloid can be scant	Lymphoma PTC	Lymphoma— predominance of monotonous proliferation, concerning clinical / imaging features PTC—look for classic nuclear features
De Quervain (sub-acute granulomatous) thyroiditis	Tender enlarged thyroid gland, multinucleated giant cells (frequent) and inflammatory cells. Well-formed granulomas and histiocytes with elongated pale nuclei can be seen	Palpation thyroiditis Thyroiditis (infectious) PTC	Palpation thyroiditis— patchy, lack neutrophils Infectious thyroiditis— clinical history, AFB/ GMS stains PTC—classic nuclear features
Riedel thyroiditis	Bland spindle cells, fibrous tissue fragments, Myofibroblast-like cells, inflammatory cells, lack atypia and mitosis [12]	Fibrosing Hashimoto's thyroiditis (FHT) [13] Paucicellular variants of anaplastic carcinoma (ATC) [14] Solitary fibrous tumor (SFT) [15]	FTH—Oncocytic/Hurthle cells, lymphocytes, and plasma cells [13] SFT— Immunohistochemical stains (STAT6) ATC—should have nuclear atypia, necrosis, and mitosis
Papillary hyperplasia	Papillary architecture usually lacking nuclear features of PTC. Focal atypia can be seen, and cautious evaluation is required to avoid over interpretation [16]	PTC	PTC—should have well-formed classic nuclear features

(continued)

Table 7.2 (continued)

Conditions	Cytomorphologic features	Differential diagnosis	Diagnostic clues
Sarcoidosis	Non-necrotizing granulomatous inflammation, epithelioid histiocytes with elongated pale nuclei	Other thyroiditis (infectious) PTC	Infectious thyroiditis—special stains PTC—well-formed nuclear features
Amyloid goiter	Amorphous eosinophilic material, fat cells [17], chronic inflammatory cells	MTC Systemic or localized amyloidosis Hyalinizing trabecular tumor	For MTC—calcitonin stain or serum calcitonin levels For amyloid (primary vs. secondary)—Congo red stain positive [18] and under polarized light apple green birefringence Thioflavin T stain bright yellow-green fluorescence under immunofluorescence microscope [19, 20]

RAI Radioactive iodine, *PTC* Papillary thyroid carcinoma, *MTC* Medullary thyroid carcinoma

Thyroid Cystic Lesions

1. *Thyroid nodule with degenerative cystic changes:* Cystic thyroid nodules contain macrophages, watery colloid, mixed pattern follicular cells, and may be Hurthle cells. Cyst-lining cells can also be seen in flat sheets with slightly elongated nuclei but with distinct borders (Fig. 7.13) [36]. They can show Hurthloid, or spindled morphology, occasional nuclear grooves, degenerative change, rare mitosis, and reactive atypia can be seen and should be evaluated cautiously to avoid overinterpretation. Papillary thyroid carcinoma with cystic changes comes in the differential diagnosis, which should show classic nuclear features of PTC such as nuclear crowding, overlapping, nuclear grooves, pseudoinclusions, and papillary architecture.

2. *Thyroglossal duct cyst:* Thyroglossal duct cysts are usually in the midline neck and near the hyoid bone. FNA usually yield low cellularity specimen, mainly consisting of inflammatory cells, macrophages, and scant epithelial component/lining cells such as ciliated respiratory type epithelium or squamous epithelial cells. The Cyst wall may contain thyroid follicular cells. Carcinoma can arise in TGDC, which is mostly PTC [37]. The differential diagnosis of TGDC includes other cystic lesions such as dermoid cyst, which usually consists of adnexal structures, and brachial cleft cyst, primarily located in the lateral neck.

3. *Parathyroid cyst:* Parathyroid cysts are rare, mainly around the inferior parathyroid gland [38] and the left thyroid lobe. They can present in any age group, but most cases are noted between the third and sixth decade [39]. Cyst aspirate is usually clear but less cellular and consists of cyst contents and scant cuboidal epithelial cells. Cyst fluid analysis can be sent for parathyroid hormone levels analysis [40, 41]. The differential diagnosis includes thyroid follicular cells or thyroid cysts. If cell block is available, performing PTH or thyroid origin markers such as Thyroglobulin and TTF-1 would be helpful to differentiate these two entities. See Table 7.3.

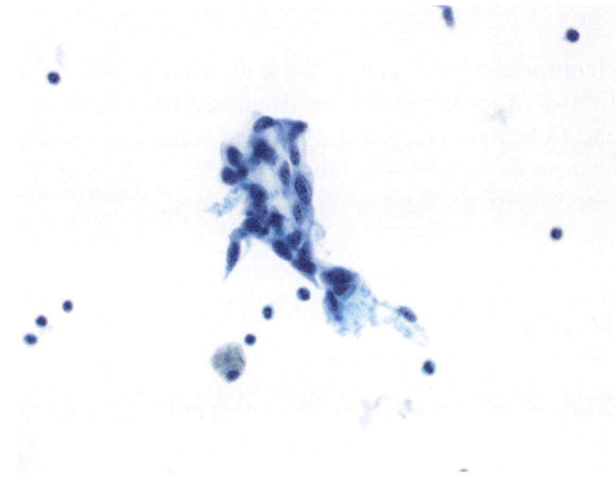

Fig. 7.13 Cyst lining cells with reactive changes and background histiocyte (ThinPrep × 400)

Table 7.3 Cystic lesions

Cystic lesions	Cytomorphologic features	Differential diagnosis
Thyroid nodule with degenerative cystic changes	Cysts contents including macrophages, follicular cells, Hurthle cells, cyst lining cells with reactive changes, watery colloid	Cystic PTC—classic nuclear features of PTC should be seen
Thyroglossal duct cyst	Cyst contents including macrophages, inflammatory cells, scant epithelial cells,	Epidermoid and dermoid cyst—mostly keratinizing squamous lining Brachial cleft cyst—lateral neck cyst
Parathyroid cyst	Clear aspirate, Hypocellular, cyst contents, scant epithelial cells	Thyroid cyst—aspirate is not clear, mostly brownish. PTH levels in aspirate are helpful

Pigments, Crystals, and Calcifications

Pigments

Pigmented material (Fig. 7.14) can be seen in thyroid parenchymal cells, including hemosiderin, lipofuscin, due to tetracycline (minocycline, Black Thyroid) and melanin.

Hemosiderin

Hemosiderin pigment is a coarse granular golden yellow to brown pigment derived from erythrocyte breakdown. Hemosiderin deposition can be seen in macrophages and follicular cells primarily due to secondary causes such as cystic degenerative changes or prior FNA or biopsy procedures. An Iron stain (Prussian blue) highlights hemosiderin as blue cytoplasmic material.

Minocycline

Oxidative changes, deposition of derivative, or degradation products of minocycline can result in dark brown granular pigmentation of follicular cells [42, 43]. It is usually seen in a long-standing history of taking tetracycline (minocycline). Pigment may stain positive for Fontana-Masson and bleach with potassium permanganate but negative for iron stain [42, 44].

Fig. 7.14 Sheet of follicular cells with granular pigment (brownish) (ThinPrep × 400)

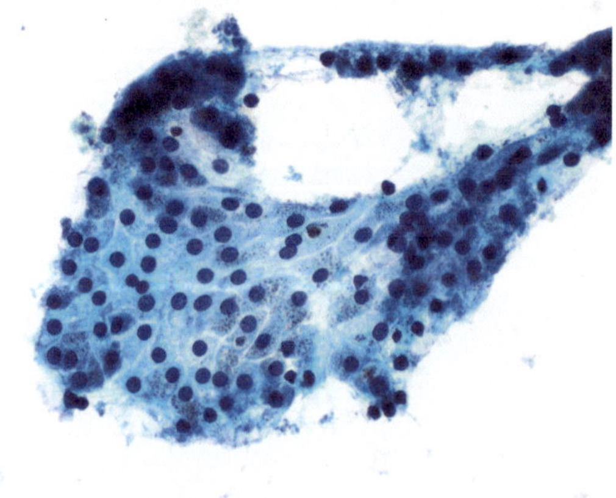

Lipofuscin

Cytoplasmic deposition of yellow to brown pigment is seen with aging and usually stain positive for lipofuscin stain and PAS-positive but negative for iron stain [44].

Melanin

Melanin is a fine granular brown-black cytoplasmic pigment. It is infrequently seen in the thyroid gland. However, rare cases of melanin-producing medullary thyroid carcinoma have been reported [45, 46]. Melanin stain with Fontana-Masson stain but negative for PAS.

Crystals

Calcium oxalate crystals are seen in the thyroid gland, specifically with colloid. They are birefringent under polarized light and can be found in all types of thyroid lesions and normal thyroid tissue [47]. They are more prevalent in goiter and adenomas [47]. the differential diagnosis includes calcifications. These crystals are rare in parathyroid tissue, and findings crystals by using polarized light microscopy would be helpful to differentiate thyroid tissue from parathyroid tissue in diagnostically challenging situations [48].

Calcifications

Dystrophic calcification: It is due to the deposition of calcified material in necrotic tissue or due to degenerative changes. They are usually coarse, dense, and irregular and do not show lamellation.

Psammoma bodies: They are basophilic and show concentric lamellation. They are often associated with papillary thyroid carcinoma. They can also be seen in benign conditions [49]. However, finding an isolated psammoma body without any atypical cells in thyroid aspirate may necessitate a comment on the presence of psammoma calcification with further correlation with clinical and imaging findings [50].

Infections

They are uncommon but can be seen due to bacterial, fungi, and mycobacterial infections.

Acute Suppurative Thyroiditis

It usually presents with fever, pain, and neck swelling due to bacterial infection, primarily by gram-positive bacteria (Staphylococcus aureus and Streptococcus species) [51]. Cytomorphologic exam may show inflammatory cells with a predominance of acute inflammation and necroinflammatory debris.

Granulomatous Thyroiditis

It can be infectious or non-infectious. Fungal (Aspergillus, Histoplasma, Candida spp., and others) [52, 53] and mycobacterial infections can cause inflammation, granuloma formation, and multinucleated giant cells reaction. Special stains and cultures are helpful for the identification and further characterization of the microorganism. Differential diagnosis includes non-infectious etiologies, including De Quervain (sub-acute) thyroiditis and sarcoidosis.

Thyroid Follicular Cells in Neck Region

Thyroid follicular cells can be seen in the central and lateral neck with associated differential diagnoses (Table 7.4).

Table 7.4 Thyroid follicular cells in the neck region

Thyroid parenchymal cells in neck region	Cytomorphologic features	Differential diagnosis	Diagnostic clues
1. Central neck [54–59]			
Thyroglossal duct cyst (TGDC)	Follicular cells, cysts contents, inflammatory cells	Papillary thyroid carcinoma (PTC)	PTC—can arise in TGDC and look for nuclear features
In lymph node	Follicular cells, lymphocytes	Metastatic PTC	PTC—if classic nuclear features of PTC are present. Presence of psammoma bodies (should be separated from dystrophic calcification)
Ectopic thyroid	Bland follicular cells and colloid	Lingual thyroid Substernal goiter PTC	Lingual thyroid—usually around base of tongue

Table 7.4 (continued)

Thyroid parenchymal cells in neck region	Cytomorphologic features	Differential diagnosis	Diagnostic clues
2. Lateral Neck [52–59]			
Parasitic nodule	Bland thyroid follicular cells, usually no lymphocytes except in Hashimoto's thyroiditis	Metastatic PTC	Evaluate for nuclear features, correlation with clinical and imaging features, any prior history of thyroid carcinoma
In lymph node	Thyroid parenchymal cells	Metastatic PTC Parasitic nodule with Hashimoto's thyroiditis	Nuclear features of PTC Additional work-up (clinical/imaging correlation) to rule out malignancy Any prior history of thyroid carcinoma

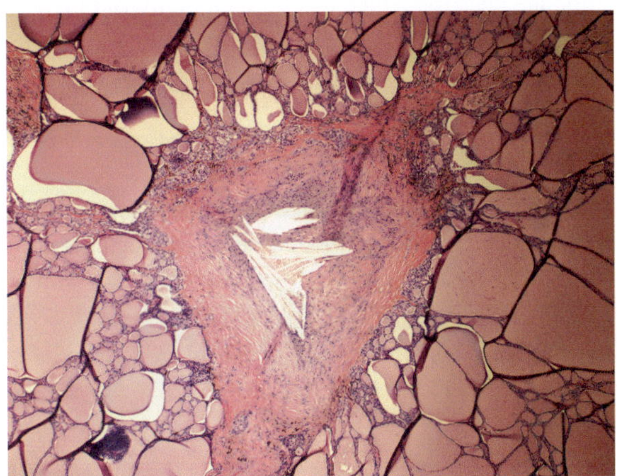

Figs. 7.15 Prior FNA-related changes with histocytes, fibrosis, cholesterol cleft formation, and surrounding follicular cells with nuclear atypia (H&E × 40)

FNA Induced Changes in Thyroid Gland and Differential Diagnosis

Fine needle aspiration (FNA) cytology helps in diagnosing thyroid lesions. However, the FNA procedure of the thyroid results in certain cytologic and histologic alterations, which are well described in the literature (Figs. 7.15). Early changes (less than 3 weeks) include the presence of hemorrhage, hemosiderin-laden macrophages, and granulation tissue. Morphologic changes that appear later include hemosiderin-laden macrophages, reactive cellular changes, fibrosis, and presence of myofibroblast cells, nuclear changes such as nuclear enlargement and clearing, metaplastic changes (squamous or oncocytic), infraction, cholesterol granuloma formation, vascular proliferation, and plumped endothelial cells [60–63]. In diagnostically challenging cases, cytomorphologic comparison with the prior FNA cytology may be helpful, if available.

Pitfalls

The presence of cytologic atypia and the above-described change in repeat thyroid FNA may pose diagnostic challenges. Nuclear atypia can stimulate features of papillary thyroid carcinoma. However, nuclear atypia due to post-FNA change is usually focal and lacks other features of PTC, such as intranuclear pseudoinclusions. The presence of spindle cells or myofibroblast-like cells, either due to reactive stromal changes or granulation tissue formation, can bring in a diagnosis of sarcoma or anaplastic thyroid carcinoma. Simultaneously, infarction due to prior procedure can stimulate necrosis which can be seen in thyroid malignancies.

Conclusion

To conclude, recognizing these cytologic changes and then the correlation with the clinical history (such as clinical/ imaging features and history of prior FNA procedure) is essential. Findings should be evaluated cautiously to avoid overinterpretation.

Acknowledgments None.

Conflict of Interest None.

References

1. Hegedüs L, Perrild H, Poulsen LR, Andersen JR, Holm B, Schnohr P, Jensen G, Hansen JM. The determination of thyroid volume by ultrasound and its relationship to body weight, age, and sex in normal subjects. J Clin Endocrinol Metab. 1983;56(2):260–3.
2. Pankow BG, Michalak J, McGee MK. Adult human thyroid weight. Health Phys. 1985;49(6):1097–103.
3. Mansberger AR Jr, Wei JP. Surgical embryology and anatomy of the thyroid and parathyroid glands. Surg Clin North Am. 1993;73(4):727–46.
4. Sinos G, Sakorafas GH. Pyramidal lobe of the thyroid: anatomical considerations of importance in thyroid cancer surgery. Oncol Res Treat. 2015;38(6):309–10.

5. Reid JD, Choi CH, Oldroyd NO. Calcium oxalate crystals in the thyroid. Their identification, prevalence, origin, and possible significance. Am J Clin Pathol. 1987;87(4):443–54.
6. Auger M. Hürthle cells in fine-needle aspirates of the thyroid: a review of their diagnostic criteria and significance. Cancer Cytopathol. 2014;122(4):241–9.
7. Cibas ES, Ali SZ. The 2017 Bethesda system for reporting thyroid cytopathology. Thyroid. 2017;27(11):1341–6.
8. Frates MC, Benson CB, Dorfman DM, Cibas ES, Huang SA. Ectopic Intrathyroidal Thymic tissue mimicking thyroid nodules in children. J Ultrasound Med. 2018;37(3):783–91.
9. Granter SR, Cibas ES. Cytologic findings in thyroid nodules after 131I treatment of hyperthyroidism. Am J Clin Pathol. 1997;107(1):20–5.
10. El Hussein S, Omarzai Y. Histologic findings and cytological alterations in thyroid nodules after radioactive iodine treatment for Graves' disease: a diagnostic dilemma. Int J Surg Pathol. 2017;25(4):314–8.
11. Centeno BA, Szyfelbein WM, Daniels GH, Vickery AL Jr. Fine needle aspiration biopsy of the thyroid gland in patients with prior Graves' disease treated with radioactive iodine. Morphologic findings and potential pitfalls. Acta Cytol. 1996;40(6):1189–97.
12. Harigopal M, Sahoo S, Recant WM, DeMay RM. Fine-needle aspiration of Riedel's disease: report of a case and review of the literature. Diagn Cytopathol. 2004;30(3):193–7.
13. Baloch ZW, Feldman MD, LiVolsi VA. Combined Riedel's disease and Fibrosing Hashimoto's thyroiditis: a report of three cases with two showing coexisting papillary carcinoma. Endocr Pathol. 2000;11(2):157–63.
14. Wan SK, Chan JK, Tang SK. Paucicellular variant of anaplastic thyroid carcinoma. A mimic of Reidel's thyroiditis. Am J Clin Pathol. 1996;105(4):388–93.
15. Rodriguez I, Ayala E, Caballero C, De Miguel C, Matias-Guiu X, Cubilla AL, Rosai J. Solitary fibrous tumor of the thyroid gland: report of seven cases. Am J Surg Pathol. 2001;25(11):1424–8.
16. Pusztaszeri MP, Krane JF, Cibas ES, Daniels G, Faquin WC. FNAB of benign thyroid nodules with papillary hyperplasia: a cytological and histological evaluation. Cancer Cytopathol. 2014;122(9):666–77.
17. Nijhawan VS, Marwaha RK, Sahoo M, Ravishankar L. Fine needle aspiration cytology of amyloid goiter. A report of four cases. Acta Cytol. 1997;41(3):830–4.
18. Ozdemir BH, Uyar P, Ozdemir FN. Diagnosing amyloid goitre with thyroid aspiration biopsy. Cytopathology. 2006;17(5):262–6.
19. Puchtler H, Waldrop FS, Meloan SN. A review of light, polarization and fluorescence microscopic methods for amyloid. Appl Pathol. 1985;3(1–2):5–17.
20. Saeed SM, Fine G. Thioflavin-T for amyloid detection. Am J Clin Pathol. 1967;47(5):588–93.
21. Wémeau JL, Klein M, Sadoul JL, Briet C, Vélayoudom-Céphise FL. Graves' disease: introduction, epidemiology, endogenous and environmental pathogenic factors. Ann Endocrinol (Paris). 2018;79(6):599–607.
22. Ralls PW, Mayekawa DS, Lee KP, Colletti PM, Radin DR, Boswell WD, Halls JM. Color-flow Doppler sonography in graves disease: "thyroid inferno". AJR Am J Roentgenol. 1988;150(4):781–4.
23. Vita R, Di Bari F, Perelli S, Capodicasa G, Benvenga S. Thyroid vascularization is an important ultrasonographic parameter in untreated Graves' disease patients. J Clin Transl Endocrinol. 2019;19(15):65–9.
24. Avs AK, Mohan A, Kumar PG, Puri P. Scintigraphic profile of thyrotoxicosis patients and correlation with biochemical and Sonological findings. J Clin Diagn Res. 2017;11(5):OC01–3.
25. Hu S, Rayman MP. Multiple nutritional factors and the risk of Hashimoto's thyroiditis. Thyroid. 2017;27(5):597–610.
26. Sostre S, Reyes MM. Sonographic diagnosis and grading of Hashimoto's thyroiditis. J Endocrinol Investig. 1991;14(2):115–21.
27. Khaled CS, Khalifeh IM, Shabb NS. Interpretive errors in Fine-needle aspiration of thyroid: a 13-year institutional experience in Lebanon. Acta Cytol. 2022;66(1):23–35.

28. Pedersen RK, Pedersen NT. Primary non-Hodgkin's lymphoma of the thyroid gland: a population-based study. Histopathology. 1996;28(1):25–32.
29. Frates MC, Marqusee E, Benson CB, Alexander EK. Subacute granulomatous (de Quervain) thyroiditis: grayscale and color Doppler sonographic characteristics. J Ultrasound Med. 2013;32(3):505–11.
30. Hennessey JV. Clinical review: Riedel's thyroiditis: a clinical review. J Clin Endocrinol Metab. 2011;96(10):3031–41.
31. Dahlgren M, Khosroshahi A, Nielsen GP, Deshpande V, Stone JH. Riedel's thyroiditis and multifocal fibrosclerosis are part of the IgG4-related systemic disease spectrum. Arthritis Care Res. 2010;62(9):1312–8.
32. Villa F, Dionigi G, Tanda ML, Rovera F, Boni L. Amyloid goiter. Int J Surg. 2008;6(Suppl 1):S16–8.
33. Yaeger KA, Hysell C, Pitman MB. Amyloid goiter. Diagn Cytopathol. 2010;38(10):742–3.
34. Ordoñez NG, Ibañez ML, Samaan NA, Hickey RC. Immunoperoxidase study of uncommon parathyroid tumors. Report of two cases of nonfunctioning parathyroid carcinoma and one intrathyroid parathyroid tumor-producing amyloid. Am J Surg Pathol. 1983;7(6):535–42.
35. Hill K, Diaz J, Hagemann IS, Chernock RD. Multiple myeloma presenting as massive amyloid deposition in a parathyroid gland associated with amyloid goiter: a medullary thyroid carcinoma mimic on intra-operative frozen section. Head Neck Pathol. 2018;12(2):269–73.
36. Faquin WC, Cibas ES, Renshaw AA. "atypical" cells in fine-needle aspiration biopsy specimens of benign thyroid cysts. Cancer. 2005;105(2):71–9.
37. Yang YJ, Haghir S, Wanamaker JR, Powers CN. Diagnosis of papillary carcinoma in a thyroglossal duct cyst by fine-needle aspiration biopsy. Arch Pathol Lab Med. 2000 Jan;124(1):139–42.
38. Cao H, Lai CK, Head CS, Sercarz JA. Cystic parathyroid presenting as an apparent thyroid goiter. Eur Arch Otorhinolaryngol. 2008;265(10):1285–8.
39. Papavramidis TS, Chorti A, Pliakos I, Panidis S, Michalopoulos A. Parathyroid cysts: a review of 359 patients reported in the international literature. Medicine (Baltimore). 2018;97(28):e11399.
40. Silva R, Cavadas D, Vicente C, Coutinho J. Parathyroid cyst: differential diagnosis. BMJ Case Rep. 2020;13(10):e232017.
41. Alvi A, Myssiorek D, Wasserman P. Parathyroid cyst: current diagnostic and management principles. Head Neck. 1996;18(4):370–3.
42. Keyhani-Rofagha S, Kooner DS, Landas SK, Keyhani M. Black thyroid: a pitfall for aspiration cytology. Diagn Cytopathol. 1991;7(6):640–3.
43. Tacon L, Tan CT, Alvarado R, Gill AJ, Sywak M, Fulcher G. Drug-induced thyroiditis and papillary carcinoma in a minocycline-pigmented black thyroid gland. Thyroid. 2008;18(7):795–7.
44. Senba M. Staining properties of melanin and lipofuscin pigments. Am J Clin Pathol. 1986;86(4):556–7.
45. Ikeda T, Satoh M, Azuma K, Sawada N, Mori M. Medullary thyroid carcinoma with a paraganglioma-like pattern and melanin production: a case report with ultrastructural and immunohistochemical studies. Arch Pathol Lab Med. 1998;122(6):555–8.
46. Kimura N, Ishioka K, Miura Y, Sasano N, Takaya K, Mouri T, Kimura T, Nakazato Y, Yamada R. Melanin-producing medullary thyroid carcinoma with glandular differentiation. Acta Cytol. 1989;33(1):61–6.
47. Katoh R, Kawaoi A, Muramatsu A, Hemmi A, Suzuki K. Birefringent (calcium oxalate) crystals in thyroid diseases. A clinicopathological study with possible implications for differential diagnosis. Am J Surg Pathol. 1993;17(7):698–705.
48. Wong KS, Lewis JS Jr, Gottipati S, Chernock RD. Utility of birefringent crystal identification by polarized light microscopy in distinguishing thyroid from parathyroid tissue on intraoperative frozen sections. Am J Surg Pathol. 2014;38(9):1212–9.
49. Ellison E, Lapuerta P, Martin SE. Psammoma bodies in fine-needle aspirates of the thyroid: predictive value for papillary carcinoma. Cancer. 1998;84(3):169–75.

50. Hunt JL, Barnes EL. Non-tumor-associated psammoma bodies in the thyroid. Am J Clin Pathol. 2003;119(1):90–4.
51. Paes JE, Burman KD, Cohen J, Franklyn J, McHenry CR, Shoham S, Kloos RT. Acute bacterial suppurative thyroiditis: a clinical review and expert opinion. Thyroid. 2010;20(3):247–55.
52. Goldani LZ, Zavascki AP, Maia AL. Fungal thyroiditis: an overview. Mycopathologia. 2006;161(3):129–39.
53. Berger SA, Zonszein J, Villamena P, Mittman N. Infectious diseases of the thyroid gland. Rev Infect Dis. 1983;5(1):108–22.
54. Barbieri A, Prasad ML, Gilani SM. Thyroid tissue outside the thyroid gland: differential diagnosis and associated diagnostic challenges. Ann Diagn Pathol. 2020;48:151584.
55. Thompson LD, Herrera HB, Lau SK. A Clinicopathologic series of 685 Thyroglossal duct remnant cysts. Head Neck Pathol. 2016;10(4):465–74.
56. Rosai J, Kuhn E, Carcangiu ML. Pitfalls in thyroid tumour pathology. Histopathology. 2006;49(2):107–20.
57. dos Santos VM, de Lima MA, Marinho EO, Marinho MA, dos Santos LA, Raphael CM. Parasitic thyroid nodule in a patient with Hashimoto's chronic thyroiditis. Rev Hosp Clin Fac Med Sao Paulo. 2000;55(2):65–8.
58. Triantafyllou A, Williams MD, Angelos P, Shah JP, Westra WH, Hunt JL, Devaney KO, Rinaldo A, Slootweg PJ, Gnepp DR, Silver C, Ferlito A. Incidental findings of thyroid tissue in cervical lymph nodes: old controversy not yet resolved? Eur Arch Otorhinolaryngol. 2016;273(10):2867–75.
59. Baloch ZW, LiVolsi VA. Post fine-needle aspiration histologic alterations of thyroid revisited. Am J Clin Pathol. 1999;112(3):311–6.
60. Recavarren RA, Houser PM, Yang J. Potential pitfalls of needle tract effects on repeat thyroid fine-needle aspiration. Cancer Cytopathol. 2013;121(3):155–61.
61. Eze OP, Cai G, Baloch ZW, Khan A, Virk R, Hammers LW, Udelsman R, Roman SA, Sosa JA, Carling T, Chhieng D, Theoharis CG, Prasad ML. Vanishing thyroid tumors: a diagnostic dilemma after ultrasonography-guided fine-needle aspiration. Thyroid. 2013;23(2):194–200.
62. Kini SR. Post-fine-needle biopsy infarction of thyroid neoplasms: a review of 28 cases. Diagn Cytopathol. 1996;15(3):211–20.
63. Batsakis JG, El-Naggar AK, Luna MA. Thyroid gland ectopias. Ann Otol Rhinol Laryngol. 1996;105(12):996–1000.

Chapter 8
Neck Lesions

Syed M. Gilani

Cystic lesions involving the neck region can be benign or malignant. Therefore, it is essential to correlate cytomorphologic features with the imaging findings as differential diagnosis varies with the location (central neck versus lateral neck cystic lesions). The non-neoplastic neck cystic lesion and their differential diagnoses are discussed below (see Table 8.1).

Table 8.1 Neck cystic lesion—differential diagnosis

Cysts	Location	Cytomorphology	Differential diagnosis
Thyroglossal duct cyst	Midline neck	Macrophages, inflammatory cells, epithelial cells (respiratory type or squamous lining) but usually scant, may have thyroid follicular cells	*Brachial cleft cyst*—lateral neck *Epidermoid cyst* and *dermoid cyst*—consist of keratinizing squamous epithelial lining *Cystic papillary thyroid carcinoma (PTC)*—classic nuclear feature of PTC
Branchial cleft cyst	Lateral neck	Macrophages, cystic debris, epithelial lining cells (mostly squamous), lymphocytes	*Thymic cyst*—mostly in pediatric age group and in lower lateral neck *Metastatic cystic squamous cell carcinoma (SCC)*—usually show atypia, mitosis, or necrosis. P16 and/or HPV positive in oropharyngeal primary type SCC

(continued)

S. M. Gilani (✉)
Department of Pathology, Albany Medical Center, Albany Medical College, Albany, NY, USA
e-mail: gilanis@amc.edu

© The Author(s), under exclusive license to Springer Nature Switzerland AG 2023
S. M. Gilani, G. Cai (eds.), *Non-Neoplastic Cytology*,
https://doi.org/10.1007/978-3-031-44289-6_8

Table 8.1 (continued)

Cysts	Location	Cytomorphology	Differential diagnosis
Cervical thymic cysts	Mostly in lateral neck	Macrophages, lymphocytes, epithelial lining cells (squamous or cuboidal), thymic tissue cells/ Hassall's corpuscles	*Brachial cleft cyst*—show lymphocytes but lack thymic tissue cells
Epidermoid and dermoid cyst	Anterior neck	Keratinizing squamous cells, debris, skin appendages (dermoid cyst)	*Branchial cleft cyst*—lateral neck *Well-differentiated SCC*— Cytologic atypia, mitosis, or stromal infiltration can be seen
Bronchogenic cyst	Midline (more) Lateral	Respiratory-type epithelial lining	*Branchial cleft cyst*—Lateral neck, usually have squamous lining and background lymphocytes

Thyroglossal Duct Cyst

Thyroglossal duct cysts (TGDC) are primarily located in the midline neck and are mostly seen in close relation to the hyoid bone [2]. TGDC arises from the embryological remnant of the thyroglossal duct and can be seen in 7% of the population [2]. Malignancy can rarely arise from TGDC, mostly papillary thyroid carcinoma [3]. However, squamous cell carcinoma has also been reported [4].

Fine needle aspiration (FNA) usually shows cyst contents, including macrophages, inflammatory cells, and cholesterol crystals. In addition, it may contain cyst-lining cells, either columnar (respiratory-type epithelium) or squamous epithelium. Thyroid follicular cells are usually in the cyst's wall and are rarely seen in the aspirates (Fig. 8.1) [3]. The differential diagnosis includes branchial cleft and epidermoid and dermoid cyst. The branchial cleft cyst is usually located in the lateral neck. Unlike TGDC, epidermoid cyst consists of squamous lining, which is keratinizing type, while dermoid cyst shows adnexal structures.

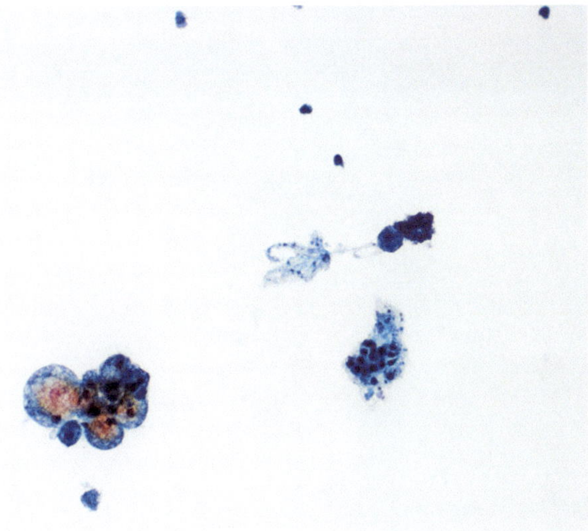

Fig. 8.1 Thyroid follicular cells and histiocytes suggestive of thyroglossal duct cyst (ThinPrep × 200)

Branchial Cleft Cyst

Branchial cleft cysts are lateral neck cysts developed from the congenital remnants of branchial cleft, mainly from the second branchial cleft and rare from the third and fourth cleft [5]. They are mostly present at the anterior border of the sternocleido-mastoid muscle and can present at any age but are typically seen in the younger age group. As these cysts present as a lateral neck mass and initial evaluation is usually performed by FNA. On cytology, the morphologic assessment shows cyst-lining cells (squamous epithelial cells), keratinous debris, and lymphocytes [6]. The differential diagnosis includes metastatic cystic squamous cell carcinoma (SCC), thymic cysts, epidermoid/dermoid cyst, lymphoceles, and laryngocele. Metastatic nonkeratinizing squamous cell carcinoma from the oropharyngeal primary is typically diffusely positive for p16-positive staining, which is not seen in branchial cleft cysts (Fig. 8.2) [7]. HPV DNA analysis could also be helpful in challenging situations [8]. On the contrary, metastatic keratinizing type SCC from other locations are usually p16 negative but can show cytologic atypia and mitosis. Cervical thymic cysts can show overlapping cytomorphologic features. Still, it is usually seen in children, and identifying thymic tissue (such as Hassall's corpuscles) can also help in morphologic differentiation. Epidermoid and dermoid cysts usually show squamous lining but lack lymphoid stroma. Lymphocele is a benign cystic structure of lymphatic origin, and on cytologic examination, it usually shows lymphocytes and macrophages (Fig. 8.3). Laryngocele is the dilatation of the laryngeal saccule, which can be external and morphologically; it shows respiratory-type epithelial lining but lacks a lymphoid component.

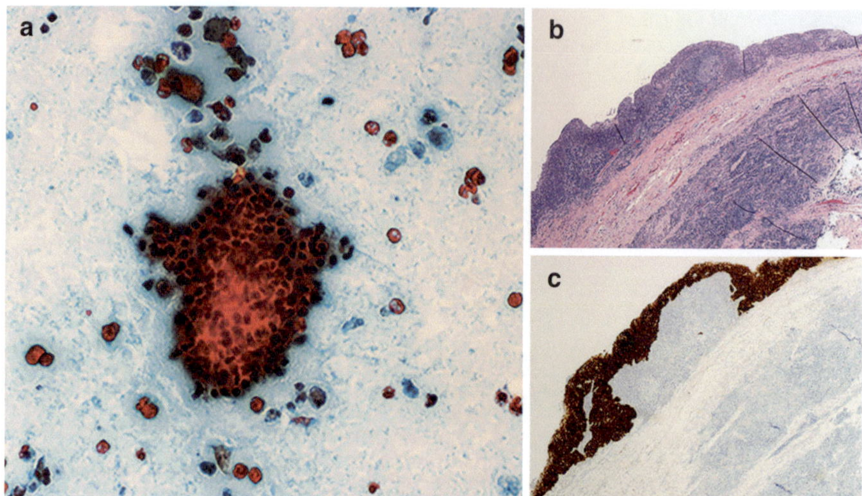

Fig. 8.2 (**a**) Cystic neck lesion FNA shows a cluster of epithelial cells in a background of histiocytes. (**b**) Resection of the cystic lesion shows a p16 positive (**c**) squamous cell carcinoma involving a lymph node ((**a**) Papanicolaou stain × 400, (**b**) H&E stain × 40, and (**c**) p16 stain × 40)

Fig. 8.3 Lymphocele with scattered lymphocyte sand macrophages (Cell block, H&E × 400)

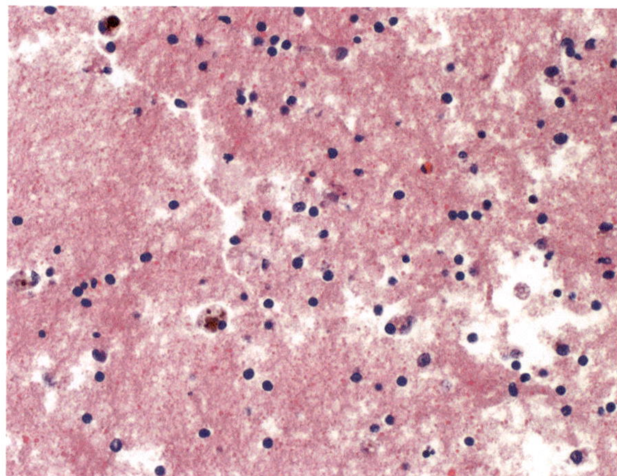

Cervical Thymic Cyst

Cervical thymic cysts are very rare and primarily seen in children. They are found in the lateral cervical region, more on the left side and usually lower neck, near the anterior aspect of the sternocleidomastoid muscle [9]. They can be unilocular or multilocular, and morphologic evaluation shows cysts contents, macrophages, cholesterol crystals, lymphocytes, and thymic tissue cells (Hassall's corpuscles) within

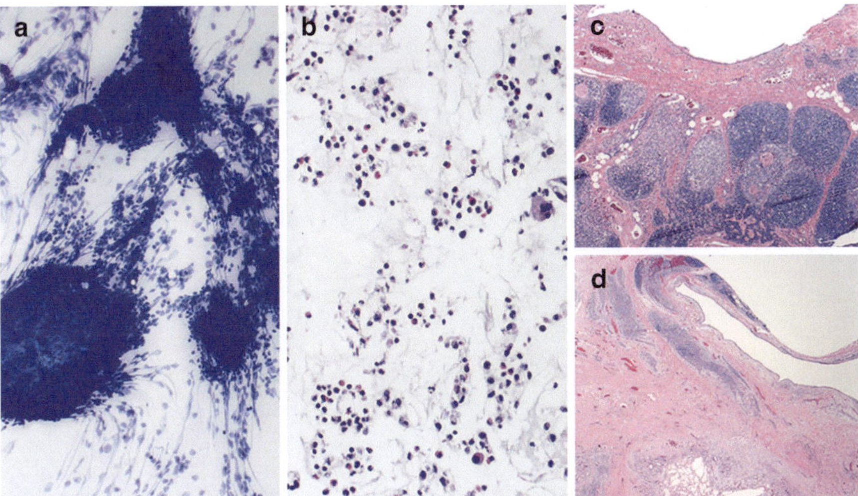

Fig. 8.4 Thymic cyst. (**a**) Crushed lymphocytes and other inflammatory cells (Diff-Quik × 100), (**b**) Mixed inflammatory cells and multinucleated giant cells (Cell block, H&E × 200), (**c** and **d**) Thymic tissue and cyst lining and background reactive changes (H&E, c × 40, and d × 20)

the cyst wall (Fig. 8.4). Cyst lining can show squamous or cuboidal cells. Differential diagnosis includes brachial cleft cyst and lymphangioma. The brachial cleft cyst is usually in the younger age group and lacks thymic tissue cells. Cystic hygroma is usually endothelial lined and can be seen in the lateral neck's anterior and posterior aspects.

Epidermoid and Dermoid Cyst

They are developmental cysts and can be seen in the anterior neck [1]. The locations in the oral cavity include the base of the tongue, floor of the mouth, and lip [1, 10]. They can be seen in any age group but are more prevalent in the younger age group [10, 11]. Cytomorphologic evaluation shows abundant keratinizing squamous epithelial cells and cystic debris (Fig. 8.5a, b). Dermoid cyst displays keratinizing squamous epithelial lining and skin appendages and rarely can also show respiratory-type epithelium [10]. Rarely, epidermoid cysts can be associated with squamous cell carcinoma [12]. The differential diagnosis includes a brachial cleft cyst and a well-differentiated keratinizing squamous cell carcinoma (SCC). Brachial cleft cysts are present in the lateral neck and show lymphoid components. Morphologic differentiation of a well-differentiated SCC from epidermoid/dermoid cysts can often be challenging. In such cases, identifying cytologic atypia, mitosis, and correlation with clinical history and imaging findings would be helpful for further differentiation.

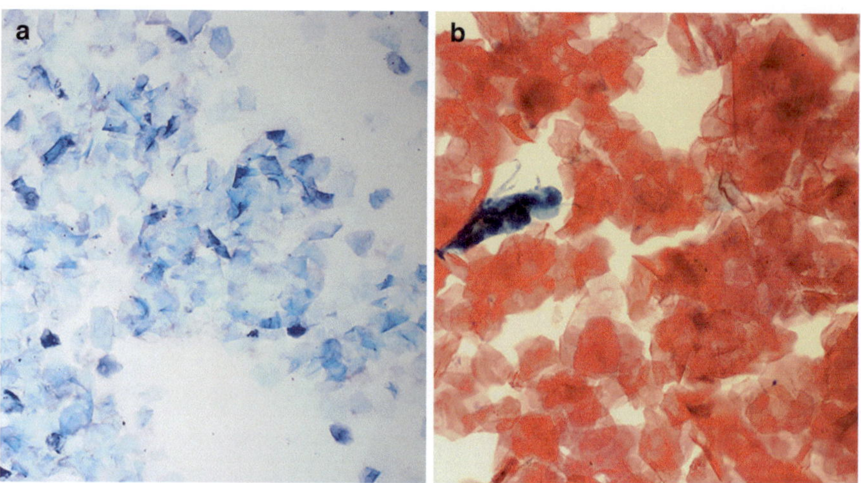

Fig.8.5 (**a**, **b**) Epidermoid cyst with anucleated squamous cells and rare multinucleated giant cells (**b**) ((**a**) Diff-Quik × 100 and (**b**) ThinPrep × 200)

Bronchogenic Cyst

Bronchogenic cysts are rare in the neck region and have been reported in adults and the pediatric population. They are primarily located in the midline neck but occasionally can be seen in the lateral neck [13]. Morphologically, they show the respiratory-type epithelial lining and cyst wall can have smooth muscle and submucous glands. The differential diagnosis includes a branchial cleft cyst typically located in the upper portion of the lateral neck [12].

Parathyroid Cyst

Parathyroid cysts are rare in the neck region and can be seen near the lower parathyroid and thyroid gland [14]. They are primarily paucicellular and contain scant epithelial cells. Measurement of PTH levels in fine needle aspiration (FNA) can be helpful. (See the thyroid chapter for details).

Lymphadenopathy

Cervical lymph node enlargement can be due to non-neoplastic or neoplastic processes. The non-neoplastic process includes Castleman disease, Kimura, Rosai-Dorfman disease, and others, and these entities are discussed in Chap. 9 (lymph node) with additional detail. The neoplastic processes include lymphoproliferative disorders/lymphoma and other metastatic malignancies.

Cystic Mass Due to Infectious Etiology or an Abscess

The infectious causes include mycobacterial infections and other infectious etiologies [15–17]. Cytologic features are variable and may show a granulomatous inflammatory reaction histiocytes (Fig. 8.6), mixed inflammatory infiltrate, or abundant acute inflammatory cells (abscess formation). In addition, the role of clinical history is significant, which often helps to include infectious causes in the differential diagnosis. In such cases, collecting an additional FNA pass for microbiologic cultures is helpful if there is any rapid onsite evaluation. In addition, special stains such as GMS and AFB on cell block material are also very helpful for identifying fungal organisms and acid-fast bacilli, respectively.

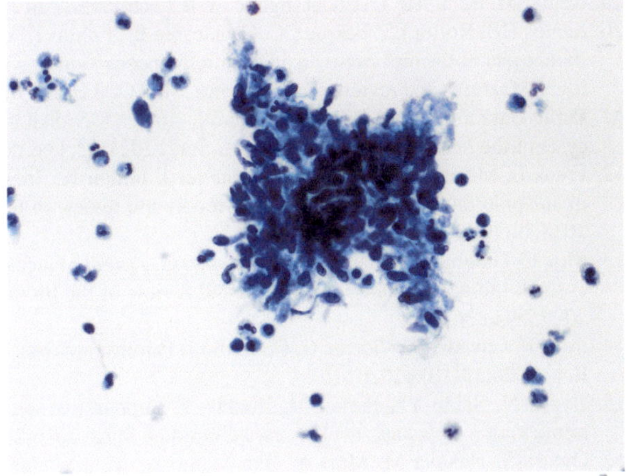

Fig.8.6 A loosely cohesive aggregate of histiocytes and surrounding inflammatory cells (ThinPrep × 400)

Acknowledgments None.

Conflict of Interest None.

References

1. Patel S, Bhatt AA. Thyroglossal duct pathology and mimics. Insights Imaging. 2019;10(1):12.
2. Ellis PD, van Nostrand AW. The applied anatomy of thyroglossal tract remnants. Laryngoscope. 1977;87(5 Pt 1):765–70.
3. Wei S, LiVolsi VA, Baloch ZW. Pathology of thyroglossal duct: an institutional experience. Endocr Pathol. 2015;26(1):75–9.
4. Henry L, Mignone R, Pepek J, Julien C, Rajasekaran K. Squamous cell carcinoma of a Thyroglossal duct cyst and the role of a level IA neck dissection. ORL J Otorhinolaryngol Relat Spec. 2020;82(3):163–7.
5. Prosser JD, Myer CM 3rd. Branchial cleft anomalies and thymic cysts. Otolaryngol Clin N Am. 2015;48(1):1–14.
6. Begbie F, Visvanathan V, Clark LJ. Fine needle aspiration cytology versus frozen section in branchial cleft cysts. J Laryngol Otol. 2015;129(2):174–8.
7. Pai RK, Erickson J, Pourmand N, Kong CS. p16(INK4A) immunohistochemical staining may be helpful in distinguishing branchial cleft cysts from cystic squamous cell carcinomas originating in the oropharynx. Cancer. 2009;117(2):108–19.
8. Sivars L, Landin D, Rizzo M, Haeggblom L, Bersani C, Munck-Wikland E, Näsman A, Dalianis T, Marklund L. Human papillomavirus (HPV) is absent in branchial cleft cysts of the neck distinguishing them from HPV positive cystic metastasis. Acta Otolaryngol. 2018;138(9):855–8.
9. Reiner M, Beck AR. Cervical thymic cysts in children. Am J Surg. 1980;139(5):704–7.
10. Santos HB, Rolim LS, Barros CC, Cavalcante IL, Freitas RD, Souza LB. Dermoid and epidermoid cysts of the oral cavity: a 48-year retrospective study with focus on clinical and morphological features and review of main topics. Med Oral Patol Oral Cir Bucal. 2020;25(3):e364–9.
11. Pupić-Bakrač J, Pupić-Bakrač A, Bačić I, Kolega MŠ, Skitarelić N. Epidermoid and dermoid cysts of the head and neck. J Craniofac Surg. 2021;32(1):e25–7.
12. Frank E, Macias D, Hondorp B, Kerstetter J, Inman JC. Incidental squamous cell carcinoma in an epidermal inclusion cyst: a case report and review of the literature. Case Rep Dermatol. 2018;10(1):61–8.
13. Moz U, Gamba P, Pignatelli U, D'Addazio G, Zorzi F, Fiaccavento S, Milesi F. Bronchogenic cysts of the neck: a rare localization and review of the literature. Acta Otorhinolaryngol Ital. 2009;29(1):36–40.
14. Silva R, Cavadas D, Vicente C, Coutinho J. Parathyroid cyst: differential diagnosis. BMJ Case Rep. 2020;13(10):e232017.
15. Bozan N, Sakin YF, Parlak M, Bozkuş F. Suppurative cervical tuberculous lymphadenitis mimicking a metastatic neck mass. J Craniofac Surg. 2016;27(6):e565–7.
16. Omura S, Nakaya M, Mori A, Oka M, Ito A, Kida W, Inayoshi Y, Inoue A, Fuchigami T, Takamori M. A clinical review of 38 cases of cervical tuberculous lymphadenitis in Japan—the role of neck dissection. Auris Nasus Larynx. 2016;43(6):672–6.
17. Melenotte C, Edouard S, Lepidi H, Raoult D. Diagnostic des adénites infectieuses [diagnosis of infectious lymphadenitis]. Rev Med Interne. 2015;36(10):668–76.

Chapter 9
Lymph Node

Omar Al-Rusan and Saja Asakrah

Introduction

Non-neoplastic lymph nodes are often sampled to rule out lymphoproliferative disorders or metastatic malignancy in cases of persistently enlarged lymph nodes and concerning imaging findings. Non-neoplastic lymph nodes are often characterized by an overall intact nodal architecture including intact follicles, preserved capsule, and patent sinuses, as well as preserved normal compartmentalization of T-lymphocytes and B-lymphocytes at different maturing stage that can be demonstrated by immunostains (Fig. 9.1). Benign lymphadenopathy may be due to infectious causes or non-infectious inflammatory/autoimmune causes. Some entities show mainly follicular pattern while others present as interfollicular/parafollicular expansion. Some inflammatory cells may be more prominent in certain entities versus others, for example, eosinophils in Kimura disease and plasma cells in IgG4-related disease. Granulomas raise a wide range of differential diagnosis including infection, foreign body reaction, sarcoidosis, and even lymphoma. Necrosis is a key feature in Kikuchi-Fujimoto disease but also raise the concern of a high-grade malignancy. Solely, these morphological features are insufficient for a final diagnosis and need to be correlated with the clinical features and specific ancillary test results.

Cytopathologic evaluation of an enlarged lymph node, although has its limitation (see Table 9.1), has been accepted as an initial diagnostic method in distinguishing between benign and malignant lymph nodes, particularly when combined with ancillary testing, such as flow cytometry and molecular studies to exclude clonality,

O. Al-Rusan · S. Asakrah (✉)
Department of Pathology and Laboratory Medicine, Emory University School of Medicine, Atlanta, GA, USA
e-mail: oalrusa@emory.edu; saja.asakrah@emory.edu

S. M. Gilani, G. Cai (eds.), *Non-Neoplastic Cytology*,
https://doi.org/10.1007/978-3-031-44289-6_9

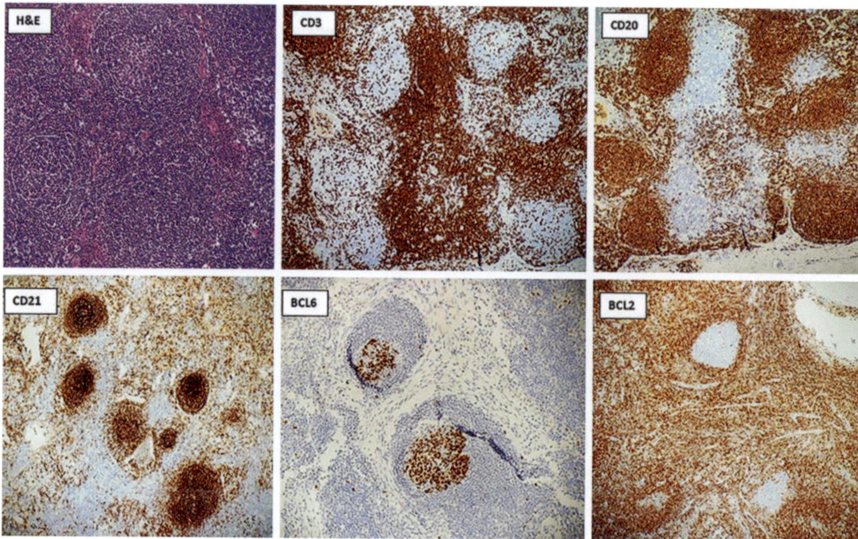

Fig. 9.1 Benign lymph node with intact architecture (40X). H&E section shows reactive germinal centers with well-defined mantle zone and normal distributed B- and T-lymphocytes. CD20 highlights B-cells arranged within CD21-positive follicular dendritic meshwork. CD3 stains properly highlight interfollicular T-cells. Germinal centers are appropriately BCL6 positive and BCL2 negative. BCL2 is also expressed by T-cells and mantle zone B-cells

Table 9.1 Limitation of fine needle aspiration in lymph node evaluation

- Lack key architectural features that distinguish certain benign lymphoid entities particularly Castleman disease, progressive transformation of lymphadenopathy (PTGC) and dermatopathic lymphadenopathy
- Limited sample with a potential risk of missing focal/partial lymphoid lesions, in-situ lymphoid neoplasm, and lymphomas that typically present with low neoplastic cells and a rich inflammatory background such as classic Hodgkin lymphoma
- Potential low cellular yield in fibrotic and necrotic lesions leading to false-negative result

and microbiology culture/staining when infection is suspected. However, further classification of benign lymph nodes is often precluded due to the lack of architecture evaluation. Additionally, one should keep in mind that ancillary testing also has limitations and may be misleading in certain instances, for example, flow cytometry usually shows negative findings in Hodgkin lymphoma, while on the other hand it may detect small clonal B-cells in reactive lymph nodes (see Table 9.2).

In this chapter, we will discuss key cytomorphological features of certain benign lymphoid lesions, the role and choice of ancillary testing to further characterize these lesions, differential diagnosis, and pitfalls. We think it useful to separate the topics that will be covered in this chapter by cause, topography, and key morphologic features (see Table 9.3).

Table 9.2 Limitation and pitfalls of flow cytometry

- A negative flow cytometry result does not exclude lymphoma particularly those with rich inflammatory background and limited neoplastic lymphoid cells
- A negative flow cytometry result may be due to sampling error of focal and partial lesions
- Identification of a monotypic B-cell population does not serve as definitive evidence of B-cell lymphoma, particularly if it is small and identified in tandem with polytypic B-cells. Small monotypic CD5 positive B-cells can be seen in chronic reactive lymph nodes and in situ mantle cell neoplasm, and small monotypic CD10 positive B-cells can be seen in lymph nodes with reactive follicular hyperplasia and in situ follicular neoplasm
- Fibrotic and necrotic samples may result in low yield cellularity leading to a non-diagnostic flow cytometry result

Table. 9.3 Classification of non-neoplastic lymphoid lesions

Infectious	Non-infectious/ reactive disorders
• Ebstein-Barr virus (EBV) (IM or IM-like hyperplasia) • Cytomegalovirus (CMV) • Human immunodeficiency virus (HIV) • Herpes simplex virus (HSV) • Cat-scratch disease • Toxoplasmosis • Mycobacterial infections	***Follicular:*** • Non-specific follicular hyperplasia • Progressive transformation of germinal center (PTGC) • Castleman disease • Kimura disease • SLE lymphadenopathy ***Parafollicular/interfollicular:*** • Dermatopathic lymphadenopathy ***Sinus:*** • Rosai-Dorfman disease ***Necrotic:*** • Kikuchi-Fujimoto disease ***Fibrotic:*** • IgG4-related lymphadenopathy ***Granulomatous:*** • Sarcoidosis

EBV Lymphadenitis (Infectious Mononucleosis)

The classic cases of infectious mononucleosis (IM) are associated with EBV, a member of the *Herpesviridae* family (HHV-4). Patients with IM will often present with typical symptoms, such as sore throat, fever, splenomegaly, and cervical or generalized lymphadenopathy [1]. To reach a proper diagnosis, clinicians will often correlate with cardinal laboratory findings, including leukocytosis, circulating atypical/reactive lymphocytes (Downey cells), a positive Monospot test and/or the presence of circulating antibodies by serology [2, 3]. Therefore, a lymph node biopsy is generally not needed. In fact, it is often discouraged as the histomorphologic features can easily mimic a neoplastic process. It is only when the patient presents with atypical signs and symptoms do healthcare professionals elect to perform a biopsy [4, 5].

Histological Findings:

Microscopically, the disease typically shows subtotal effacement of normal lymph node architecture, reactive follicular hyperplasia, and paracortical expansion mostly by a "polymorphous" B-cell infiltrate composed of immunoblasts, plasma cells, plasmacytoid B-cells, and small to medium sized B-cells [6, 7]. Focal necrosis is not an uncommon finding. Some of these features might be notably more prominent or exaggerated in immunocompromised individuals.

Cytological Findings

Lymph node aspirates will often contain small to medium sized lymphocytes mixed with a variable number of immunoblasts. Early in the disease course, immunoblasts might be scarce and difficult to detect. With more advanced stages of the disease, the immunoblast population becomes more visible and larger Reed-Sternberg like immunoblasts may start to appear (Fig. 9.2a). Although it is exceedingly rare to find multi/binucleated immunoblasts that would mimic the characteristic Reed-Sternberg cells seen in Classic Hodgkin Lymphoma (Fig. 9.2b) [8].

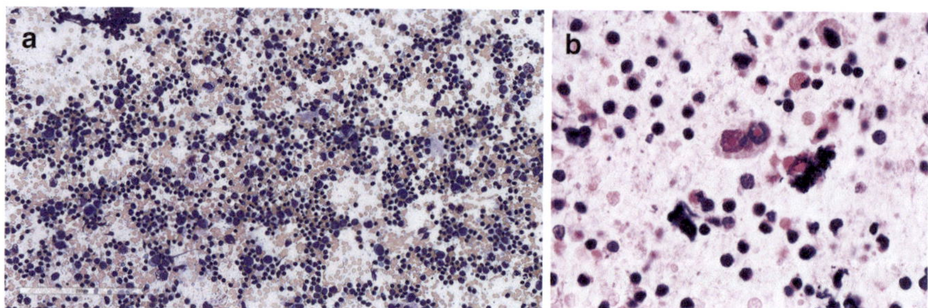

Fig. 9.2 EBV infection with immunoblasts: (**a**) Cytology smear (diff-quick stain 60X) demonstrating a mixture of variably sized cells including small lymphocytes, plasma cells, and large immunoblasts. (**b**) Cytology cell block section (H&E, 100X) showing typical Reed-Sternberg Hodgkin cells (binucleated with prominent red cherry nucleoli)

Differential Diagnosis:

Classic Hodgkin Lymphoma (CHL)

As mentioned above, IM can mimic CHL, especially when there are large Hodgkin-like immunoblasts. In such cases, the following features might help in supporting one versus the other. Nevertheless, definitive diagnosis can only be made on adequate histological sections.

- In contrast to CHL, reactive immunoblasts are CD45 positive and often retain B-cell markers expression including CD20 and strong PAX5. Reactive immunoblasts are negative for CD15 and may show variable staining with CD30. In contrast, Hodgkin cells show strong staining with CD30, partially or completely loss of B-cell markers expression and may or may not show CD15 co-expression.
- EBV (Epstein-Barr Virus) status can be determined by immunohistochemistry or in situ hybridization and could be positive in both CHL and EBV lymphadenitis. However, it is worth noting that EBV positivity tends to be in the small and large cells in IM (as opposed to only Hodgkin cells in CHL).

Other Viral-Induced Lymphadenitis

Alternative causes of viral lymphadenitis, HSV, CMV, and early HIV infections, share a lot of histologic and cytomorphologic features with IM; including having a mixed population of variably sized lymphocytes, immunoblasts, and histiocytes. In these situations, serological testing becomes necessary to make the diagnosis.

CMV Lymphadenitis

Like EBV, CMV is a member of the *Herpesviridae* family (HHV-5) and can cause infections in both immunocompetent and immunocompromised patients [9]. Healthy adult hosts are usually either asymptomatic or have an IM-like disease, whereas immunosuppressed hosts can experience a broad spectrum of disease manifestations, ranging from generalized constitutional symptoms to severe and potentially life-threatening infections [10]. In the vast majority of cases, performing a lymph node biopsy is deemed unnecessary and often avoided [11].

Histological Findings

The histomorphologic features of CMV lymphadenitis have been well documented [12, 13] and microscopic examination typically shows follicular hyperplasia, monocytoid B-cell proliferation, prominent vasculature, and paracortical expansion. These changes are parallel to those seen in other viral infections. Immunoblasts are also readily visible with some even resembling Reed-Sternberg cells.

Cytological Findings

Lymph node and fluid aspirate smears can show a mixture of small lymphocytes and proliferating immunoblasts as well as the distinctive viral cytopathic change seen in some of the infected cells; the so-called owl-eye eosinophilic inclusion body surrounded by a clear halo [14]. A CMV immunohistochemical stain or in situ hybridization may be used to highlight those intranuclear inclusions when necessary [15].

Differential Diagnosis

Infectious Mononucleosis (IM)

As mentioned above CMV lymphadenitis can resemble IM both clinically and microscopically, but IM is different in that:

- Laboratory testing will yield positive results for serum EBV IgM and heterophilic antibodies, especially in the acute phase.
- In situ hybridization for EBV-encoded RNA (EBER) will be positive.
- Will be negative for CMV (by in situ hybridization or immunohistochemistry).
- Will not have the characteristic "owl-eye" inclusion bodies.

HSV Lymphadenitis

Follicular hyperplasia is often present in HSV, and lymph nodes can show prominent monocytoid B-cell hyperplasia as well as extensive necrosis (similar to CMV lymphadenitis). Although the following features of HSV lymphadenitis will be helpful in making the distinction:

- Large multinucleated cells and chromatin margination.
- Nuclear molding (best appreciated by cytology).

- Ground-glass eosinophilic intranuclear inclusion bodies (Cowdry A).
- Positive serological testing for HSV.
- No "owl-eye" inclusion bodies.

Cat-Scratch Disease

Cat-scratch disease is a self-limited infection caused by facultative-intracellular, Gram-negative bacteria, *Bartonella henselae*. As the name implies, the disease is transmitted via asymptomatic feline carriers (primarily cats), usually after a scratch or a bite. In most instances, patients are younger than 18 years of age and typically present with tender lymphadenopathy localized to axillary, neck, or inguinal regions, which may be associated with mild constitutional symptoms, such as fever, fatigue, or generalized joint pains [16, 17]. The infection usually spontaneously resolves within 2 months in immunocompetent hosts. Although treatment may be indicated in more persistent cases or in patients with suppressed immune response [16].

Histological Findings

Initially, lymph nodes show proliferation of monocytoid cells and neutrophils as well as the characteristic amorphous eosinophilic deposits within germinal centers. As the inflammation progresses, small foci of necrosis start to appear, which eventually enlarge and coalesce to form necrotizing granulomas *"Stellate granulomas"* [18]. An immmunohistochemical stain or a modified silver stain (Warthin-Starry) is often used to detect *B. henselae*, with some studies suggesting combining the two methods for a higher sensitivity [19].

Cytological Findings

Smears show aggregates of epithelioid histiocytes with many interspersed neutrophils, and a varying number of medium sized monocytoid lymphocytes (Fig. 9.3). The number of neutrophils can be so high that it obscures the smaller granulomas [20]. These findings can be seen in other causes of granulomatous lymphadenitis (e.g., tuberculosis), which is why cytologic diagnosis must be suggestive at best, or confirmatory in cases with tangible clinical suspicion.

Fig. 9.3 Suppurative granuloma in cat-scratch infection: Cytology smear (Papanicolaou (PAP) stain 60X) showing granuloma with necrosis and numerous neutrophils

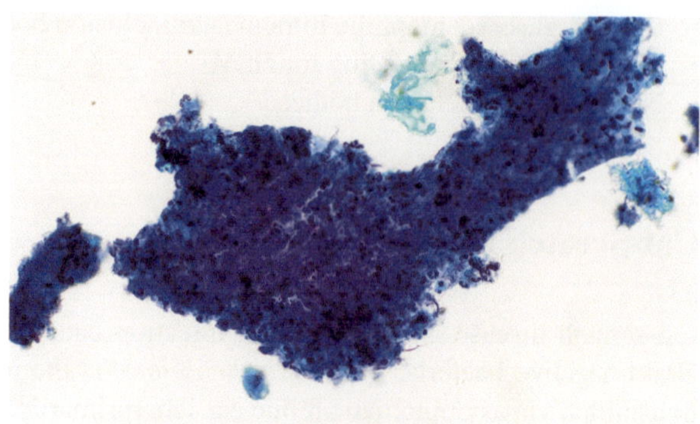

Differential Diagnosis

Mycobacterial Lymphadenitis

Some of the features that would support the diagnosis of mycobacterial lymphadenitis over cat-scratch disease are the following:

- Clinically, patients will often present with bilateral hilar lymphadenopathy, respiratory symptoms, and might have cavitary pulmonary lesions.
- Mycobacterial infections will cause caseating (not stellate) granulomas.
- Acid-fast staining may highlight the causative microorganism.
- Tuberculin skin testing, interferon gamma release assays (IGRA), and PCR molecular testing can be used for identification.

Fungal Lymphadenitis

The following are some helpful key features:

- Fungal elements, such as hyphae and yeast forms, may be appreciated on routine H&E stains.
- Definitive identification with culture study is necessary.
- GMS or PAS stains can be used to highlight the causative agent.

Classic Hodgkin Lymphoma (CHL)

Granulomas can occasionally be seen in CHL, particularly the mixed cellularity subtype. The granulomatous inflammation might be so exuberant that it may mask the neoplastic process and be misinterpreted as an infectious one [21]. In such cases, the following features help distinguish it from cat-scratch disease:

- The presence of Hodgkin/Reed-Sternberg cells with the classic immuno-phenotype.
- Mixed inflammatory background, including eosinophils and plasma cells.

Follicular Hyperplasia (FH) with Progressive Transformation of Germinal Center (PTGC)

PTGC is a benign reactive lymphoid lesion of unclear etiology commonly identified in the head and neck region. PTGC is usually self-resolved but may last more than 6 months.

Histological Findings

PTGC is characterized by large germinal centers with ill-defined mantle zone and dense small mantle B-cells occupying and disrupting the germinal centers. Florid reactive follicular hyperplasia is often present. Such morphology may resemble follicular lymphoma (FL) and nodular lymphocyte predominant Hodgkin lymphoma (NLPHL); therefore, both should be excluded. Of note, a small percentage PTGC are proceeded by or concomitantly associated with NLPHL.

Cytological Findings

The diagnosis of PTGC cannot be made in fine needle aspiration samples as it requires the identification of key architectural features described above. The cytology smear of a lymph node with florid follicular hyperplasia with or without PTGC is usually cellular with dense lymphoid population thus often triaged for flow cytometry when evaluated on site. The lymphocytes are heterogenous and include small mature lymphocytes with scant cytoplasm and dense nuclear chromatin, large centroblasts with vesicular nuclear chromatin and multiple membrane bound nucleoli, and immunoblasts with prominent central nucleoli. Tingible-body macrophages and fragments of follicular dendritic meshwork are frequently present (Fig. 9.4). Follicular dendritic cells (FDCs) show delicate nuclear membranes, vesicular nuclear chromatin, and ill-defined cytoplasmic membranes.

Differential Diagnosis

Mainly includes B-cell lymphoma. Features that distinguish FH/PTGC from B-cell lymphoma include the following:

- Heterogenous lymphoid population supports FH/PTGC, while a monomorphic lymphoid population, particularly if it constitutes of large B-cells, is concerning for large B-cell lymphoma. It is important to keep in mind that FL may not present as a monomorphic smear, and it usually shows a mixture of small centrocytes

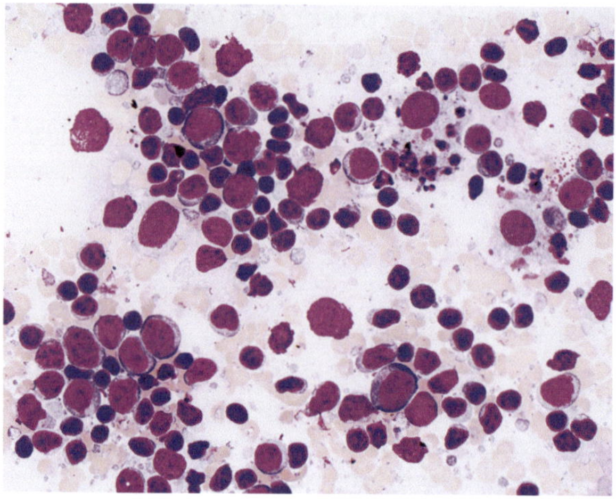

Fig. 9.4 Florid follicular hyperplasia with frequent centroblasts: Cytology smear (diff-quick stain 60X) showing mixture of large centroblasts and small centrocytes and tingible body macrophages

and large centroblasts in variable ratios depending on the cytological grade. Tingible body macrophages although less frequent, can be seen in FL.

- Flow cytometry in FH/PTGC show polytypic B-cells. However, one should always consider the limitations and pitfalls of flow cytometry (see Table 9.2).

Castleman Disease

Castleman Disease (CD) is a lymphoproliferative disorder that usually affects adults in the third decade of life. The etiology is still largely unknown, but is believed to be related to immune dysregulation, genetic factors, or infections in some cases. CD is divided into two types: unicentric (UCD) and multicentric (MCD). The extent of disease manifestation varies depending on the type. Patients with UCD are mostly asymptomatic or have localized lymphadenopathy found incidentally by imaging. Whereas the MCD type will often be found in immunocompromised (IC)/HIV-infected patients driven by HHV8 infection. MCD also can be HHV8 negative classified as "idiopathic" or associated with rare multisystemic diseases (i.e., POEMS syndrome, TAFRO syndrome) [22]. Patients with MCD present with generalized lymphadenopathy, and severe systemic features caused by high cytokine levels notably IL6. Fever, night sweats, pleural effusions, leukocytosis, and weight loss are common clinical features [23].

Histological Findings

CD is histologically divided into the "hyaline vascular" and the "mixed/plasmacytic" variants. The hyaline vascular CD variant is more frequent in UCD and shows many atrophic follicles with concentric layering of the mantle zones, commonly referred to as the "onion skin" appearance. The germinal center in these regressed follicles will often be penetrated by a hyalinized blood vessel that if tangentially cut, will demonstrate the characteristic "lollipop" sign. Some follicles will also have two germinal centers, a feature commonly described as "twinning" [24]. Moreover, the interfollicular area will be expanded with high endothelial venules that may obliterate the sinuses. The mixed/plasmacytic variant is more common in MCD and shows a mixture of atrophic and hyperplastic follicles with interfollicular polytypic plasmacytosis. In some cases, particularly those associated with HIV and HHV8 infection, small clusters of HHV8-positive plasmablasts located primarily in the mantle zone can be seen. These plasmablasts are lambda restricted.

Cytological Findings

Findings on aspirate smears are non-specific and may reveal branching or fragmented blood vessels with a variable number of plasma cells in a background of a polymorphous cell population. Low frequency of plasmablasts and immunoblasts can also be seen (Fig. 9.5). The plasmablast are large in sized with abundant

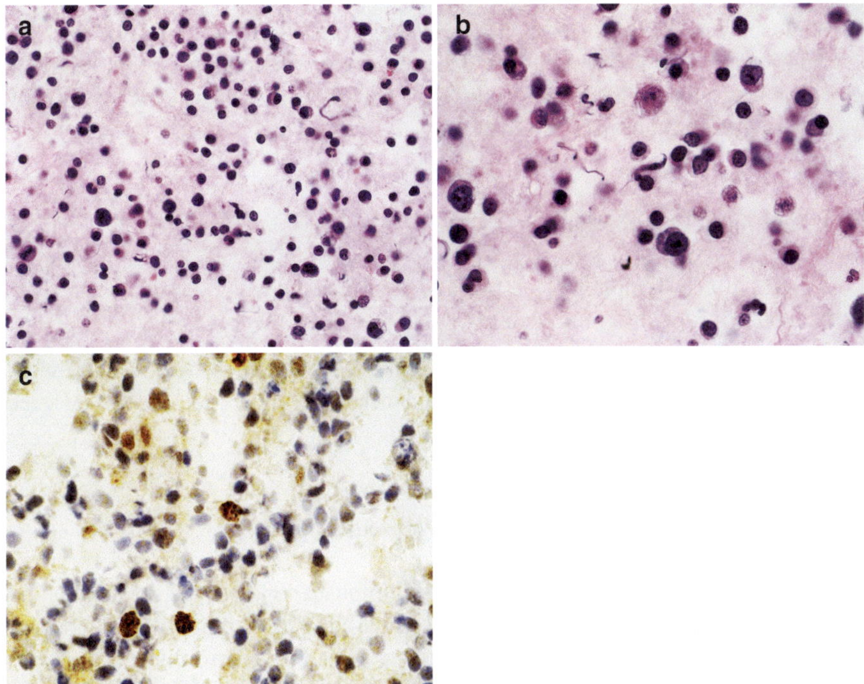

Fig. 9.5 Multicentric Castleman disease in HIV-infected patient: (**a**) Cytology smear (Papanicolaou (PAP) stain 60X) showing a mixture of small lymphocytes, plasma cells, and plasmablasts. (**b**) A large plasmablast with prominent nucleoli. (**c**) Few scattered plasma blasts are positive for HHV8 immunostain with typical nuclear dot-like pattern

basophilic cytoplasm and eccentric nucleus with prominent nucleoli (Fig. 9.5b). The immunoblasts are intermediate to large lymphoid cells with prominent nucleoli. Nonetheless, a lymph node excision is imperative for a certain diagnosis [25, 26].

Differential Diagnosis

HHV8-Positive Plasmablastic Malignancy, Primarily Include Primary Effusion Lymphoma (PEL) and HHV8-Positive Diffuse Large B-Cell Lymphoma (DLBCL)

Clinical features (HIV/IC patient, LAD, systemic disease), inflammatory blood tests (high IL6), and cytological findings (HHV8-positive plasmablasts) are found in PEL, HHV8-DLBCL, and MCD; therefore, the distinction between these entities is often challenging. Features that are in favor of a malignancy are the following:

- HHV8-positive plasmablasts are the prominent population in PEL and HHV8-DLBCL, while they are usually not frequent in multicentric CD specimen (Fig. 9.5c).
- While plasmablasts are lambda restricted in HHV8-DLBCL and MCD; PEL usually lacks surface/cytoplasmic light chain expression (small subset might be kappa restricted). Also, clonality by *IGH* gene rearrangement PCR test is only observed in PEL and HHV8-DLBCL.

Marginal Zone Lymphoma

Low-grade B-cell lymphomas, especially marginal zone lymphoma, can show marked plasmacytic differentiation but will also exhibit the following:

- Evidence of a monotypic and monoclonal B-cell population by flow cytometry, immunohistochemical stains for kappa and lambda light chain, and *IGH* gene rearrangement PCR test.

Systemic Lupus Erythematosis (SLE) lymphadenopathy

SLE as well as other autoimmune-related lymphadenopathies (e.g., rheumatoid arthritis, IgG4-related disease) are often considered in the differential diagnosis of CD, as they can also show prominent plasmacytosis [27]. Performing appropriate serological testing and knowing the patient's clinical presentation is crucial in such cases.

Kimura Disease

Kimura disease (KD) is a rare chronic inflammatory disorder of unknown etiology that involves the subcutaneous tissue and lymph nodes of the head and neck region. The pathogenesis is still poorly understood but is thought to be related to infectious causes although a definite correlation with a pathogen has yet to be identified. Other proposed causes include allergic conditions and various other immune-related phenomena [28]. It predominately occurs in young adult Asian males and presents as subcutaneous nodules in the head and neck area associated with regional lymphadenopathy. Patients may also have renal manifestations [29]. Peripheral blood eosinophilia and elevated serum immunoglobulin E (IgE) levels are essentially always detected [30], but systemic symptoms are not common.

Histological Findings

Microscopic examination often reveals a preserved, although somewhat distorted, lymph node architecture that is characterized by reactive follicular hyperplasia with marked eosinophilia, focally forming eosinophilic microabscesses [31]. The eosinophils can be seen trickling into the germinal centers, which in many cases, can have proteinaceous IgE deposits as well as Warthin-Finkeldey type prokaryocytes [31].

Cytological Findings

When carried out, fine needle aspirations yield a polymorphous cell population including many eosinophils and occasional interspersed Warthin-Finkeldey cells, the giant cells with multiple grape-like clustering of nuclei. Endothelial fragments and fibrinous strands can also be identified [32, 33]. However, establishing a diagnosis solely based on these cytomorphologic features is difficult and a biopsy is always strongly recommended to make a definite diagnosis [34].

Differential Diagnosis

Angiolymphoid Hyperplasia with Eosinophilia (ALHE)

The main differential diagnosis of KD is ALHE, also known as epithelioid hemangioma. Histologically similar although it has distinctive clinical and laboratory findings:

- No racial predilection and patients are predominantly female (as opposed to Asian males in KD).
- Typically presents with superficial skin nodules or papules without lymphadenopathy.

Peripheral eosinophilia and elevated serum IgE levels are not usually detected [35].

Drug Related or Non-Specific Follicular Hyperplasia

Knowing the patient's medication history and correlating it with the onset of lymphadenopathy is always important whenever there is obvious eosinophilia. The possibility of parasitic infections should also be investigated.

Systemic Lupus Erythematosus (SLE) Lymphadenopathy

SLE is a multisystemic autoimmune connective tissue disorder that predominantly affects young females. The etiology of this disease remains unknown, although numerous studies have set forth multiple potential mechanisms; namely those of dysregulation of the innate and/or adaptive immune system [36]. A specific constellation of symptoms, signs, and laboratory findings are required for fulfilling the criteria to diagnose SLE. Patients will have many clinical presentations with varying degrees of severity, ranging from mild fever and joint pains to possibly lethal multi-organ failure. Localized (e.g., cervical) or generalized lymphadenopathy is common in SLE, especially in the setting of high antibody titers [37].

Histological Findings

Histologically, lymph nodes will show abundant polytypic plasma cells and paracortical hyperplasia with varying degrees of coagulative necrosis, especially in the acute phase of the disease. The most specific finding is the presence of Hematoxylin bodies; amorphous basophilic material formed from necrotic nuclei [38]. Another classically identified feature, is when this basophilic material is deposited within the walls of the small blood vessels in the necrotic areas, which is termed the "Azzopardi phenomenon" [39]. It is important to note that some of these histopathologic features might be concealed by the effects of immunosuppressive therapy. Immunophenotypically, plasma cells and B-cells will be polytypic and a predominantly CD8-positive T-cells population will be present. Although not common, EBV has been detected using in situ hybridization in some cases of SLE lymphadenopathy [40].

Cytological Findings

The cytomorphologic appearance of SLE lymphadenopathy is mostly that of non-specific reactive hyperplasia with plasmacytosis, with some plasma cells having cytoplasmic inclusion bodies (Russell bodies). Acellular necrotic debris can also be identified.

Differential Diagnosis

Kikuchi-Fujimoto Disease

The major differential diagnostic consideration is Kikuchi-Fujimoto disease, which can be histologically and immunophenotypically indistinguishable from SLE lymphadenopathy, particularly in the absence of Hematoxylin bodies [41]. Moreover, patient demographics are similar between these two entities and generalized lymphadenopathy can be the first presenting symptom in SLE.

- A well-demarcated wedge-shaped pattern of necrosis is seen more in Kikuchi-Fujimoto disease.
- If present, Hematoxylin bodies and vascular fibrinoid necrosis can help favor SLE lymphadenopathy.
- Fulfilling the diagnostic criteria for SLE, such as detecting anti-dsDNA antibodies and other autoantibodies is necessary to make the distinction.

Other entities that can be considered in the differential diagnosis are IM, cat-scratch disease, and mycobacterial lymphadenitis.

Dermatopathic Lymphadenopathy

This is a distinctive type of lymph node reaction commonly involving inguinal and axillary lymph nodes and associated with chronic skin disorders such as eczema, psoriasis, mycosis fungoides among others. Occasionally, it has been reported in cases with no discernable skin diseases and in unusual sites [42].

Histological Findings

Dermatopathic LAD is mainly characterized by nodal paracortical expansion comprising a mixture of inflammatory cells with variable densities including dendritic cells, macrophages, melanophages, hemosiderin laden macrophages, and

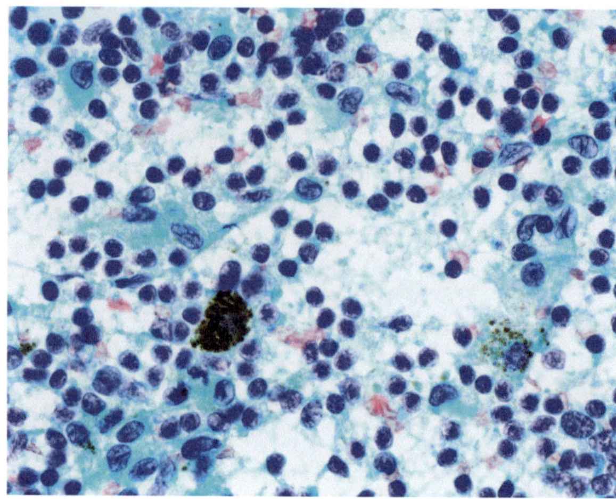

Fig. 9.6 Dermatopathic lymphadenopathy: Cytology smear (Papanicolaou (PAP) stain 60X) showing Langerhans cells with coffee-bean-like nuclei and melanopahges with coarse brown cytoplasmic granules. Eosinophils are not seen

variably-sized lymphocytes. The dendritic cells include mainly Langerhans cells (LCs), interdigitating dendritic cells (IDCs), and plasmacytoid dendritic cells (PDCs). LCs are characterized by moderate amount of vacuolated eosinophilic cytoplasm, ill-defined borders, and vesicular nuclei with twisted/grooved contour (Fig. 9.6). The lymphocytes are mainly small with mature condensed nuclear chromatin and scant cytoplasm. Scattered non-sheeting immunoblasts (large lymphocytes with prominent nucleoli) and atypical intermediate lymphocytes with twisted nuclear contours are also present in limited numbers. Plasma cells and eosinophils are present but usually not prominent.

Cytological Findings

Cytological smears demonstrate non-cohesive and polymorphous inflammatory cell population with similar constituents [43].

The evaluation of nodal architecture (precluded in cytology specimen) is essential to exclude other diagnostic mimickers. Ancillary studies including flow cytometry, immunohistochemical stains, and molecular testing that can be carried out on cytological specimens may help in certain instances.

Differential Diagnosis

Main diagnostic possibilities that come to mind with somewhat similar cytological findings include the following:

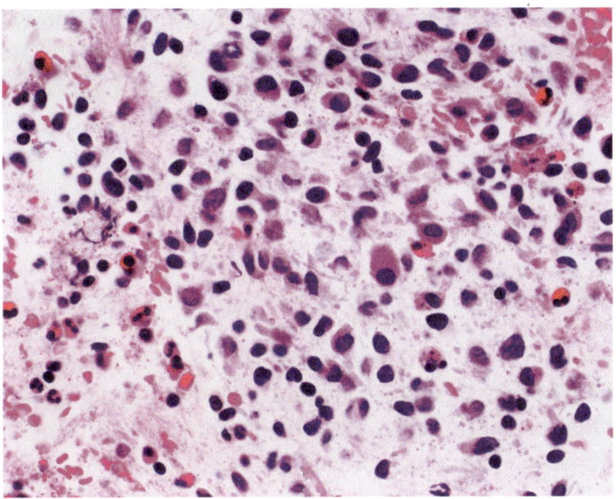

Fig. 9.7 Langerhans cell histiocytosis: Cytology cell block section (H&E, 60X) showing Langerhans cells with coffee-bean-like nuclei and frequent eosinophils

Langerhans Cell Histiocytosis (LCH)

Both dermatopathic LAD and LCH show a prominent population of Langerhans cell histocytes with characteristic coffee bean nuclei expressing S100, CD1a, and langerin immunostains [42]. Features that distinguish LCH from dermatopathic LAD are the following:

- Eosinophils are more prominent in LCH (Fig. 9.7).
- LCH show sinusoidal expansion as opposed to paracortical expansion in dermatopathic LAD (a feature evaluated only in excisional biopsies).
- LCH may harbor BRAF V600E gene mutation (50%) or genes involving mitogen-activated protein (MAP) kinase pathway (35%) [44]. These mutations can be detected by mutational analysis testing (e.g., NGS, pyrosequencing) or immunostain for BRAF V600E mutation. Additionally, strong and diffuse expression of cyclin D1 immunostain supports LCH. Cyclin D1 is a downstream transcription factor of MAPK pathway thus upregulated and overexpressed in LCH [45].

Mycosis Fungoides (MF)

It can be very challenging to distinguish dermatopathic lymphadenopathy from a lymph node that is partially involved by mycosis fungoides/sezary syndrome as both may show atypical intermediate size lymphocytes with irregular/grooved nuclear contours. Ancillary testing including flow cytometry and molecular test for TCR gamma gene rearrangement PCR test is vital in this situation; results that supports mycosis fungoides over dermatopathic LAD are the following:

- Flow cytometry shows distinct T-cell population with phenotypic features characteristic of MF (typically CD4 T-helper cells with major loss of CD7 and CD26). Other less frequent atypical immunoprofile have been reported [46].
- TCR gamma gene rearrangement PCR test show a clonal T-cell peak particularly if identical to peaks previously identified in other samples (e.g., skin and/ or blood).

Classic Hodgkin lymphoma

Dermatopathic LAD can harbor frequent large immunoblasts with prominent nucleoli that may raise the concern for Hodgkin lymphoma. The constellation of clinical features, morphology, and the immunoprofile of these large cells may distinguish between these two entities. Features that support classic Hodgkin lymphoma:

- The identification of multi-nucleated large Reed-Sternberg cells is more concerning for CHL.
- CD30 is positive in both immunoblasts and Hodgkin cells; however, aberrant immunostains that support CHL include loss of B-cell markers (CD20, CD79a, OCT2, BOB1), dim PAX5 staining, co-expression of CD15, and lack of CD45.
- Dendritic cells are typically not present in CHL.

Rosai-Dorfman Disease

Rosai-Dorfman disease (RDD), formerly known as sinus histiocytosis with massive lymphadenopathy, is a rare benign histiocytic disorder that has a wide age range but primarily affects children and young adolescents. Patients often present with bilateral cervical lymphadenopathy although other lymph nodes can also be involved. Extranodal disease is common and has been documented in up to 40% of patients [47]. Frequently involved sites include the skin, bone, kidney, and upper respiratory tract. Despite being idiopathic in many cases, the etiology of RDD is thought to be multifactorial, with mutually exclusive *MAP2K1* and *KRAS* mutations found in approximately one third of cases [48].

Histological Findings

In RDD, lymph nodes will have a distorted architecture and markedly distended sinusoids containing large histiocytes with pale eosinophilic cytoplasm. Plasma cells will also be abundant between the sinuses, while eosinophils are scarce if present. Most importantly, histiocytes often exhibit "emperipolesis"; the presence of

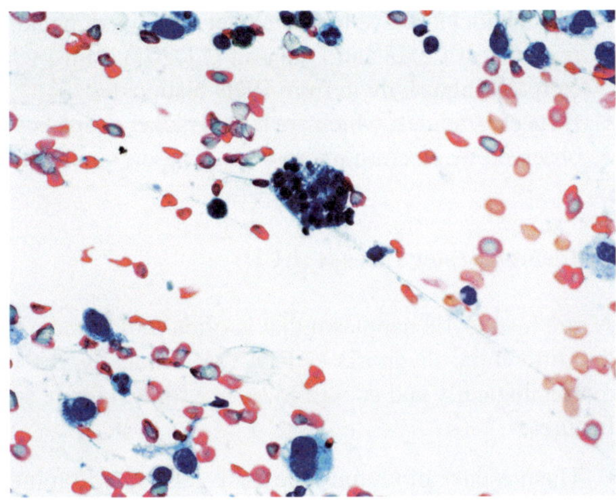

Fig. 9.8 Rosai-Dorfman disease (RDD). Cytology smear (Papanicolaou (PAP) stain 60X) showing a large histiocyte in the middle of the image with emperipolesis (lymphocytes and plasma cells within the cytoplasm borders)

intact small lymphocytes and plasma cells within the cytoplasm [47]. This feature might be inconspicuous in extranodal disease, where prominent stromal fibrosis may also be seen. S100 immunohistochemical stain is positive in the RDD histiocytes and will often demonstrate the emperipolesis phenomenon. In more challenging cases, OCT2 and Cyclin-D1 stains can also be used to highlight the cells.

Cytological Findings

Histiocytes with emperipolesis can also be identified by cytologic examination of RDD cases as the cells will have round nuclei, ample cytoplasm, and contain small viable inflammatory cells (Fig. 9.8). A mixed population composed of small lymphocytes, plasma cells, and immunoblasts can also be seen in the background, typically with no eosinophils [49].

Differential Diagnosis

Langerhans Cell Histiocytosis (LCH)

The main differential diagnosis of RDD is LCH, a neoplastic histiocytic disorder that typically occurs in the bone, skin, and to a much lesser extent, lymph nodes of younger children. In LCH,

- Smears will show a higher cellularity than in RDD and eosinophils are commonly increased in the background (Fig. 9.7) [50].

- The histiocytes have folded nuclei with linear nuclear grooving, and they will be positive for CD1a and Langerin (CD207) stains, which will immunophenotypically distinguish them from RDD histiocytes [51].
- Birbeck granules, which are tennis racket-shaped cytoplasmic organelles, can be observed by electron microscopy. These granules are not seen in RDD.

Erdheim-Chester Disease (ECD)

A rare histiocytic neoplasm that is often multisystemic, ECD can be considered in the differential diagnosis of RDD. Additionally, the two may potentially overlap morphologically and coexist [52]. The following are some of ECD's distinguishing features:

- The presence of touton-type giant cells and prominent fibrosis.
- Classic RDD histiocytes and emperipolesis are not seen.
- Immunophenotypically, the cells will be positive for CD68, CD163, and Factor XIII. While negative for S100 and OCT2.
- The histiocytes will also be negative for CD1a and Langerin (CD207), which will distinguish it from LCH.

Kikuchi-Fujimoto Disease (Histiocytic Necrotizing Lymphadenitis)

Kikuchi-Fujimoto disease (KFD) is a rare and benign self-limiting condition that typically occurs in young women; commonly in those of Asian descent. It often presents with tender cervical lymphadenopathy accompanied by mild fever and night sweats. The etiology is still unknown but it has been suggested to be related to viral or autoimmune-related causes [53] and the pathogenesis is driven by an exaggerated cytotoxic (CD8-positive) T-cell response.

Histological Findings

There are three histologic phases (or patterns) described in KFD that may overlap based on the timing of the lymph node biopsy. In early stages, a mixed population of histiocytes, plasmacytoid dendritic cells (PDCs), and immunoblasts start to proliferate with little to no necrosis. This phase is aptly named the "proliferating" phase. In the "necrotic" phase, a well-demarcated area of necrosis, containing numerous apoptotic bodies, karyorrhectic debris, and scattered fibrin thrombi are seen. This distinct area of necrosis is arguably the most classic feature of the disease and what most diagnoses rely on. Eventually, it progresses into the "Xanthomatous/ foamy cell" phase, where the histiocytes phagocytize the debris and start to align around the periphery of the necrotic areas forming a rim [54, 55]. Immunohistochemical stains, such as CD123 and TCL-1, highlight the PDCs well, and flow cytometry can also be helpful by identifying the CD123-positive PDC population.

Cytological Findings

Fine needle aspiration samples obtained from patients with KFD will have distinctive cytomorphologic features that can be diagnostic in the proper clinical context. Smears often show a gritty background full of necrotic matter and histiocytes with eccentric and crescentic nuclei, with some having phagocytized karyorrhectic debris [56]. Tingle-body macrophages are larger and have round nuclei, which can help distinguish them from the characteristic histiocytes seen in KFD. Other cell populations are also seen, including plasmacytoid monocytes and immunoblasts [57]. Although there will be hardly any neutrophils or plasma cells present.

Differential Diagnosis

As previously mentioned, SLE lymphadenopathy is the main entity to be excluded when considering the diagnosis of KFD (see section "SLE Lymphadenopathy"). Other causes of necrotizing lymphadenopathy can also be considered in the differential diagnosis, including herpes simplex lymphadenitis, IM, cat-scratch disease, mycobacterial or fungal infections.

IgG4-Related Lymphadenopathy

IgG4-related disease is an immune-mediated inflammation associated with various degrees of fibrosis and IGG4-positive plasmacytosis clinically presenting as an insidious tumor [58]. Clinical symptoms are mostly related to the obliterative effect of fibrosis, the organ involved, and the extent of organ damage. Commonly, it is asymptomatic and identified incidentally. Sites typically affected are the salivary glands, orbits, pancreas, retroperitoneum, lacrimal glands, kidneys, lungs, aorta, and meninges. IgG4-related lymphadenopathy usually occurs along with the extranodal disease and infrequently by itself.

Histological Findings

Histologically, lymph nodes involved by IgG4-related disease show variable histological patterns that mimic other entities such as CD, PTGC, non-specific follicular hyperplasia, inflammatory pseudotumor, and RDD [59, 60]. A common finding among these histological variants is the expansion of IgG4-positive plasma cells with an IgG4/IgG ratio exceeding 40%. Eosinophils are also commonly found in IgG4-related LAD and may further support this entity over its mimickers. Nevertheless, the diagnosis of IgG4-related disease cannot be rendered based on morphology alone.

Cytological Findings

Cytologically, the fine needle aspiration smears may show an expanded plasma cell population with a variable cellular yield depending on the density of fibrosis in the sampled lesion. This finding is non-specific at all; however, it may raise some diagnostic consideration and trigger further work up such as flow cytometry to rule out clonal B-cells and plasma cells, immunohistochemical stains, for example, IgG4, Treponemal, HHV8, and kappa and lambda light chain immunostains or in situ hybridization (ISH).

Differential Diagnosis

Elevated IgG4-positive plasma cells in a cytological and surgical lymph node specimen is a non-specific finding and has been reported in many other entities, such as marginal zone lymphoma, RDD, MCD, infections, among others [61]. Features that support IgG4-related disease are as follows:

- The presence of typical extranodal manifestation of IgG4-related disease.
- The exclusion of other entities associated with elevated IgG4-positive plasma cells as mentioned above.
- The rapid and sustained response to glucocorticoid therapy.

Features that support marginal zone lymphoma is the identification of monotypic B-cell and plasma cell populations by flow cytometry, or kappa and lambda light chain immunostains or in situ hybridization, or evidence of clonality by *IGH* gene rearrangement PCR testing. Features that support MCD is the identification of positive HHV8-positive plasmablasts in HIV and immunosuppressed patients, elevated IL6 and C-reactive protein (CRP) in serum, and severe systemic inflammatory symptoms that are typically not seen in IgG4-related disease. Features that support RDD is the identification of histiocytes with emperipolesis with expression of S100, OCT2, and Cyclin-D1 immunostains [62].

Sarcoidosis

Sarcoidosis is a multisystemic granulomatous disease that more commonly affects African-American females. It is primarily immune mediated, but the exact etiology is unknown. Patients present with bilateral hilar lymphadenopathy and will frequently have pulmonary manifestations, often as interstitial lung disease. However, some patients may be asymptomatic with the enlarged lymph nodes being incidentally found on routine imaging (e.g., chest X-ray) [63]. Hypercalcemia, elevated angiotensin-converting enzyme (ACE) serum levels, and increased CD4+/CD8+ T-cell ratio in bronchoalveolar lavage specimens (can be assessed by flow cytometric immunophenotyping), might be helpful in making the diagnosis of sarcoidosis, although it is still a diagnosis of exclusion in most cases, as other causes of a granulomatous inflammatory response must be ruled out.

Histological Findings

The lymph node architecture will be predominantly effaced and densely occupied by well-formed granulomas, which will sometimes be referred to as "naked" granulomas; meaning devoid of any lymphocytes. The granulomas in sarcoidosis will mostly be non-caseating but can be necrotic in some cases [64]. Other findings that can be observed include asteroid bodies (stellate structures within granulomas, mostly containing calcium), Schaumann bodies (laminated concentric inclusions, composed of calcium and iron), and Hamazaki-Wesenberg bodies (large yellow-brown lysosomes) [64]. All of which are non-specific for sarcoidosis and can be seen in other diseases (e.g., berylliosis).

Cytological Findings

Smears usually show multinucleated giant cells and small aggregates of epithelioid histiocytes with elongated, spindle-shaped nuclei, and inconspicuous nucleoli [65]. The background will have a mixed population of lymphocytes and necrotic debris should be minimal if present.

Differential Diagnosis

As stated above, other causes of granulomatous inflammation must be thoroughly investigated before rendering a diagnosis of sarcoidosis. Fungal and mycobacterial infectious are among the most common entities to be excluded, which will have key defining characteristics (see the differential diagnosis in section "Cat Scratch Disease").

References

1. Nowalk A, Green M. Epstein-Barr Virus. Microbiol Spectr. 2016;4(3):10–128. https://doi.org/10.1128/microbiolspec.DMIH2-0011-2015.
2. Niller HH, Bauer G. Epstein-Barr virus: clinical diagnostics. Methods Mol Biol. 2017;1532:33–55. https://doi.org/10.1007/978-1-4939-6655-4_2.
3. Lesesve JF, Troussard X. Apoptotic cells in a peripheral blood smear in the context of EBV infection. Am J Hematol. 2001;67(2):148–9. https://doi.org/10.1002/ajh.1096.
4. Kanderi T, Khoory MS. Infectious mononucleosis mimicking Epstein-Barr virus positive diffuse large B-cell lymphoma not otherwise specified. Int J Hematol Oncol. 2020;9(2):IJH25. https://doi.org/10.2217/ijh-2020-0002.
5. Gerber-Mora R, VP YL, Moreno-Silva R, González-Arriagada W. Fine needle cytology features of an atypical presentation of infectious mononucleosis. J Oral Maxillofac Pathol. 2020;24(Suppl 1):S139–42. https://doi.org/10.4103/jomfp.JOMFP_80_17.
6. Jamiyan T, Nakazato Y, Kuroda H, Kojima M, Imai Y. Characteristic histological findings of asymptomatic ebv-associated lymphoproliferative disorders in tonsils. J Clin Exp Hematop. 2018;58(3):122–7. https://doi.org/10.3960/jslrt.18017.
7. Anagnostopoulos I, Hummel M, Kreschel C, Stein H. Morphology, immunophenotype, and distribution of latently and/or productively Epstein-Barr virus-infected cells in acute infectious mononucleosis: implications for the interindividual infection route of Epstein-Barr virus. Blood. 1995;85(3):744–50.
8. Louissaint A Jr, Ferry JA, Soupir CP, Hasserjian RP, Harris NL, Zukerberg LR. Infectious mononucleosis mimicking lymphoma: distinguishing morphological and immunophenotypic features. Mod Pathol. 2012;25(8):1149–59. https://doi.org/10.1038/modpathol.2012.70.
9. Krishna BA, Wills MR, Sinclair JH. Advances in the treatment of cytomegalovirus. Br Med Bull. 2019;131(1):5–17. https://doi.org/10.1093/bmb/ldz031.
10. Dioverti MV, Razonable RR. Cytomegalovirus Microbiol Spectr. 2016;4:4. https://doi.org/10.1128/microbiolspec.DMIH2-0022-2015.
11. Yu SC, Ko KY, Teng SC, Huang TC, Lo HT, Cheng CL, Yao M, Hong RL, Chen CN, Chen TC, Yang TL. A clinicopathological study of cytomegalovirus lymphadenitis and tonsillitis and their association with epstein-barr virus. Infect Dis Ther. 2021;10(4):2661–75. https://doi.org/10.1007/s40121-021-00528-1.
12. Wang SA. *"Cytomegalovirus lymphadenitis." diagnostic pathology lymph nodes and spleen with extranodal lymphomas: amirsys.* New York: Springer; 2011. p. 2–86.
13. Ioachim HL, Medeiros LJ, Ioachim HL. Chapter 10 cytomegalovirus lymphadenitis. In: Ioachim's lymph node pathology. 4th ed. Philadelphia/London: Lippincott Williams & Wilkins; 2009. p. 83–6.
14. Miranda RN, Khoury JD, Medeiros LJ. "Cytomegalovirus Lymphadenitis". Atlas of Lymph Node Pathology. 1st ed. New York: Springer-Verlag. p. 71–3.
15. Lu DY, Qian J, Easley KA, Waldrop SM, Cohen C. Automated in situ hybridization and immunohistochemistry for cytomegalovirus detection in paraffin-embedded tissue sec-

tions. Appl Immunohistochem Mol Morphol. 2009;17(2):158–64. https://doi.org/10.1097/PAI.0b013e318185d1b5.

16. Biancardi AL, Curi AL. Cat-scratch disease. Ocul Immunol Inflamm. 2014;22(2):148–54. https://doi.org/10.3109/09273948.2013.833631.

17. Shinall EA. Cat-scratch disease: a review of the literature. Pediatr Dermatol. 1990;7(1):11–8. https://doi.org/10.1111/j.1525-1470.1990.tb01066.x. Erratum in: Pediatr Dermatol 1990 Jun;7(2);165.

18. Miranda RN, Khoury JD, Medeiros LJ. "Cat-Scratch Lymphadenitis". Atlas of Lymph Node Pathology. 1st ed. New York: Springer-Verlag. p. 35–6.

19. Peng J, Fan Z, Zheng H, Lu J, Zhan Y. Combined application of immunohistochemistry and Warthin-starry silver stain on the pathologic diagnosis of cat scratch disease. Appl Immunohistochem Mol Morphol. 2020;28(10):781–5. https://doi.org/10.1097/PAI.0000000000000829.

20. Stastny JF, Wakely PE Jr, Frable WJ. Cytologic features of necrotizing granulomatous inflammation consistent with cat-scratch disease. Diagn Cytopathol. 1996 Aug;15(2):108–15. https://doi.org/10.1002/(SICI)1097-0339(199608)15:2<108::AID-DC5>3.0.CO;2-E.

21. Du J, Zhang Y, Liu D, Zhu G, Zhang Q. Hodgkin's lymphoma with marked granulomatous reaction: a diagnostic pitfall. Int J Clin Exp Pathol. 2019;12(7):2772–4.

22. Dispenzieri A, Fajgenbaum DC. Overview of Castleman disease. Blood. 2020;135(16): 1353–64. https://doi.org/10.1182/blood.2019000931.

23. Szalat R, Munshi NC. Diagnosis of Castleman disease. Hematol Oncol Clin North Am. 2018;32(1):53–64. https://doi.org/10.1016/j.hoc.2017.09.005.

24. Nishimura MF, Nishimura Y, Nishikori A, Yoshino T, Sato Y. Historical and pathological overview of Castleman disease. J Clin Exp Hematop. 2022;62(2):60–72. https://doi.org/10.3960/jslrt.21036.

25. Singh N, Chowdhury N, Pal S, Goyal JP, Bhakhri BK, Rao S. Hyaline vascular type of Castleman disease: diagnostic pitfalls on cytology and its clinical relevance. Cureus. 2021;13(8):e17174. https://doi.org/10.7759/cureus.17174.

26. Deschênes M, Michel RP, Tabah R, Auger M. Fine-needle aspiration cytology of Castleman disease: case report with review of the literature. Diagn Cytopathol. 2008;36(12):904–8. https://doi.org/10.1002/dc.20934.

27. Kojima M, Nakamura S, Itoh H, Yoshida K, Asano S, Yamane N, Komatsumoto S, Ban S, Joshita T, Suchi T. Systemic lupus erythematosus (SLE) lymphadenopathy presenting with histopathologic features of Castleman' disease: a clinicopathologic study of five cases. Pathol Res Pract. 1997;193(8):565–71. https://doi.org/10.1016/S0344-0338(97)80015-5.

28. Wang X, Ma Y, Wang Z. Kimura's disease. J Craniofac Surg. 2019 Jul;30(5):e415–8. https://doi.org/10.1097/SCS.0000000000005430.

29. Chen H, Thompson LD, Aguilera NS, Abbondanzo SL. Kimura disease: a clinicopathologic study of 21 cases. Am J Surg Pathol. 2004;28:505–13.

30. Fan L, Mo S, Wang Y, Zhu J. Clinical, pathological, laboratory characteristics, and treatment regimens of Kimura disease and their relationships with tumor size and recurrence. Front Med (Lausanne). 2021;8:720144. https://doi.org/10.3389/fmed.2021.720144.

31. Hui PK, Chan JK, Ng CS, Kung IT, Gwi E. Lymphadenopathy of Kimura's disease. Am J Surg Pathol. 1989;13(3):177–86. https://doi.org/10.1097/00000478-198903000-00001.

32. Sahu P, Jain S, Kaushal M. Kimura's disease: a short study of cytomorphologic features with its differential diagnosis and review of literature. Cytojournal. 2022;19:50. https://doi.org/10.25259/Cytojournal_77_2020.

33. Chow LT, Yuen RW, Tsui WM, Ma TK, Chow WH, Chan SK. Cytologic features of Kimura's disease in fine-needle aspirates. A study of eight cases. Am J Clin Pathol. 1994;102(3):316–21. https://doi.org/10.1093/ajcp/102.3.316.

34. Sherpa M, Lamichaney R, Roy AD. Kimura's disease: a diagnostic challenge experienced with cytology of postauricular swelling with histopathological relevance. J Cytol. 2016;33(4):232–5. https://doi.org/10.4103/0970-9371.190453.

35. Zou A, Hu M, Niu B. Comparison between Kimura's disease and angiolymphoid hyperplasia with eosinophilia: case reports and literature review. J Int Med Res. 2021;49(9):3000605211040976. https://doi.org/10.1177/03000605211040976.

36. Pan L, Lu MP, Wang JH, Xu M, Yang SR. Immunological pathogenesis and treatment of systemic lupus erythematosus. World J Pediatr. 2020;16(1):19–30. https://doi.org/10.1007/s12519-019-00229-3.

37. Soares L, Rebelo Matos A, Mello Vieira M, Cruz R, Caixas U. Generalized lymphadenopathy as the first manifestation of systemic lupus erythematosus. Cureus. 2022;14(10):e30089. https://doi.org/10.7759/cureus.30089.

38. Kojima M, Motoori T, Asano S, Nakamura S. Histological diversity of reactive and atypical proliferative lymph node lesions in systemic lupus erythematosus patients. Pathol Res Pract. 2007;203(6):423–31. https://doi.org/10.1016/j.prp.2007.03.002. Epub 2007 May 30

39. Medeiros LJ, Kaynor B, Harris NL. Lupus lymphadenitis: report of a case with immunohistologic studies on frozen sections. Hum Pathol. 1989;20(3):295–9. https://doi.org/10.1016/0046-8177(89)90141-x.

40. Kojima M, Motoori T, Itoh H, Shimizu K, Iijima M, Tamaki Y, Murayama K, Ohno Y, Yoshida K, Masawa N, Nakamura S. Distribution of Epstein-Barr virus in systemic rheumatic disease (rheumatoid arthritis, systemic lupus erythematosus, dermatomyositis) with associated lymphadenopathy: a study of 49 cases. Int J Surg Pathol. 2005;13(3):273–8. https://doi.org/10.1177/106689690501300307.

41. Hu S, Kuo TT, Hong HS. Lupus lymphadenitis simulating Kikuchi's lymphadenitis in patients with systemic lupus erythematosus: a clinicopathological analysis of six cases and review of the literature. Pathol Int. 2003;53(4):221–6. https://doi.org/10.1046/j.1320-5463.2003.01458.x.

42. Garces S, Yin CC, Miranda RN, Patel KP, Li S, Xu J, Thakral B, Poppiti RJ, Medina AM, Sriganeshan V, Castellano-Sánchez A, Khoury JD, Garces JC, Medeiros LJ. Clinical, histopathologic, and immunoarchitectural features of dermatopathic lymphadenopathy: an update. Mod Pathol. 2020;33(6):1104–21. https://doi.org/10.1038/s41379-019-0440-4.

43. Srinivasamurthy BC, Saha K, Senapati S, Saha A. Fine needle aspiration cytology of dermatopathic lymphadenitis in an asymptomatic female: a case report. J Cytol. 2016;33(1):49–51. https://doi.org/10.4103/0970-9371.175523.

44. Badalian-Very G, Vergilio JA, Degar BA, MacConaill LE, Brandner B, Calicchio ML, Kuo FC, Ligon AH, Stevenson KE, Kehoe SM, Garraway LA, Hahn WC, Meyerson M, Fleming MD, Rollins BJ. Recurrent BRAF mutations in Langerhans cell histiocytosis. Blood. 2010;116(11):1919–23. https://doi.org/10.1182/blood-2010-04-279083.

45. Chatterjee D, Vishwajeet V, Saikia UN, Radotra B, De D, Bansal D. CyclinD1 is useful to differentiate Langerhans cell Histiocytosis from reactive Langerhans cells. Am J Dermatopathol. 2019;41(3):188–92. https://doi.org/10.1097/DAD.0000000000001250.

46. Horna P, Wang SA, Wolniak KL, Psarra K, Almeida J, Illingworth AJ, Johansson U, Craig FE, Torres R. Flow cytometric evaluation of peripheral blood for suspected Sézary syndrome or mycosis fungoides: international guidelines for assay characteristics. Cytometry B Clin Cytom. 2021;100(2):142–55. https://doi.org/10.1002/cyto.b.21878.

47. Foucar E, Rosai J, Dorfman R. Sinus histiocytosis with massive lymphadenopathy (Rosai-Dorfman disease): review of the entity. Semin Diagn Pathol. 1990;7(1):19–73.

48. Tang M, Gu XZ, Wu PC, Yang XT. Clinicopathological and gene mutation analysis of 27 cases with Extranodal Rosai-Dorfman disease. J Inflamm Res. 2022;15:2775–87. https://doi.org/10.2147/JIR.S365098. Erratum in: J Inflamm Res 2022;15:3769–3770.

49. Rajyalakshmi R, Akhtar M, Swathi Y, Chakravarthi R, Bhaskara Reddy J, Beulah PM. Cytological diagnosis of rosai-dorfman disease: a study of twelve cases with emphasis on diagnostic challenges. J Cytol. 2020;37(1):46–52. https://doi.org/10.4103/JOC.JOC_4_19.

50. Shabb N, Fanning CV, Carrasco CH, Guo SQ, Katz RL, Ayala AG, Raymond AK, Cangir A. Diagnosis of eosinophilic granuloma of bone by fine-needle aspiration with concurrent

institution of therapy: a cytologic, histologic, clinical, and radiologic study of 27 cases. Diagn Cytopathol. 1993;9(1):3–12. https://doi.org/10.1002/dc.2840090103.

51. Rodriguez-Galindo C, Allen CE. Langerhans cell histiocytosis. Blood. 2020;135(16):1319–31. https://doi.org/10.1182/blood.2019000934.

52. Razanamahery J, Diamond EL, Cohen-Aubart F, Plate KH, Lourida G, Charlotte F, Hélias-Rodzewicz Z, Goyal G, Go RS, Dogan A, Abdel-Wahab O, Durham B, Ozkaya N, Amoura Z, Emile JF, Haroche J. Erdheim-Chester disease with concomitant Rosai-Dorfman like lesions: a distinct entity mainly driven by *MAP2K1*. Haematologica. 2020;105(1):e5–8. https://doi.org/10.3324/haematol.2019.216937.

53. Kucukardali Y, Solmazgul E, Kunter E, Oncul O, Yildirim S, Kaplan M. Kikuchi-Fujimoto disease: analysis of 244 cases. Clin Rheumatol. 2007;26(1):50–4. https://doi.org/10.1007/s10067-006-0230-5.

54. Perry AM, Choi SM. Kikuchi-Fujimoto disease: a review. Arch Pathol Lab Med. 2018;142(11):1341–6. https://doi.org/10.5858/arpa.2018-0219-RA.

55. Tsang WY, Chan JK, Ng CS. Kikuchi's lymphadenitis. A morphologic analysis of 75 cases with special reference to unusual features. Am J Surg Pathol. 1994;18(3):219–31.

56. Tsang WY, Chan JK. Fine-needle aspiration cytologic diagnosis of Kikuchi's lymphadenitis. A report of 27 cases. Am J Clin Pathol. 1994;102(4):454–8. https://doi.org/10.1093/ajcp/102.4.454.

57. Tong TR, Chan OW, Lee KC. Diagnosing Kikuchi disease on fine needle aspiration biopsy: a retrospective study of 44 cases diagnosed by cytology and 8 by histopathology. Acta Cytol. 2001;45(6):953–7. https://doi.org/10.1159/000328370.

58. Perugino CA, Stone JH. IgG4-related disease: an update on pathophysiology and implications for clinical care. Nat Rev Rheumatol. 2020;16(12):702–14. https://doi.org/10.1038/s41584-020-0500-7.

59. Bookhout CE, Rollins-Raval MA. Immunoglobulin G4-related lymphadenopathy. Surg Pathol Clin. 2016;9(1):117–29. https://doi.org/10.1016/j.path.2015.09.005.

60. Wick MR, O'Malley DP. Lymphadenopathy associated with IgG4-related disease: diagnosis & differential diagnosis. Semin Diagn Pathol. 2018;35(1):61–6. https://doi.org/10.1053/j.semdp.2017.11.006.

61. Ebbo M, Grados A, Bernit E, Vély F, Boucraut J, Harlé JR, Daniel L, Schleinitz N. Pathologies associated with serum IgG4 elevation. Int J Rheumatol. 2012;2012:602809. https://doi.org/10.1155/2012/602809.

62. Ravindran A, Goyal G, Go RS, Rech KL. Mayo Clinic Histiocytosis working group. Rosai-Dorfman disease displays a unique monocyte-macrophage phenotype characterized by expression of OCT2. Am J Surg Pathol. 2021;45(1):35–44. https://doi.org/10.1097/PAS.0000000000001617.

63. Spagnolo P, Rossi G, Trisolini R, Sverzellati N, Baughman RP, Wells AU. Pulmonary sarcoidosis. Lancet Respir Med. 2018;6(5):389–402. https://doi.org/10.1016/S2213-2600(18)30064-X.

64. Welter SM, DeLuca-Johnson J, Thompson K. Histologic review of sarcoidosis in a neck lymph node. Head Neck Pathol. 2018;12(2):255–8. https://doi.org/10.1007/s12105-017-0847-5.

65. Mehrotra R, Dhingra V. Cytological diagnosis of sarcoidosis revisited: a state-of-the-art review. Diagn Cytopathol. 2011;39(7):541–8. https://doi.org/10.1002/dc.21455.

Chapter 10
Breast

Osvaldo Hernandez and Aylin Simsir

Introduction

The use of fine needle aspiration (FNA) as a diagnostic tool has been around since the mid-nineteenth century. Initially, FNA biopsy was performed predominantly in European countries. It wasn't until the 1930s, however, that the technique started to be widely used in the United States [1]. Since that time, FNA has been applied successfully to diagnose breast masses. Early reports in the literature highlight the use of FNA in diagnosing palpable breast cysts and carcinoma [2]. With the advent of improved imaging techniques, breast FNA was no longer limited to palpable lesions. Breast masses that were detected by sonogram could also undergo aspiration biopsy with ultrasound guidance [3]. The use of breast FNA in the United States has declined in the past three decades. A survey published in 2000 by the Papanicolaou Society of Cytopathology reported an increase in the use of core needle biopsies and a parallel decrease in FNAs for diagnosing breast masses [4]. A similar result was noted in a 2019 survey the College of American Pathologists (CAP) [5]. The CAP survey reported the volume changes for FNA and core needle biopsy (CNB) specimens in 494 laboratories. The results were as follows: no change in volume (FNA: 40.5% vs. CNB: 20.3%); a decrease in volume (FNA: 31.8% vs. CNB: 6.8%); an increase in volume (FNA: 7.9% vs. CNB: 53.8%); and did not know the volume change (FNA: 19.8% vs. CNB: 19.1%) [5].

There are several reasons for the decline in breast FNAs and parallel increase in CNBs in the United States. Core biopsies are better able to diagnose borderline breast lesions and yield less unsatisfactory specimens [6]. In addition, a core biopsy can distinguish between in situ carcinoma and invasive carcinoma [7].

O. Hernandez (✉) · A. Simsir
Department of Pathology, NYU Langone Health, New York, NY, USA
e-mail: osvaldo.hernandez@nyulangone.org; aylin.simsir@nyulangone.org

© The Author(s), under exclusive license to Springer Nature Switzerland AG 2023
S. M. Gilani, G. Cai (eds.), *Non-Neoplastic Cytology*,
https://doi.org/10.1007/978-3-031-44289-6_10

However, there are numerous well-known advantages to performing an FNA. FNA is a rapid and safe technique to evaluate breast lesions, with a rapid turnaround time and low cost [7, 8]. An FNA can be performed in an outpatient setting without the need for anesthesia. FNA specimens can be evaluated while the patient is still present and, if required, additional samples may be obtained for ancillary tests. Complications from an FNA are minor when they occur, and most commonly consist of bruising, hematoma, or pain at the FNA site.

Interpretation of FNA specimens of breast lesions has to take place in the context of the triple test: correlating clinical findings, radiologic imaging studies, and cytologic results [9]. It is especially important that a benign FNA be interpreted in the context of the clinical and imaging findings. In the setting of suspicious clinical or radiologic findings, a benign FNA is discordant and a repeat FNA or core biopsy is warranted for further evaluation [10]. If the clinical, radiologic, and cytologic findings are all concurrent for a benign lesion, patients may return for a follow-up ultrasound to assess stability of the lesion.

As demonstrated by the triple test, a multidisciplinary approach is crucial to interpreting breast FNAs. Proper communication with breast surgeons and radiologists is key to ensuring that the triple test is concordant in every case [7].

The preparation of aspirated material is important for accurate evaluation of specimens [11]. While it is ideal to have a cytopathologist perform breast FNAs, in many clinical settings a radiologist performs the procedure under ultrasound guidance. In other instances, surgeons perform FNAs by palpation in the outpatient setting. Several factors can lead to inadequate specimen in these scenarios. Having a cytopathologist present for rapid on-site evaluation (ROSE) can lead to a decreased percentage of non-diagnostic samples, as well as a decrease of atypical diagnoses [12]. The skill of the aspirator is critical for obtaining and preparing adequate specimens [6]. The aspirator must have adequate training in smear preparation to avoid crushing artifact during the smearing technique. In addition, injection of large amounts of lidocaine in the tissue surrounding the mass may lead to poor preservation of cellular material.

In 2016, the International Academy of Cytology (IAC) gathered a group of international cytopathologists, surgical pathologists, radiologists, oncologists, and surgeons to develop best-practice guidelines for breast fine needle aspiration specimens [11]. The meeting led to the 2019 publication of the IAC Yokohama System for Reporting Breast Cytopathology which created a standardized and reproducible reporting system for breast FNA specimens similar to that found for other organ systems [9]. In addition, the system provides indications for performing breast FNAs, guidelines for specimen preparation and ancillary testing, and correlation with management guidelines [11]. The IAC Yokohama System for Reporting Breast Cytopathology consists of five categories: category 1—insufficient material for a diagnosis; category 2—benign; category 3—atypical, probably benign; category 4—suspicious for malignancy; and, category 5—malignant. Each category lists specific diagnostic criteria and management recommendations [9]. The interobserver reproducibility of the different categories is high, especially if the suspicious and malignant categories are combined [13].

Breast FNA has been shown to be an accurate method to evaluate breast masses. A large meta-analysis of studies published prior to the implementation of the Yokohama System calculated the overall breast FNA sensitivity of 96.3%, specificity of 98.8%, positive predictive value (PPV) of 98.7%, negative predictive value (NPV) of 95.3%, false-negative rate of 3.7%, and false-positive rate of 1% [10]. Most false-negative cases are a result of sampling issues, rather than interpretative errors [10]. Other studies published using the Yokohama System have reported similar rates. Chauhan et al. reported a sensitivity of 98.9%, specificity of 99.16%, PPV of 97.82%, NPV of 99.58%, and a diagnostic accuracy of 99.09% [14].

In addition, each category is associated with a risk of malignancy (ROM) based on two large retrospective studies by Montezuma et al. and Wong et al. The ROM ranges from 2.6% to 4.8% for category 1 (unsatisfactory), 1.4–1.7% for category 2 (benign), 13–15.7% for category 3 (atypical), 84.6–97.1% for category 4 (suspicious for malignancy), and 99–100% for category 5 (malignant) [8, 12]. In a meta-analysis, Hoda et al. pooled the data from 27 studies published from 1997 to 2017. Overall, these studies included over 33,000 breast FNA cases, and, even though they were published prior to the IAC Yokohama System in 2019, most classified FNAs into five diagnostic categories. The ROM was 30.3% for category 1 (insufficient material), 4.7% for category 2 (benign), 51.5% for category 3 (atypical), 85.4% for category 4 (suspicious), and 98.7% for category 5 (malignant) [10].

While the vast majority of breast FNAs are performed in women, breast FNAs in male patients also show high sensitivity and specificity. Hoda et al. reported a sensitivity of 95.8% and a specificity of 100% for FNAs of palpable male breast lesions [15].

Fibrocystic Change

Fibrocystic change (FCC) is a benign breast disorder encompassing various metaplastic, hyperplastic, cystic, and fibrotic changes to the mammary epithelium and stroma. FCC has been classified as non-proliferative or proliferative. Non-proliferative FCC consists of stromal fibrosis, mild usual ductal hyperplasia, adenosis, and cysts. Cysts may be of varying sizes, and there may be apocrine metaplasia of the lining epithelial cells exhibiting a papillary growth pattern. Proliferative FCC includes moderate to florid usual ductal hyperplasia, sclerosing adenosis, radial scars, and sclerosing lesions. Apocrine metaplasia may be present in proliferative fibrocystic changes. In practice, it is not uncommon to see a mixture of non-proliferative and proliferative changes in areas of FCC (Figs. 10.1 and 10.2). Atypical changes, either cytologic or architectural, can occur in FCC (FCC with atypia).

Although non-proliferative FCC, proliferative FCC without atypia and proliferative FCC with atypia all comprise a spectrum of benign breast disease, each carries a different risk factor associated with the development of subsequent breast cancer [16]. There is no increased risk with non-proliferative FCC. Patients with

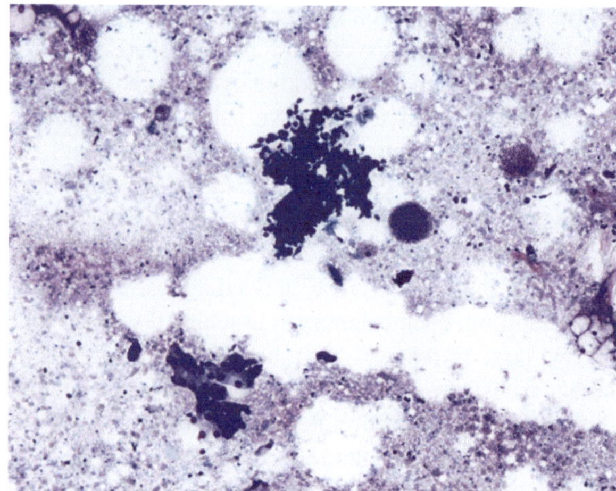

Fig. 10.1 Fibrocystic change. Fibrocystic changes showing a cluster of benign ductal cells and myoepithelial cells, a group of apocrine cells and macrophages in a background of proteinaceous fluid. (Diff Quik 10×)

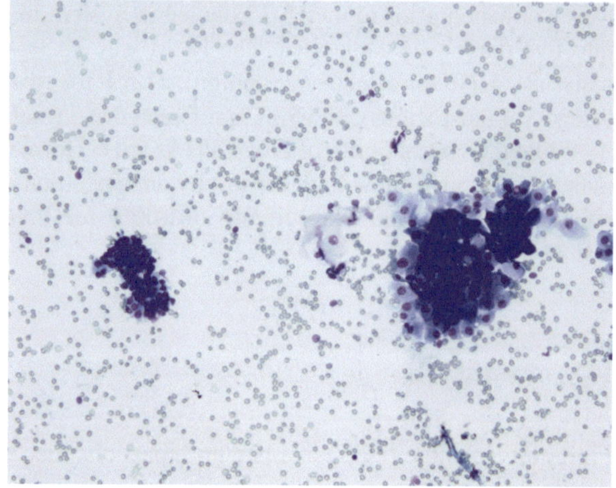

Fig. 10.2 Fibrocystic change. A small cluster of benign ductal epithelium (left side of image) and a cluster of apocrine cells (right side of image). These findings are seen in aspirates of fibrocystic change. (Diff Quik 10×)

proliferative FCC without atypia have a slight increased risk of developing subsequent breast cancer (1.5–2 times), while patients with FCC with atypia have a moderately increased risk (four to five times) [16]. The pathologic findings are only one of several factors that determines the risk of developing breast cancer. The age of the patient, family history, and genetic abnormalities must also be taken into consideration when determining risk factors for developing breast carcinoma [17].

As has been stated in the literature, it may not be possible to distinguish between non-proliferative FCC and proliferative FCC without atypia on aspiration biopsy since there may be considerable overlap in the cytologic findings [18, 19]. Ultimately, an FNA of a breast lesion should differentiate between benign and atypical or malignant changes, and the distinction between non-proliferative FCC and proliferative FCC without atypia may not be possible on aspiration specimens.

Benign epithelial breast lesions typically yield a dual population of cells consisting of ductal epithelial cells and myoepithelial cells in varying proportions. The presence of this dual cell population is an important finding in differentiating benign from malignant breast lesions. On cytology, myoepithelial cells appear as oval nuclei that lack cytoplasm ("bare oval nuclei"). The nuclei of myoepithelial cells are hyperchromatic compared to the nuclei of ductal epithelial cells and lack nucleoli. Myoepithelial cells may be present admixed with the ductal epithelium or may be found in the background of the smears separate from the epithelial cells. Pattari et al. found that the number of myoepithelial cells identified on aspiration smears is one helpful criterion in differentiated benign from malignant lesions, with invasive carcinomas having absent to markedly decreased myoepithelial cells [20].

Non-proliferative FCC

The nature of aspirates from non-proliferative FCC will vary depending on the degree of fibrosis and the amount of cystic component present. When there is extensive fibrosis, smears will have a clean background and low cellularity with scant monolayered groups of cohesive ductal epithelial cells lacking cytologic atypia [16, 21] (Figs. 10.3 and 10.4). Paucicellular specimens may be compatible with non-proliferative FCC due to extensive fibrosis; however, correlation with the clinical and imaging studies must be done (triple test) [22]. An FNA of a radiologically suspicious mass that yields scant benign epithelial cells represents a discordant finding and must undergo histologic evaluation [23].

When cysts are aspirated, fluid of varying quality may be obtained. The cyst fluid may be watery or viscous, clear or straw-colored, or serosanguinous. Benign cysts should not yield bloody fluid. The clinical history is crucial in cases of cyst FNAs since the aspirates may yield only acellular fluid. Most cyst aspirates, however, will

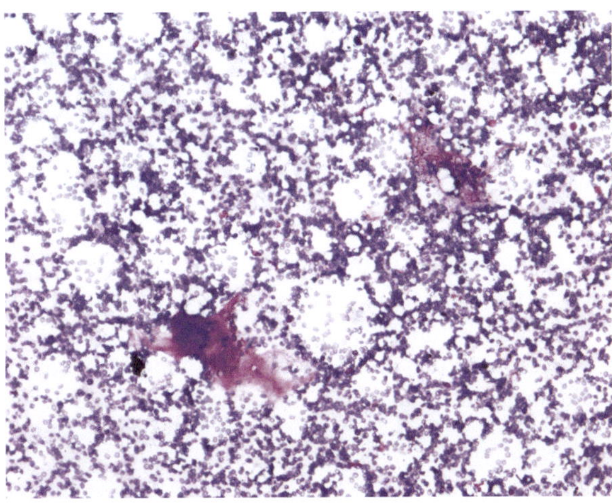

Fig. 10.3 Non-proliferative fibrocystic change showing fibrous stroma (Diff Quik 10×)

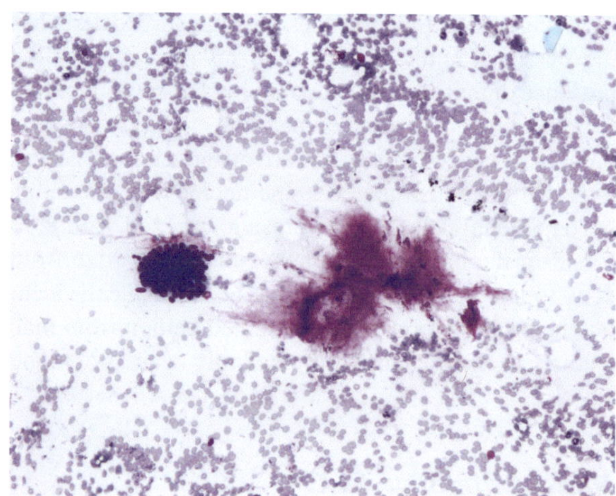

Fig. 10.4 Non-proliferative fibrocystic change showing a stromal fragment and one small group of ductal epithelium (Diff Quik 10×)

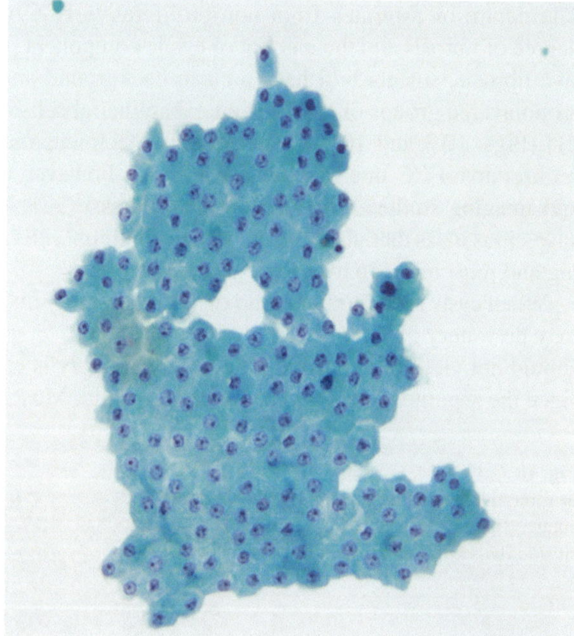

Fig. 10.5. A flat sheet of apocrine cells in a ThinPrep specimen. The apocrine cells have well-defined cell borders, abundant granular cytoplasm, and round centrally located nuclei with prominent nucleoli (ThinPrep 20×)

show some amount of macrophages. Apocrine cells may also be present and may be seen as flat sheets, single cells, or as papillary clusters (Fig. 10.5.). Crystals may also be seen within the proteinaceous fluid (Figs. 10.6 and 10.7).

Cysts, as well as dilated ducts, may contain mucinous material. FNA smears may yield abundant extracellular mucin with minimal cellularity [24]. If epithelial cells

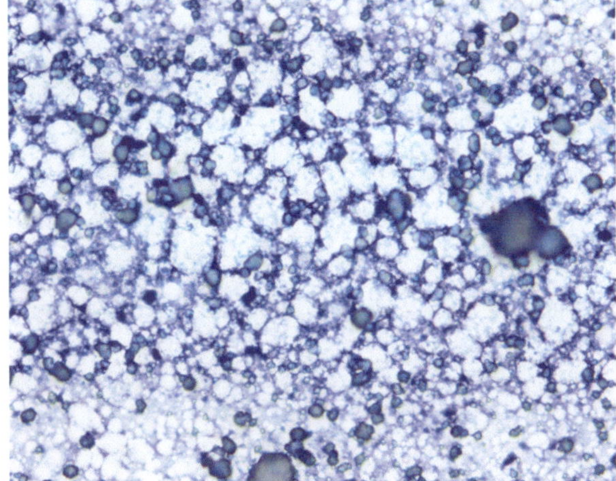

Fig. 10.6 Cyst contents showing proteinaceous material with numerous refractile crystals (Diff Quik 20×)

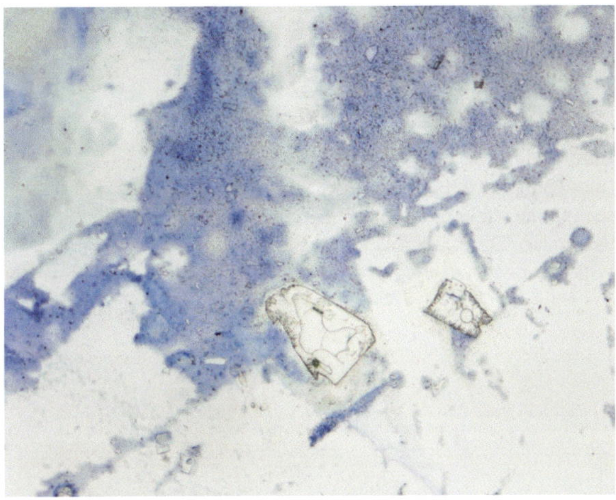

Fig. 10.7 Aspirate of a cyst with proteinaceous debris and flat crystals (Diff Quik 20×)

are present, they are found in clusters with little to no dissociated cells. The epithelial cells lack cytologic atypia and bare oval nuclei are also identified with the mucinous material [24].

Proliferative FCC

Aspirates of usual ductal hyperplasia show moderate to high cellularity, with variably sized and tightly cohesive groups of epithelial cells (Figs. 10.8, 10.9, 10.10 and 10.11). The groups of epithelium may be flat or three-dimensional with overlapping

Fig. 10.8 Proliferative fibrocystic change showing large groups of ductal epithelial cells. Apocrine cells are present in the lower left of the image and scattered bare oval nuclei are present in the background of the smear (Diff Quik 4×)

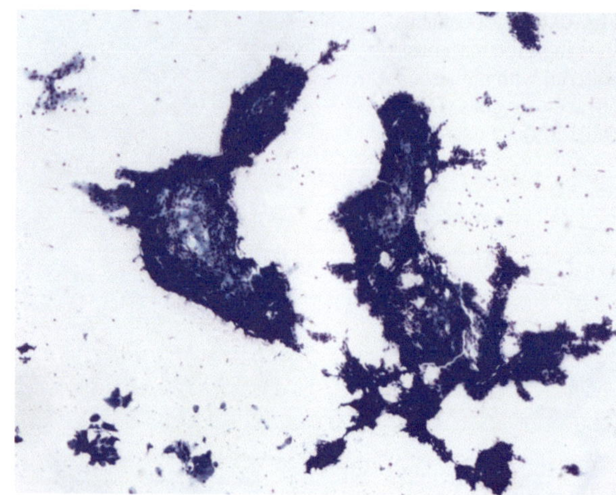

Fig. 10.9 Fibrocystic change, proliferative. Aspirate shows groups of benign ductal epithelium and myoepithelial cells. Bare oval nuclei (myoepithelial cells) are seen in the background of the smear. (Diff Quik 4×)

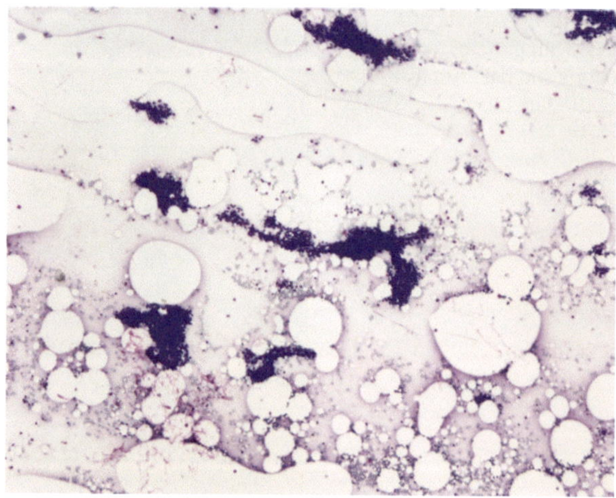

Fig. 10.10 A benign group of ductal epithelium. Myoepithelial cells are present admixed with the benign epithelial cells and as bare oval nuclei in the background of the smear (ThinPrep 40×)

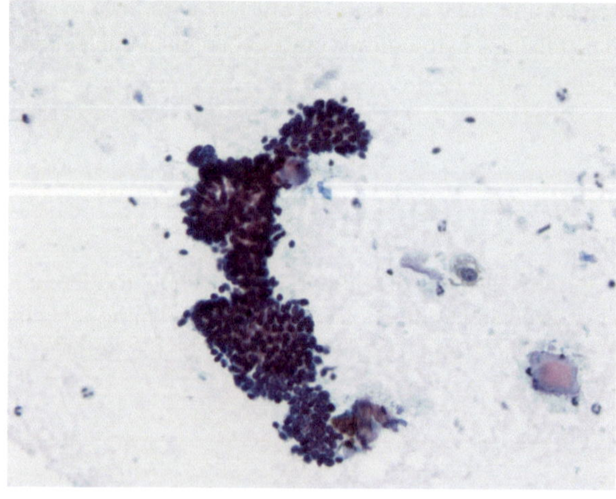

Fig. 10.11. A group of
benign ductal epithelial
cells and myoepithelial
cells in a ThinPrep
specimen (ThinPrep 20×)

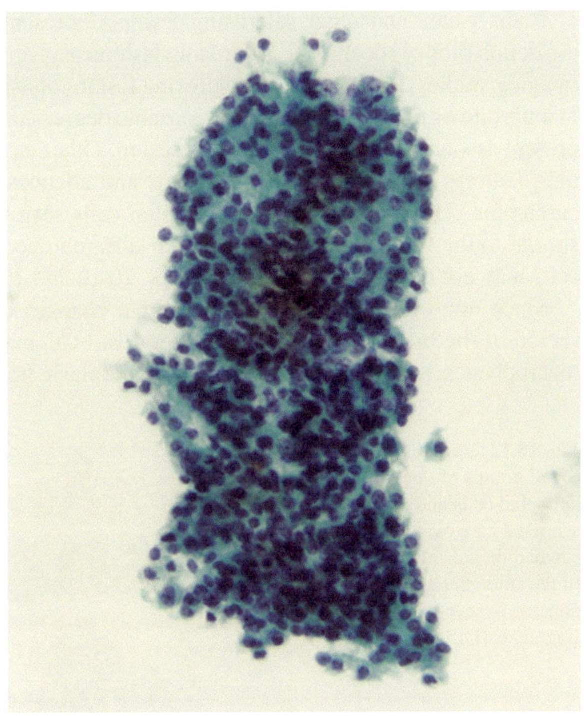

epithelial cells admixed with myoepithelial cells. In some cases, irregular lumen formations may be seen. Overall, there is variability in the appearance of the epithelial cells. The cells may appear round or elongated with slightly enlarged nuclei and small nucleoli [16, 21]. On histology, the epithelial cells of usual ductal hyperplasia have some variation in the cellular and nuclear size and shape. There is a haphazard arrangement of epithelial cells with admixed myoepithelial cells. These histologic features can be in cytologic specimens of proliferative FCC. Scattered bare oval nuclei, representing myoepithelial cells, may be seen in the background of the smears. A fibroadenoma, rather than FCC, should be favored if there are numerous bare oval nuclei [16].

Proliferative fibrocystic changes can also produce hyperplastic epithelial clusters that exhibit a branching, or pseudopapillary appearance, on cytologic smears [25, 26]. These clusters lack fibrovascular cores, and therefore are not true papillae. Care must be taken not to overinterpret these groups as papillary lesions.

FNA specimens of sclerosing adenosis yield cellular specimens. Reviewing cases of sclerosing adenosis that had prior FNA biopsies, Cho et al. reported finding small acinar groups of ductal and myoepithelial cells, scattered individual epithelial cells without atypia, and small fragments of hypocellular and hyalinized stroma in all cases [27]. In addition, the small stromal fragments were tightly attached to the acinar groups of epithelial cells.

Radial scars and other sclerosing lesions represent a diagnostic challenge on aspiration biopsy specimens. Sclerosing lesions may appear as spiculated masses on imaging studies. Histologically, sclerosing lesions consist of small glands entrapped in a fibrotic or fibroelastotic stroma. Variable degrees of fibrocystic changes may be present associated with the sclerosing lesion. Other authors have reported overlapping features between sclerosing lesions and adenocarcinoma, especially tubular carcinoma. The small clusters of epithelial cells seen in sclerosing lesions appear similar to the tubular groups seen in well-differentiated carcinomas. Myoepithelial cells may not be prominent [28, 29] (Figs. 10.12 and 10.13).

Since non-proliferative and proliferative changes can be present in the same region of the breast, aspirates of proliferative FCC may also show apocrine cells, macrophages, and cyst fluid, along with hyperplasic findings [16].

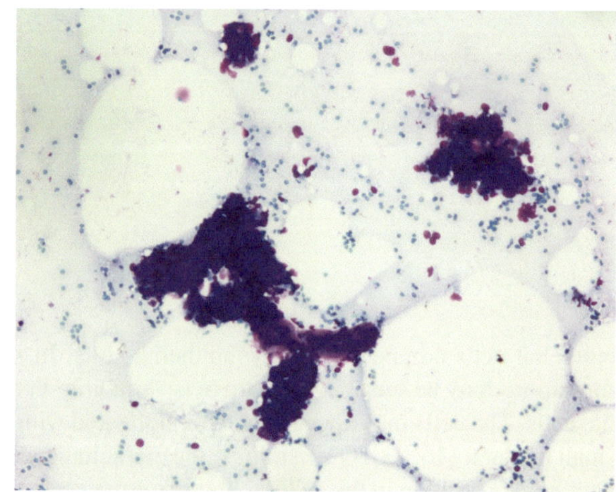

Fig. 10.12 Radial scar. Small groups of ductal epithelial cells and scattered bare oval nuclei (myoepithelial cells). Some of the epithelial groups are adhered to stromal fragments (Diff Quik 10)

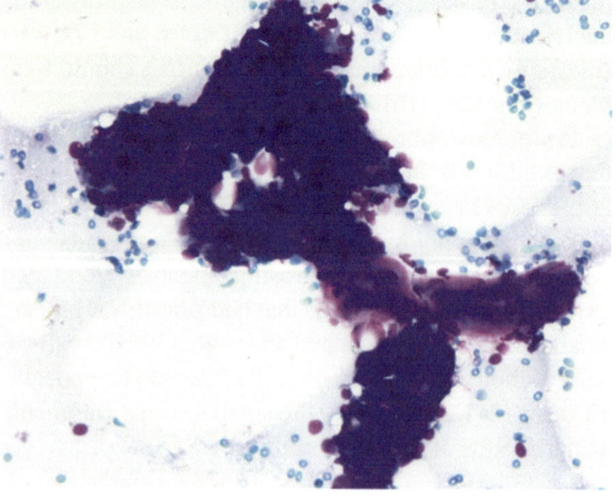

Fig. 10.13 Radial scar. Higher magnification of prior image (Diff Quik 20×)

Proliferative FCC with Atypia

The definition epithelial atypia in breast FNA specimens has not been well established and is subject to interobserver variability [30]. The presence of atypical cells in cases of FCC must be recognized since there is an increased risk of malignancy on excisional specimens. Lim et al. reported a malignancy rate of 37% following surgical resection of FNA cases diagnoses as atypical. The malignancies included both invasive and in situ carcinomas. Aspirates of proliferative FCC with atypia show moderate to high cellularity. Atypical findings include dissociation of epithelial groups with an increased number of dispersed and intact epithelial cells, absence of myoepithelial cells, loss of polarity of the epithelial cell groups, enlarged hyperchromatic nuclei that are larger than three to four times the size of a red blood cell, irregular nuclear contours, and a coarse chromatin pattern. Myoepithelial cells may still be seen within the epithelial groups [16, 23] (Figs. 10.14 and 10.15). Dispersed

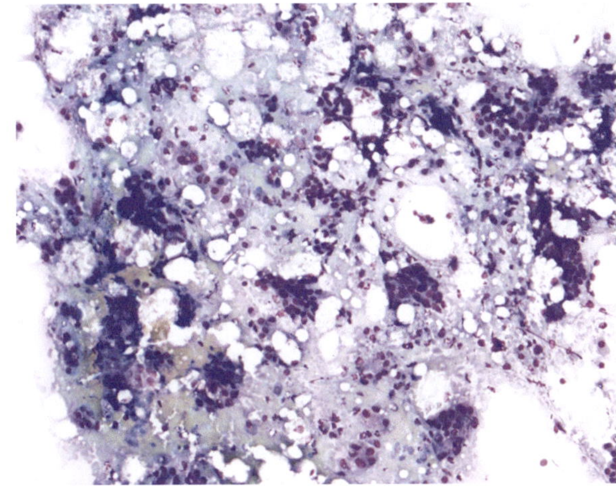

Fig. 10.14 FCC with atypia. Groups of ductal epithelium with dissociation of epithelial cells. Some of the dissociated epithelial cells have enlarged nuclei. The excisional specimen revealed a complex sclerosing lesion (Diff Quik 10)

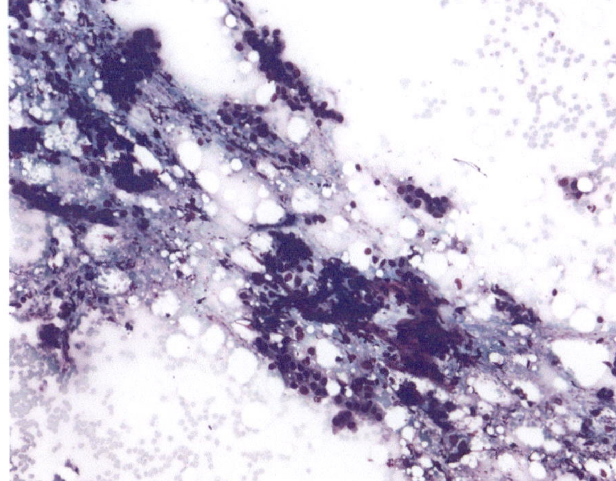

Fig. 10.15 FCC with atypia. Same case as above. Groups of ductal epithelium with slight dissociation if the epithelial cells. A stromal fragment is present. The excisional specimen revealed a complex sclerosing lesion (Diff Quik 10)

epithelial cells may also have cytoplasmic mucin vacuoles. Cytologic atypia can also be defined as the presence of a population of epithelial cells with a monomorphic and uniform appearance, without nuclear overlap and absence of myoepithelial cells [21]. Monomorphic, evenly-spaced round nuclei are histologic features seen in cases of atypical ductal hyperplasia.

Even with the above criteria of cytologic atypia it should be recognized that there is significant overlap between cases that are benign and those that are malignant [30].

The atypical findings are focal and are usually found in a background of benign changes [23]. If there is marked atypia or if the atypical findings are extensive, a diagnosis of suspicious for carcinoma or positive for carcinoma should be considered.

While there is an increased risk of malignancy on surgical resection specimens, the majority of cases diagnosed as atypical on breast FNA are benign on surgical follow-up. The histologic spectrum of proliferative breast lesions is wide, and this translates directly to the variability seen on cytologic specimens. Sclerosing lesions, florid usual ductal hyperplasia, papillary lesions, apocrine changes, and even fibroadenomas can produce atypia on aspiration biopsy [30, 31]. Other causes of atypia may be due to post-radiation changes, (Figs. 10.16 and 10.17), inexperience in evaluating breast FNA specimens, poor preservation of cells due to lidocaine artifact and reactive changes due to inflammation.

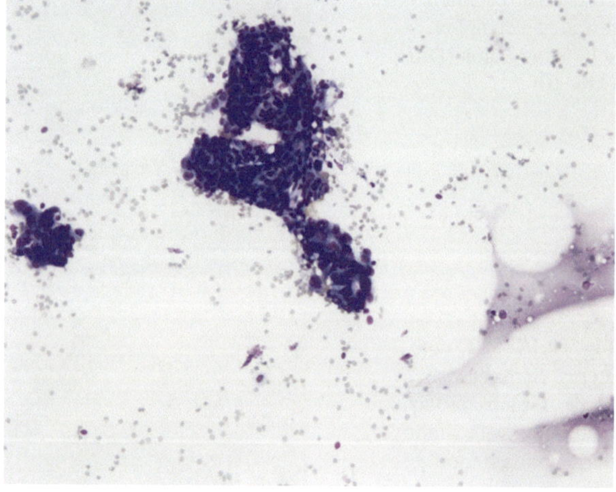

Fig. 10.16 Radiation atypia. Cohesive groups of ductal epithelium and myoepithelial cells. Some of the epithelial cells display enlarged nuclei (Diff Quik 10×)

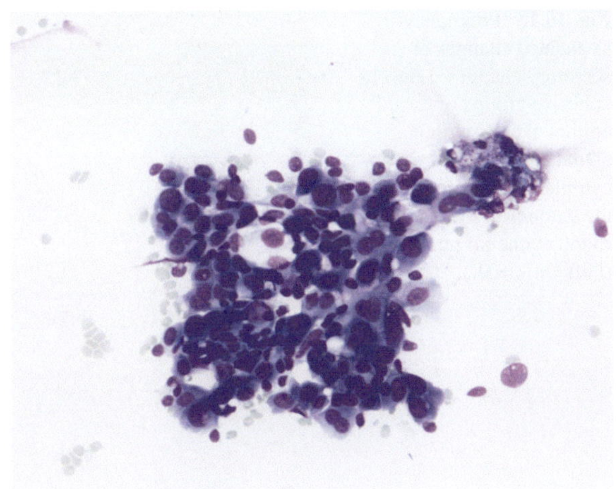

Fig. 10.17 Radiation atypia. Cohesive group of ductal epithelium and myoepithelial cells. Some of the epithelial cells display markedly enlarged nuclei (Diff Quik 20×)

Pregnancy-Related Changes

During pregnancy and lactation, the mammary epithelium undergoes physiologic changes leading to an increase in the number and size of acini and terminal duct lobular units. The epithelial cells also undergo secretory or lactational changes. On cytology, these changes consist of enlarged epithelial cells with abundant finely vacuolated cytoplasm, enlarged round nuclei, and prominent nucleoli [32]. Epithelial cells with secretory or lactational changes have delicate cytoplasm that tends to fray during the smearing process, leading to the presence of bare round epithelial nuclei. These bare nuclei still maintain smooth nuclear contours. The background of the smears consists of lipid-rich and proteinaceous material (Figs. 10.18 and 10.19).

The vast majority of breast masses in pregnant women are benign; the most common being lactating adenomas, galactoceles, and fibroadenomas. Carcinomas occurring during pregnancy or the immediate post-partum period account for approximately 3% of breast cancers; however, it has been reported that pregnancy-related breast cancers are more aggressive and present at a higher stage, with lymphovascular invasion and lymph node involvement, compared to carcinomas arising in non-pregnant women [33]. Clinically and radiologically, it may be difficult to evaluate a mass occurring during pregnancy due to the increased breast volume and increased density of breast tissue. Pathologic evaluation, therefore, is essential and an FNA is a rapid and safe diagnostic tool to make a diagnosis and determine if additional management is warranted.

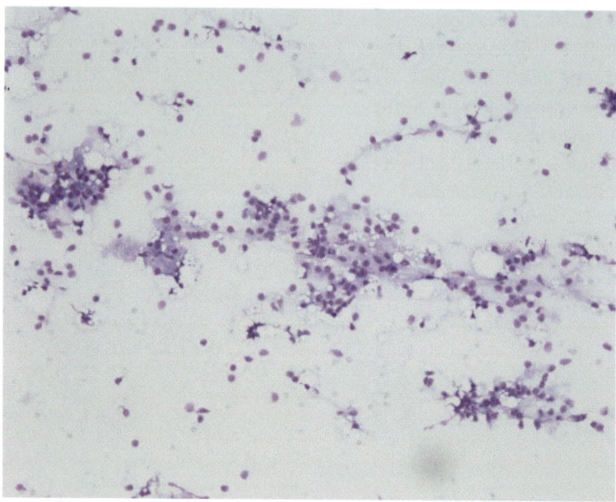

Fig. 10.18 Pregnancy-associated changes or secretory changes. Loosely cohesive groups of ductal epithelial cells with abundant fragile cytoplasm. Dissolution of the cytoplasm leads to bare round epithelial nuclei (Diff Quik 10X)

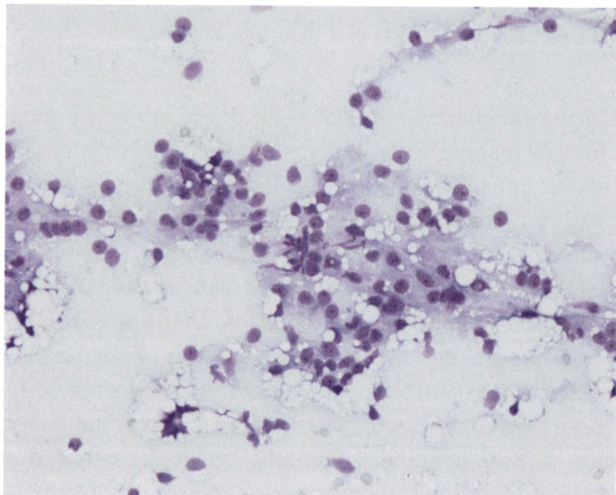

Fig. 10.19 Pregnancy-associated changes or secretory changes. Nuclei are round with prominent nucleoli (Diff Quik 20X)

Galactocele

A galactocele is a cystic collection of milk occurring most commonly in the third trimester of pregnancy, during lactation or after cessation of breastfeeding. Galactoceles in pregnant or lactating women are thought to arise as a result of duct obstruction leading to altered milk flow, stagnation, and the formation of a cystic mass lined by flattened cuboidal epithelium. The duct obstruction may be secondary to a mass, such as a fibroadenoma or implant, inflammation or post-surgical scar tissue, such as in patients' status post-mammoplasty [34]. Rare cases of galactoceles have been reported in male infants and in nulliparous women secondary to hyperprolactinemia.

A galactocele typically presents as a painless, mobile mass in the subareolar or periareolar region, although it can occur anywhere along the milk line. Unusual cases have been reported in the axilla [35]. While most galactoceles have benign clinical features, on occasion they may present as firm, fixed masses with overlying skin erythema due to the presence of inflammation.

An ultrasound is the initial and best imaging modality to evaluate a breast mass in pregnant women. By sonogram galactoceles may have a characteristic appearance of a benign cyst: a well-circumscribed anechoic mass with posterior acoustic enhancement. However, most galactoceles appear as hypoechoic masses with a fluid-fat level or internal echoic foci depending on the proportions of fluid, fat, and protein [36–38]. A galactocele on mammography will appear as radiolucent mass, a cystic mass with a fluid-fat level or as a mass with heterogeneous density [35, 39, 40].

FNAs can be both a diagnostic and a therapeutic procedure. FNA yields milky-white or cloudy fluid of varying viscosity. A significant decrease in the size of or complete resolution of the galactocele may occur after aspiration. Smears show granular or foamy secretory fluid consisting of lipid and proteinaceous material. This milky fluid is best seen on Diff Quik stained smears and may not be evident in liquid-based preparations. Admixed within the milky fluid are macrophages containing lipid vacuoles; the number of macrophages may be numerous (Figs. 10.20 and 10.21). Ductal epithelial cells with secretory changes are rarely seen. If present, epithelial cells may be intact and show secretory changes consisting of finely vacuolated cytoplasm and prominent nucleoli, or they may have lost their cytoplasm and appear as round, bare epithelial cell nuclei with prominent nucleoli [32, 41]. Crystals may form within longstanding galactoceles due to precipitation of inspissated material (crystallizing galactocele). FNA will yield numerous refractile, polarizable, and birefringent crystals of varying sizes and shapes [42–44].

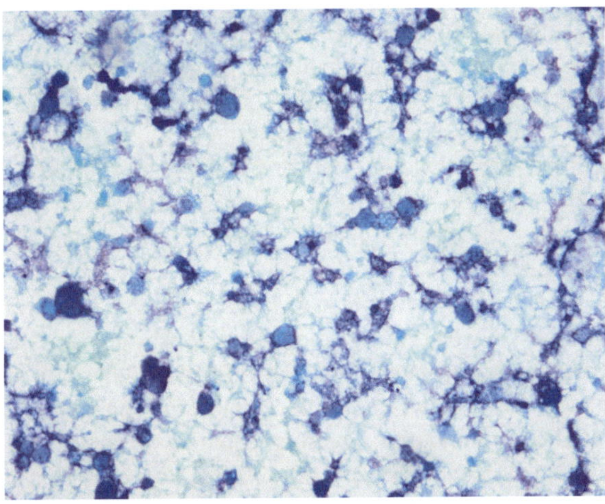

Fig. 10.20 Galactocele. Lipo-proteinaceous material and crystals in an aspirate of a galactocele (Pap 20X)

Fig. 10.21 Galactocele. Lipo-proteinaceous material and histiocytes (Diff Quik 20X)

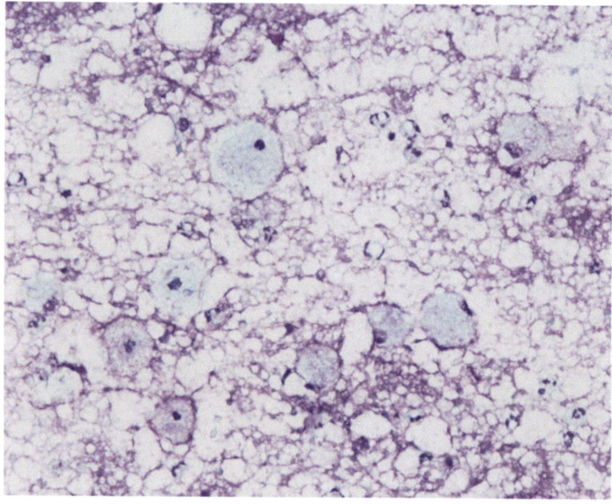

With an adequate clinical history, the cytologic diagnosis of a galactocele is straightforward. It is important to recognize secretory changes in epithelial cells, when present on the smears and be aware that enlarged nuclei with prominent nucleoli are typical features.

Lactating Adenoma

A lactating adenoma is a benign breast mass that occurs during pregnancy, typically in the third trimester, and in the post-partum period. It is currently unknown whether a lactating adenoma is a true neoplasm or whether it represents a localized, hyperplastic response due to the physiologic effects of pregnancy [41]. One study assessing genetic alterations in different types of adenomas did not detect any genetic mutations in lactating adenomas, including mutations in the exon 2 of the MED12 gene that are characteristically found in fibroadenomas [45]. Histologically, a lactating adenoma consists of nodular aggregates of hyperplastic acini showing secretory changes that coalesce with little intervening stroma. This nodular aggregate will form a discrete, palpable mass that is distinct from the surrounding breast tissue. A lactating adenoma typically presents as a circumscribed, mobile mass that is non-tender.

The distinction between a lactating adenoma and a fibroadenoma with lactational changes may be difficult clinically and pathologically. Fibroadenomas may be present prior to pregnancy, while lactating adenomas will first be identified during pregnancy or lactation. A fibroadenoma will maintain an underlying fibroepithelial architecture and the secretory changes of ductal epithelium are typically focal. Lactating adenomas typically resolve after cessation of breastfeeding. Ultimately, the distinction between a lactating adenoma and a fibroadenoma with lactational changes may not be clinically important.

Ultrasound is the preferred imaging study to evaluate a lactating adenoma [46]. Sonographic findings are suggestive of a benign lesion and include a well-circumscribed mass with homogeneous echotexture and posterior acoustic enhancement [47].

Aspiration of a lactating adenoma reveals a moderately to highly cellular specimen consisting of ductal epithelium showing secretory changes. The epithelial cells may be present as flat sheets, three-dimensional clusters or as intact, hyperplastic lobular units. Single, bare epithelial nuclei may also be seen. The epithelial cells show secretory changes, including abundant vacuolated cytoplasm, enlarged round nuclei, and prominent nucleoli. The background of the smears shows granular or proteinaceous material consistent with milk (Figs. 10.22, 10.23, 10.24, 10.25 and 10.26).

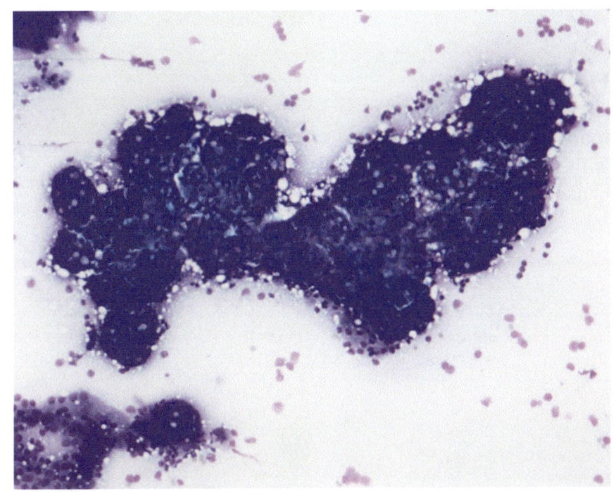

Fig. 10.22 Lactating adenoma. Aspirate of a lactating adenoma showing intact lobular clusters. The ductal cells within the acini show secretory changes (Diff Quik 10×)

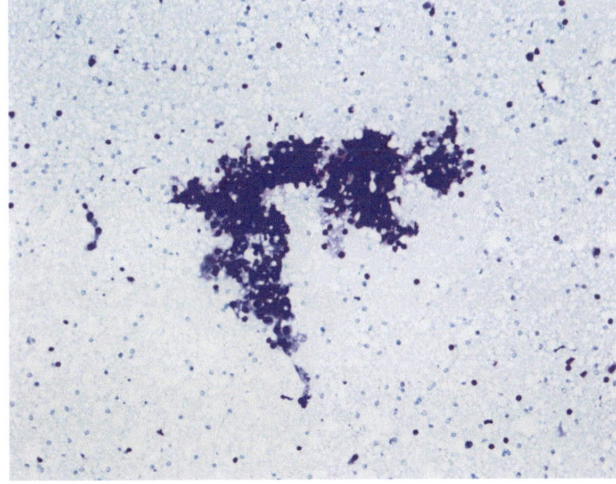

Fig. 10.23 Lactating adenoma. Group of ductal epithelial cells with secretory changes in a background of proteinaceous fluid (Diff Quik 10×)

Fig. 10.24 Lactating adenoma. Group of ductal epithelial cells with secretory changes in a background of proteinaceous fluid (Diff Quik 20×)

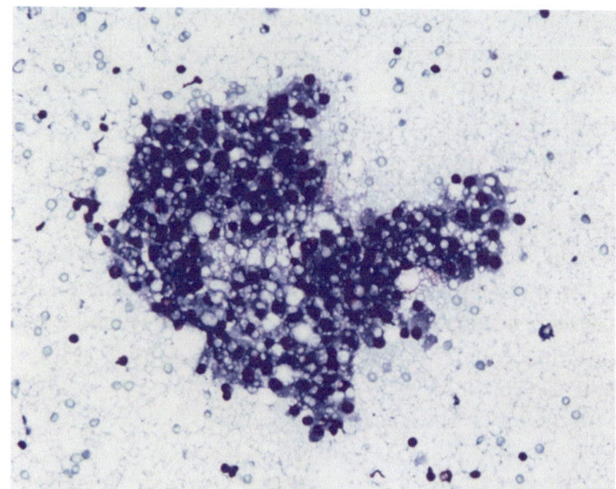

Fig. 10.25 Lactating adenoma. Numerous bare, round epithelial nuclei with small nucleoli (Diff Quik 20×)

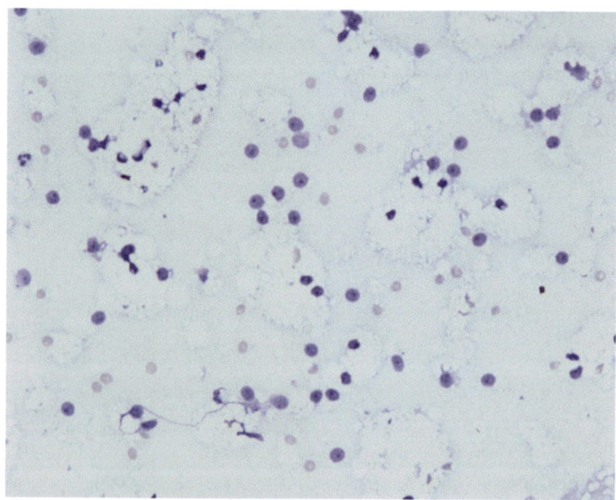

Fig. 10.26 Lactating adenoma. A stromal fragment in a lactating adenoma (Diff Quik 20X)

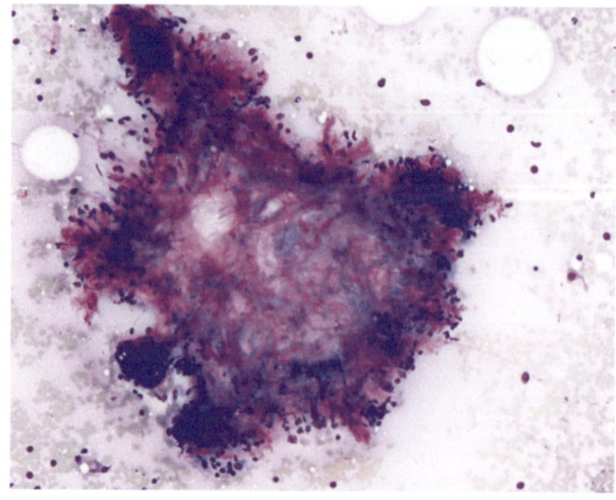

Mammary Duct Ectasia

Mammary duct ectasia is a benign, inflammatory process that primarily affects large, extra-lobular ducts in the retroareolar region in perimenopausal and post-menopausal women. The histologic appearance has been well documented and characteristically consists of dilated, ectatic ducts, periductal fibrosis, and periductal chronic inflammation. The ectatic ducts are lined by a layer of flattened ductal epithelium without epithelial hyperplasia. Rarely, squamous metaplasia may occur. The duct lumen typically contains granular, lipid-laden debris that contains crystals and macrophages. The luminal secretion may be viscous and resemble comedo necrosis. Periductal chronic inflammation consists of lymphocytes, plasma cells, and macrophages, including macrophages containing cytoplasmic lipofuscin pigment (termed ochrocytes) [48–50]. Histiocytes may also be present within the epithelial layer of the ectatic ducts. These intraepithelial histiocytes stain for histiocytic markers, such as CD68, and their presence should not be confused for Paget's disease. End-stage MDE presents as fibrotic ducts with the residual lumen appearing as a peripheral layer of small spaces ("garland sign") surrounding a sclerotic central zone.

The etiology of MDE is unknown. The walls of large subareolar ducts may weaken with age due to loss of elastin, a process that leads to duct ectasia and stasis of secretions. Rupture of the duct with leakage of secretions into the surrounding stroma leads to a chronic inflammatory response and periductal fibrosis. However, some studies have suggested that periductal inflammation (periductal mastitis) is the initiating event that subsequently leads to duct stasis and dilatation. Some believe that smoking is a risk factor although reports in the literature are contradictory. MDE has rarely been reported in childhood and in men [51, 52].

Some patients with MDE may be asymptomatic, while others may present with a variety of symptoms. Nipple discharge may occur and can be clear, bloody or consist of thick, inspissated material. The nipple discharge may be multiductal and bilateral. Patients may also present with a palpable mass in the retroareolar region. The presence of extensive periductal fibrosis may cause a firm mass fixed to the overlying skin and cause nipple or skin retraction, signs that may mimic a carcinoma clinically [53]. Pain may be associated with the retroareolar mass although overlying skin erythema is not a clinical feature.

Mammography has a low sensitivity for the evaluation of intraductal masses and may not be diagnostic in patients with MDE who present with nipple discharge. If a mass is present on physical exam, increased density in the retroareolar region may be seen due to periductal fibrosis. Calcifications may also be present in a linear and branching distribution, a sign that may be mistaken for DCIS. Ultrasound has higher sensitivity and specificity for evaluating intraductal lesions [54]. By ultrasound, large dilated anechoic branching ducts without blood flow may be seen in the retroareolar region. The ducts may be filled with echogenic material representing luminal secretions, or they appear as anechoic cystic masses [53, 54]. MRI is useful in evaluating for the presence of enhancing masses within dilated ducts that may be worrisome for a neoplastic process, such as a papilloma. No abnormal enhancing masses should be noted on MRI in the ducts or in the periductal region in cases of MDE [55].

FNA of mammary duct ectasia is non-specific and may overlap with other benign and inflammatory disorders [48]. Aspirates yield granular, proteinaceous material comprising intraluminal secretions. Crystals or macrophages may be present admixed within the proteinaceous debris. Depending on the degree of periductal inflammation present, lymphocytes and plasma cells may also be seen. Ductal epithelial cells are usually scant to absent. When present the epithelial cells are found in clusters although some single cells may also be seen (Figs. 10.27, 10.28, 10.29 and 10.30). The epithelial cells may show reactive changes, such as enlarged, overlapping nuclei and small prominent nucleoli. Nuclear contours should be smooth

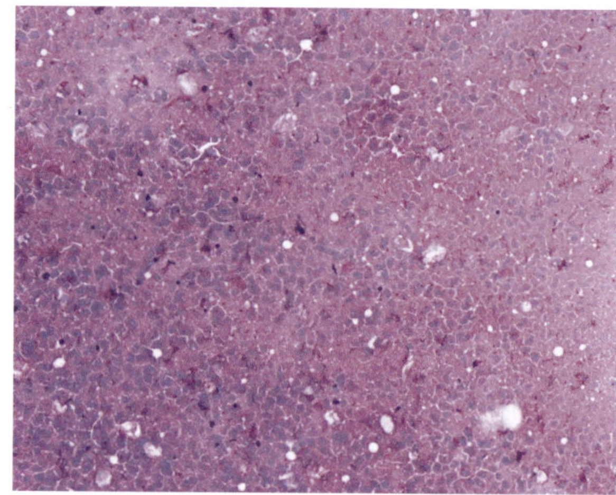

Fig. 10.27 Mammary duct ectasia. Thick, acellular proteinaceous material representing luminal secretion. It is critical not to confuse this amorphous, granular material for necrosis (Diff Quik 10×)

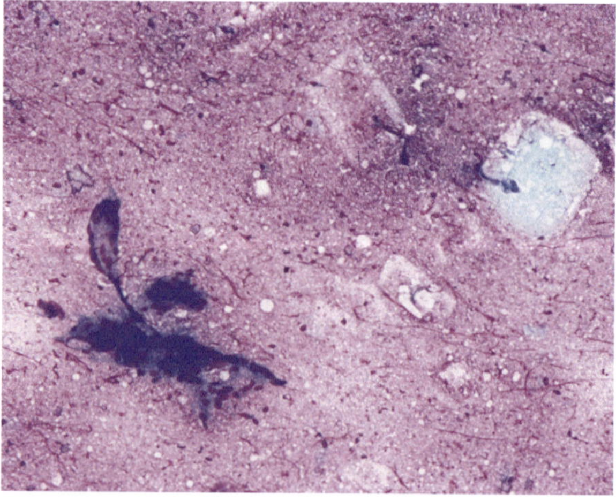

Fig. 10.28 Mammary duct ectasia. Granular debris, crystals, and a multinucleated giant cell (Diff Quik 10×)

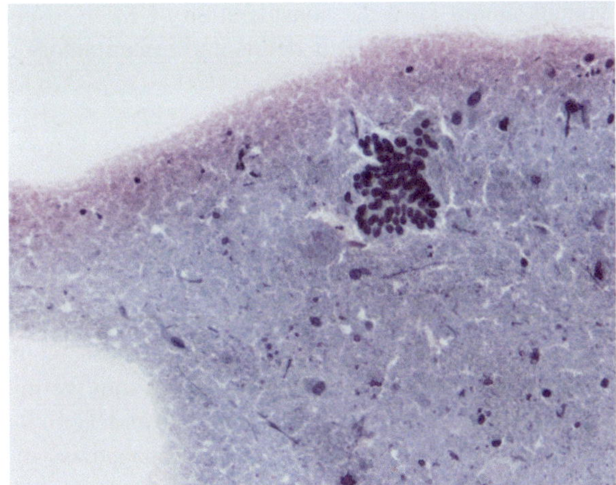

Fig. 10.29 Mammary duct ectasia. Granular debris and a small cluster of benign ductal epithelium. (Pap 20×)

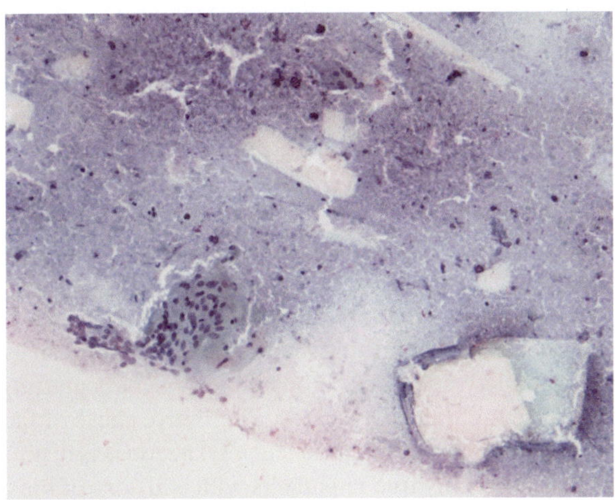

Fig. 10.30 Mammary duct ectasia. A multinucleated giant cell and crystals in a background of granular debris (Pap 20×)

and the nuclei should have an even chromatin pattern. A unique finding is the presence of histiocytes within the epithelial clusters. These histiocytes are large mononuclear cells with abundant vacuolated cytoplasm and standout from the surrounding epithelial cells [48]. If there is prominent periductal fibrosis, FNA samples may not yield much material. Squamous metaplasia of the ductal epithelium lining the ducts may rarely occur, and reactive squamous cells may be present in FNA samples, although this is a rare finding [56]. The presence of numerous squamous cells, especially in the presence of keratin debris and acute inflammation, is most likely the secondary to squamous metaplasia of lactiferous ducts (SMOLD), not due to duct ectasia [48, 50].

While a specific diagnosis of MDE may be difficult, the presence of a dilated cystic mass located behind the nipple in a perimenopausal or postmenopausal woman should raise the consideration of MDE, especially in FNA samples that yield mostly proteinaceous debris and inflammatory cells with little to no ductal epithelium.

Fat Necrosis

Mammary fat necrosis is a benign, inflammatory process that results from injury to the breast and subsequent degeneration of adipose tissue. The clinical, radiologic, and pathologic findings vary depending on the stage of the lesion [57]. In the early stages of fat necrosis, there is hemorrhage into the injured area, leading to edema and the destruction of adipocytes by tissue and blood lipases. Foamy histiocytes and multinucleated giant cells infiltrate the damaged tissue, and fibroblasts proliferate at the edge of the lesion, beginning the healing process that will lead to the formation of scar tissue or a loculated area of liquefactive necrotic fat surrounded by fibrosis (oil cyst). Dystrophic calcifications may also form in the chronic stages, including peripheral ("eggshell") calcifications surrounding the oil cyst [58, 59].

Fat necrosis can mimic breast carcinoma both clinically and radiologically [58, 60]. Fine needle aspiration (FNA) has been shown to be a useful tool to diagnose fat necrosis, thereby eliminating the need for more invasive biopsies or surgical procedures [57].

The causes of mammary fat necrosis are numerous. Fat necrosis most often occurs as a result of direct injury to the breast, such as after physical trauma, radiation therapy or after an FNA, core biopsy or surgical procedure, such as lumpectomy or mammoplasty. Other less common causes include ruptured cysts, duct ectasia, abscess, periductal mastitis, infection, pacemaker insertion, use of the internal mammary artery for coronary artery bypass grafting, and anticoagulant therapy [58, 59, 61–65]. In some cases, a definitive cause of fat necrosis is not identified.

The main clinical importance of fat necrosis is distinguishing it from a neoplasm. This is especially true in patients with a history of breast carcinoma who are status post therapy and a recurrence must be ruled out. On physical exam, fat necrosis typically presents as a painless, round, or ill-defined mass. However, in a small percentage of patients' worrisome clinical findings may be present, and these include a firm, fixed mass with associated nipple retraction, erythema, and skin dimpling [57, 63]. Patients with a history of trauma may report overlying skin ecchymosis. The clinical signs of fat necrosis may occur months to several years after the initiating event [59].

Mammary fat necrosis most commonly occurs in perimenopausal women; however, it may also occur in men [57, 66]. In a study looking at FNAs of breast masses in men, 21 cases out of 614 (3.4%) were diagnosed as fat necrosis [67].

Mammary fat necrosis has a wide spectrum of appearance on different imaging modalities based on the time frame of the lesion, the amount of inflammation present and the degree of calcification, fibrosis, and cystic degeneration [68]. Mammographic findings may include features that are indistinguishable with malignancy, including asymmetries in the breast parenchyma, spiculated masses, and calcifications [59]. The calcifications may have benign features or have a suspicious appearance, with pleomorphism and a branching configuration [69]. If cystic degeneration has occurred, a benign-appearing radiolucent mass (oil cyst) that may contain peripheral calcifications will be seen [70]. Sonographic features include a solid mass that may be circumscribed or ill-defined with a variable echogenic appearance [70]. Masses that appear echogenic or as anechoic cysts with posterior enhancement are less worrisome; while masses that are ill-defined, hypoechoic or of mixed echogenicity have more suspicious findings [69, 70]. The presence of an oil cyst will yield a hypointense T1-weighted signal on MRI. With the presence of prominent inflammation, there will be enhancement on MRI following the administration of MRI, leading to features indistinguishable from a neoplasm [69]. The presence of acute and chronic inflammatory cells in fat necrosis may result in increased FDG uptake on PET/CT scan, thereby leading to suspicious findings and misinterpretation as a neoplasm [68, 71].

Since the clinical and radiologic findings may overlap with those of a breast carcinoma, fine needle aspiration (FNA) is a useful tool to exclude malignancy and provide a definitive diagnosis [57]. FNA specimens are typically hypocellular with an oily background consisting of lipid droplets or a granular background of cellular debris (Figs. 10.31, 10.32, 10.33, 10.34 and 10.35). In the early stages of fat necrosis, FNA shows degenerated fibroadipose tissue with adipocytes showing loss of nuclei. Hemorrhage and acute inflammation may also be seen. Red blood cells may coalesce to form myospherulosis [72]. During the intermediate stage, lipid-laden macrophages and multinucleated giant cells will predominate [60]. As the fat necrosis heals, fibroblasts deposit collagen, leading to the formation of a scar. FNA at this stage may yield reactive fibrohistiocytic cells. Chronic inflammation, hemosiderin-laden macrophages, and calcifications may also be present. Healing, which may occur months to years after the initiating event, may also occur in the form of a cystic cavity containing liquified adipose tissue and a fibrous wall. FNA may yield

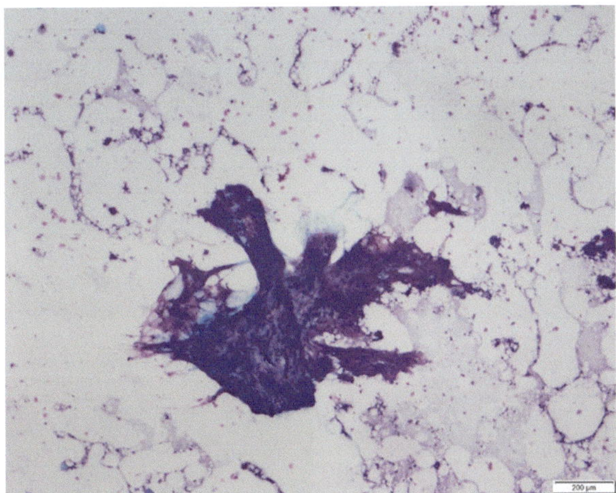

Fig. 10.31 Fat necrosis. A stromal fragment in a background of macrophages (Diff Quik 20×)

Fig. 10.32 Fat necrosis showing a background of lipid (Diff Quik 20×)

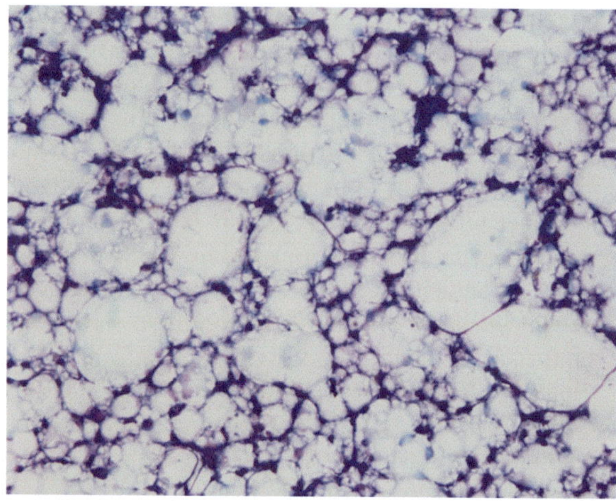

Fig. 10.33 Fat necrosis. The aspirate shows macrophages, inflammatory cells, and lipid (Diff Quik 40×)

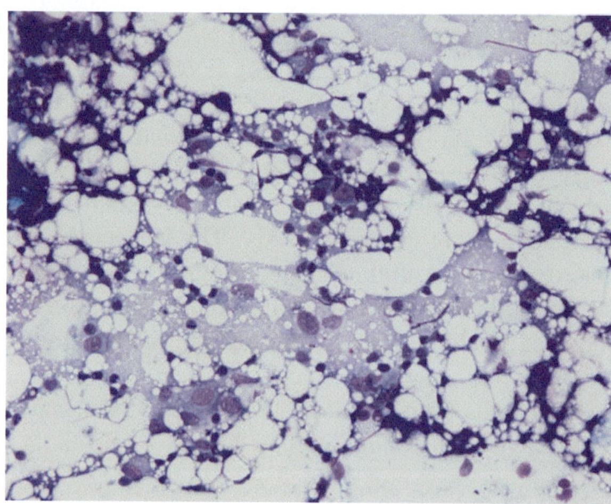

Fig. 10.34 Fat necrosis. Fragments of degenerated fibroadipose tissue (Pap stain 4×)

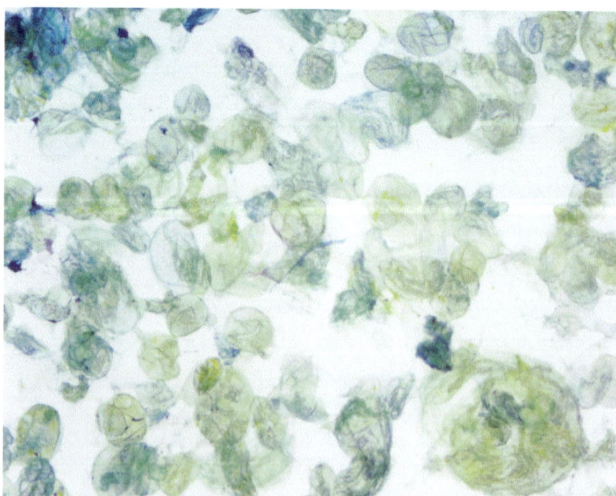

Fig. 10.35 Fat necrosis. Aspirate of myospherulosis and degenerated fibroadipose tissue (Pap stain 40×)

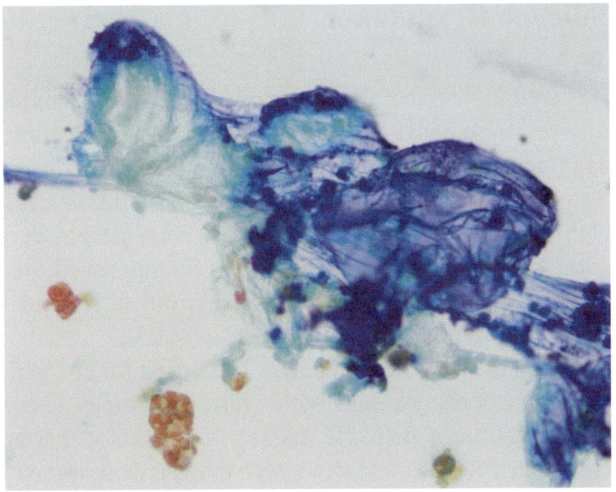

only acellular oily material representing liquified adipose tissue (liquefied fat necrosis or oil cyst). The FNA may remove most or all of the oily material in the cyst, thereby being a therapeutic, as well as a diagnostic, procedure. Oil cysts may be lined by peripheral calcifications, and tough, gritty calcification may be felt during the aspiration. The cytologic findings of fat necrosis are easily identified on conventional smears; however, essential diagnostic findings, such as background oily material, inflammation, and adipocytes, may be lost with liquid-based preparations [73].

The cytologic diagnosis of fat necrosis is usually straightforward; however, there may be some pitfalls. Some cases yield cellular specimens consisting of numerous macrophages which may have reactive features, such as enlarged nuclei and prominent nucleoli. This may be mistaken for epithelial cells, and granular cell tumor. Reactive fibrohistiocytic cells may also be present that may mimic a stromal or a spindle cell lesion.

While epithelial cells are usually not aspirated in a significant number, scant groups of ductal epithelial cells may be seen. It is important to distinguish reactive epithelial cells from neoplastic cells, especially in patients with a prior history of carcinoma and chemoradiation. Differentiating reactive ductal cells secondary to radiotherapy from recurrent tumor may be challenging. Some of these cases may be called atypical or suspicious on cytology.

It is important to remember that mammary fat necrosis may occur in the presence of a malignancy and the cytologic findings of fat necrosis on FNA may mask an underlying neoplastic process. Care must be taken to evaluate for the presence of neoplastic cells.

Silicone Granuloma

It is well known that the presence of free silicone in the breast elicits an inflammatory response consisting of a foreign-body giant cell reaction (silicone granuloma). Mammary prostheses filled with silicone may rupture or there be leakage of silicone into the surrounding breast parenchyma without evidence of implant rupture. In addition, injection of free silicone has been used as a cosmetic procedure. The Food and Drug Administration (FDA) has not approved the use of free silicone for cosmetic purposes in the United States; however, silicone injection for breast augmentation is common in other countries [74, 75].

Silicone breast implants have been used for cosmetic breast augmentation or for reconstruction in patients with a history of breast cancer [76]. Silicone may lead to the formation of palpable masses in the breast that are firm, irregular, fixed, and sometimes painful, features which may be worrisome for a carcinoma and for which an FNA is indicated [77]. Palpable axillary lymphadenopathy may also be present [78]. In addition, patients with implants may develop a fibrous capsule surrounding the implant that leads to contracture and deformity of the breast. Clinical findings typically occur many years after the implant placement or silicone injections [75].

When silicone ruptures beyond the capsule and spreads into the mammary parenchyma, it can form a density on mammography. Calcifications may be present. On sonogram, free silicone appears as bright, echogenic foci with posterior acoustic shadowing ("snow storm sign") [79]. MRI is the most sensitive imaging study to evaluate for implant rupture. Free silicone shows variable signal intensity, with low signal intensity on T1-weighted images and hyperintense on T2-weighted images [71]. MRI also shows type 1 kinetic enhancement, compatible with a benign lesion [74]. Due to the underlying inflammatory reaction, silicone granulomas may appear as PET-avid lesions [71]. Image guided is best to avoid implant rupture.

FNA of can definitely diagnose a silicone granuloma and evaluate for the presence of an underlying carcinoma. Aspirates of silicone granulomas may be scant or moderately cellular. The characteristic findings are variable numbers of histiocytes and multinucleated giant cells with cytoplasmic vacuoles [78] (Figs. 10.36 and 10.37). Histiocytes may coalesce to form loose aggregates [77]. The nuclei of the histiocytes and multinucleated giant cells show benign or reactive features, with smooth nuclear membranes, open chromatin, and small or inconspicuous nucleoli. The cytoplasmic vacuoles may appear empty or may have crystals within them. The crystals represent free silicone and are birefringent and refractile. Extracellular amorphous material may also be present and likely represents extracellular silicone. This acellular material is seen only on air-dried smears but is not identified on fixed smears [77]. A mixed inflammatory infiltrate, with a predominance of chronic inflammation, may be seen in some cases [77]. Reactive ductal epithelial cells have been reported, but when identified are usually present in small numbers [78]. However, it has been reported that carcinoma may occur in the association with silicone granulomas, so care must be taken to evaluate for the presence of an underlying neoplasm.

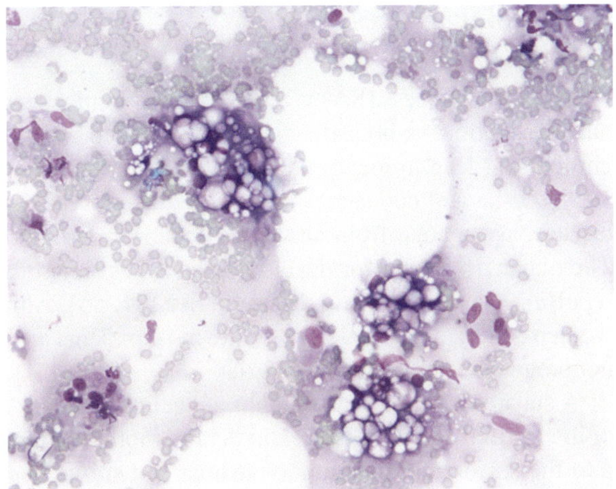

Fig. 10.36 Silicone granuloma. Multinucleated giant cells with numerous clear vacuoles (Diff Quik 20X)

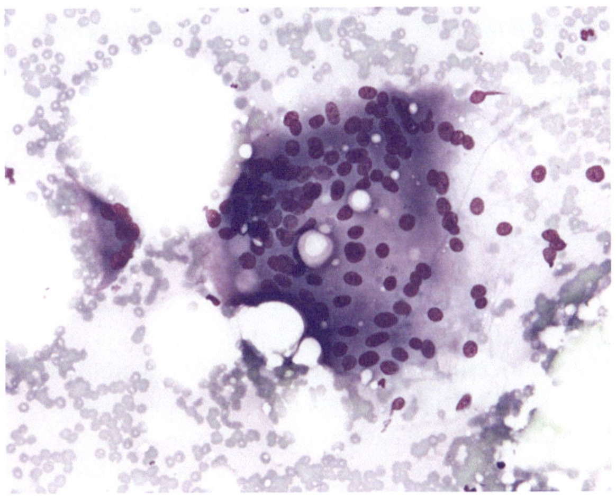

Fig. 10.37 Silicone granuloma. A multinucleated giant cell with several clear vacuoles (Diff Quik 20X)

While the term silicone granuloma is used to describe the inflammatory response, epithelioid granulomas with elongated nuclei like those seen in sarcoidosis or certain infectious diseases are not present. Necrosis is also not a feature of silicone reaction in the breast.

The fibrous capsule surrounding an implant is typically not sampled with an aspiration biopsy. Sampling the capsule would yield low cellularity due to the presence of fibrosis [77].

Free silicone can migrate via lymphatics from the breast to extra-mammary sites, the most common location being axillary lymph nodes [80]. Other reported extra-mammary sites include cervical lymph nodes, liver, spleen, dermis, and lung [79, 81, 82].

Subareolar Abscess

A subareolar abscess (SA) is a well-defined clinical entity that is unrelated to pregnancy, lactation, or breastfeeding. If not treated properly, this disorder can become chronic and lead to recurrent abscesses, fistula formation, and draining sinuses. In 1951, Zuska and colleagues described this entity, known eponymously as Zuska's disease, as separate from abscesses occurring at other sites in the breast [83, 84]. The major risk factor for developing an SA is smoking, with a majority of patients reporting chronic or heavy cigarette use [84, 85]. Although SA can occur in both women and men in a wide age range, most patients are women in their 30 s who are not pregnant or breastfeeding [84].

A subareolar abscess is thought to occur secondary to obstruction and dilatation of the lactiferous ducts by keratin debris, rupture of the duct with leakage of keratin into the surrounding mammary stroma and subsequent inflammation. Lactiferous ducts are lined by a double layer of cuboidal epithelium from the level of the acini (lobular unit) until the ampulla. The ampulla, located at the nipple-areolar complex, and the remaining portion of the duct that opens onto the nipple surface are lined by squamous epithelium [85, 86]. Squamous metaplasia of the normal cuboidal epithelium leads to the production of keratin that is sloughed into the lumen of the lactiferous duct and eventually leads to plugging, obstruction, inspissation of secreted material, and dilatation of the duct [84–86]. These pathologic findings are also referred to as squamous metaplasia of lactiferous ducts (SMOLD) [84, 87, 88]. Rupture of the duct and the release of keratin elicits an inflammatory reaction composed of neutrophils and foreign-body giant cells. Superimposed bacterial infection will lead to abscess formation. The abscess may drain spontaneously, leading to purulent nipple or areolar discharge. If an SA is left untreated or if treatment is ineffective, a chronic fistula opening onto the areola will develop [84, 88]. The most common bacterial organism in the acute abscess stage is *Staphylococcus aureus*. In later chronic stages, anaerobic organisms, or mixed flora may be cultured [89, 90].

Patients with SA present with a subareolar or periareolar mass that is associated with pain and overlying skin erythema. Nipple discharge that is purulent or hemopurulent may be present. In the chronic stage of the disease, a fistulous tract may be seen, typically located at the border of the areola [84, 85]. The diagnosis of an SA is usually made based on the clinical findings, and imagining studies may not be warranted to make the diagnosis. A mammogram may be normal or show nonspecific findings, such as skin thickening or asymmetry [91]. An ultrasound is more useful, especially to identify an abscess and assist with the aspiration of the abscess. Sonographic findings include hypoechoic, heterogeneous masses that may be circumscribed or ill-defined [91]. In the early stages of the disorder when an abscess is present, aspiration or incision and drainage, along with antibiotic therapy may be an effective treatment [84]. However, SA tends to recur, leading to recurring abscesses and chronic fistulous tracts. Surgical excision of the involved duct, ampulla and, if present, fistulous tract, is the definitive treatment [85, 92].

The cytologic findings of SA on fine needle aspiration have been described in both women and men [93–98]. The findings are similar in all cases. Aspiration will yield purulent material. Smears are cellular due to the presence of numerous neutrophils and anucleated squamous cells. In addition, metaplastic squamous cells with nuclear atypia may be seen although these cells should not be numerous. The atypia seen in the squamous cells is most likely secondary to inflammatory atypia [93]. Other findings include granulation tissue, foreign-body giant cell reaction, lymphocytes and plasma cells, and groups of ductal epithelial cells with reactive atypia [93, 95] (Figs. 10.38, 10.39, 10.40 and 10.41).

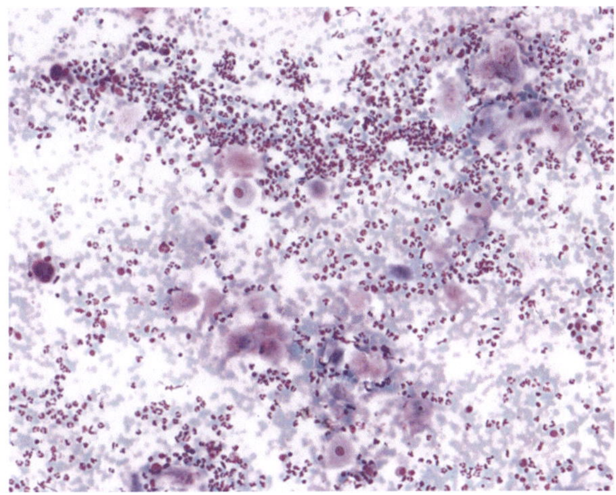

Fig. 10.38 Subareolar abscess. Squamous cells and acute inflammation (Diff Quik 10×)

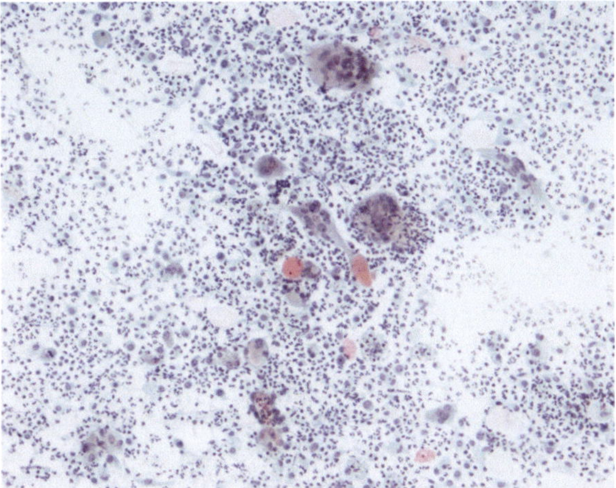

Fig. 10.39 Subareolar abscess. Squamous cells, multinucleate giant cells, and acute inflammation (Pap 10×)

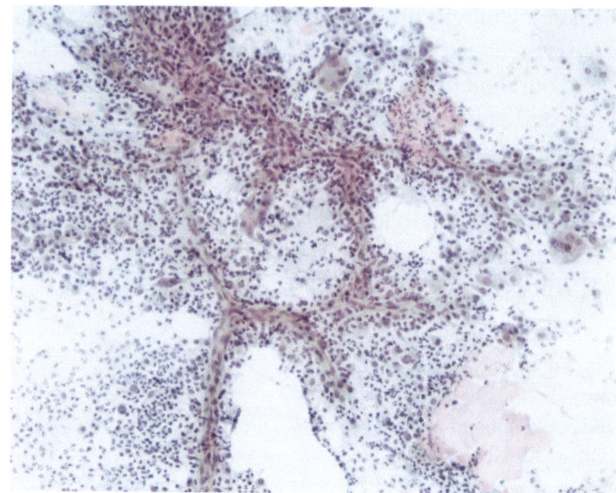

Fig. 10.40 Subareolar abscess. Granulation tissue and acute inflammation (Pap 10×)

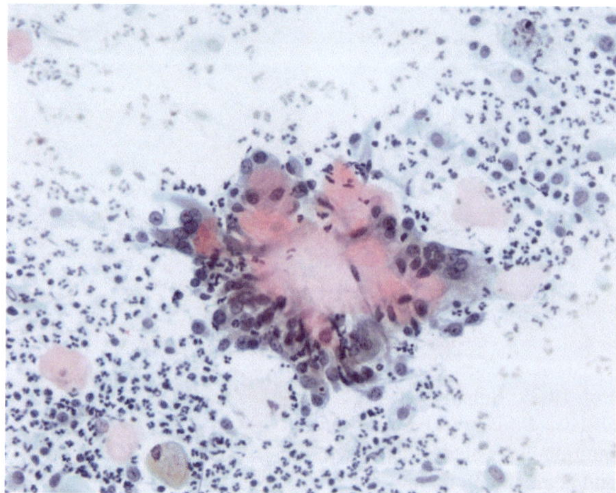

Fig. 10.41 Subareolar abscess. Keratin debris surrounded by multinucleate giant cells (Pap 20×)

Lactational Mastitis/Abscess

The most common setting of acute mastitis occurs in lactating women who are breastfeeding (lactational or puerperal mastitis) [99]. The incidence of lactational mastitis has been reported to be between 9 and 20% and most commonly occurs in the first 2–3 weeks post-partum [100, 101]. The etiology of lactational mastitis is thought to be secondary to stasis of milk within lactiferous ducts. This subsequently leads to increased pressure and leakage of milk into the surrounding breast parenchyma and an acute inflammatory reaction.

In addition, bacterial infections may play a role in the development of lactational mastitis. During nursing, bacteria from the mother's skin or the infant's oral cavity may enter the breast tissue via breaks in the skin of the nipple. The most common causative agent in cases of lactational mastitis is *Staphylococcus aureus* [102]. Other agents include Streptococcus and mixed anaerobic species [32]. Retrograde infection into the mammary ducts may be a cause of stagnation of breast milk. With persistent inflammation a localized cavity filled with necrotic cellular debris and marked acute inflammation (lactational abscess) may form. Lactational abscesses most commonly occur in the upper outer quadrant of the breast [103]. It has been estimated that less than 3% of women with lactational mastitis will develop an abscess [104]. Repeat aspiration with a large bore needle to drain the abscess or surgical incision and drainage along with antibiotic therapy is the standard treatment.

Inflammation of the breast tissue in lactating women leads to skin erythema, warmth, and tenderness in a localized area of the breast. Patients with an abscess present with a fluctuant breast mass. Systemic signs and symptoms may also be present, such as general malaise, increased peripheral blood neutrophil count and fever [99, 105]. Axillary lymphadenopathy may be present. The signs and symptoms of lactational mastitis and abscess may overlap with those of inflammatory breast carcinoma.

While lactational mastitis is usually diagnosed based on clinical findings, radiologic studies may also be performed, especially to exclude an underlying carcinoma. Ultrasound is the preferred modality to evaluate acute mastitis. Ultrasound findings include a well or ill-defined cystic mass representing an abscess, dilated subareolar ducts, or irregular hypoechoic areas [106]. Mammographic findings are non-specific and include focal or diffuse asymmetric density, an ill-defined mass, or an architectural distortion [107].

Aspirates of acute mastitis and breast abscesses show similar cytologic findings, and the distinction between the two entities is not possible on cytology. Aspirates grossly appear as yellow thick material consistent with purulent inflammation. Cytologically, the aspirates consist of abundant neutrophils and necrotic, cellular debris. With healing and organization, the smears may also show mononuclear cells consisting of macrophages, lymphocytes, and plasma cells although neutrophils still predominate [108, 109]. Granulation tissue may also be present during the latter stages of the disease (Figs. 10.42, 10.43 and 10.44).

Performing a Gram stain and submitting material for bacterial cultures should be performed whenever there is marked acute inflammation in a breast FNA. The results of the culture will help guide antibiotic treatment. Negative culture results, however, do exclude an infection [109].

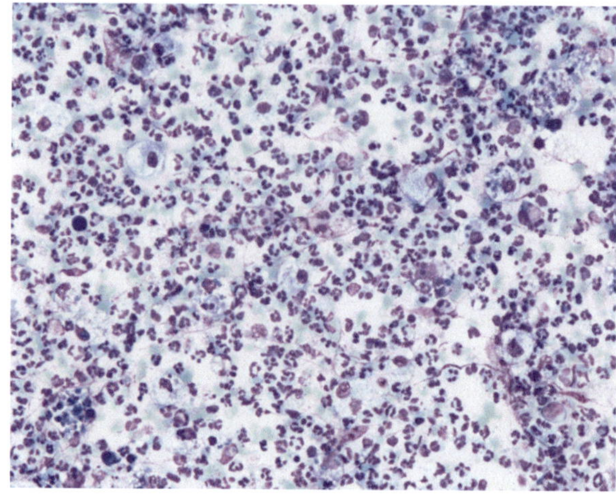

Fig. 10.42 Lactational mastitis. Marked acute inflammation and macrophages (Diff Quik 20×)

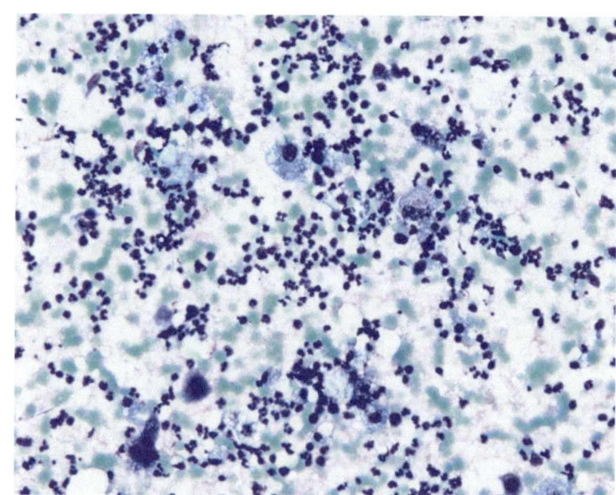

Fig. 10.43 Lactational mastitis. Marked acute inflammation and macrophages (Diff Quik 20×)

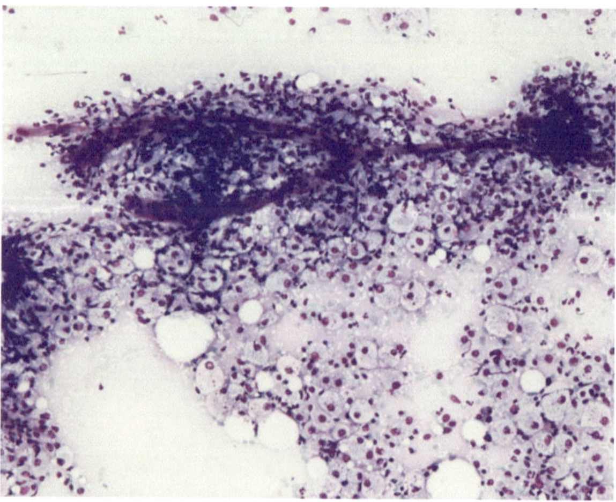

Fig. 10.44 Lactational mastitis. Acute inflammation, macrophages, and granulation tissue (Diff Quik 20×)

Idiopathic Granulomatous Mastitis

Idiopathic granulomatous mastitis, also known as idiopathic granulomatous lobular mastitis, is an inflammatory disorder of unknown etiology. Histologically, the process is centered around lobules and consists of non-caseating granulomas, microabscesses, multinucleated giant cells, lymphocytes, and plasma cells [110]. The granulomatous inflammation may be so severe that the lobulocentric distribution may not be obvious on histologic sections.

The disorder affects premenopausal women of childbearing age. Many patients have a history of pregnancy or breastfeeding within 5 years of the onset of the disease [111]. The most common presenting symptoms are a breast mass and breast pain although other signs and symptoms include breast edema and erythema, nipple retraction, nipple discharge, and draining sinus or fistula [112]. Axillary lymphadenopathy is present in up to 15% of patients [113]. These clinical findings may mimic inflammatory breast carcinoma. Imaging studies have non-specific findings and may also mimic carcinoma [114]. Ultrasound may show hypoechoic masses, tubular hypoechoic lesions, fistulae formations, or axillary lymphadenopathy [115]. Mammographic findings include a focal asymmetric density, diffuse increase in breast density and skin thickening [116]. Treatment remains controversial, with some patients undergoing surgery of the affected area of the breast while other patients are offered a course of corticosteroid therapy [112].

Aspiration biopsies are useful in demonstrating that the disease process is inflammatory, rather than neoplastic [117]. FNA samples show non-caseating granulomas, multinucleated giant cells, and a mixed inflammatory infiltrate [118, 119] (Figs. 10.45, 10.46, 10.47 and 10.48). The granulomas have the typical appearance of tightly cohesive clusters of epithelioid histiocytes with oval nuclei and abundant cytoplasm [120]. In some cases, neutrophils may be the most prominent inflammatory cell in the background of the smears, while in other cases a chronic

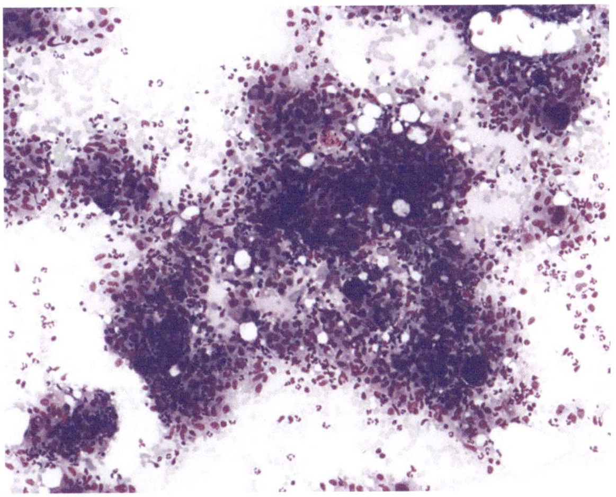

Fig. 10.45 Idiopathic granulomatous mastitis. Granulomas and acute inflammation. Necrosis is not identified (Diff Quik 10×)

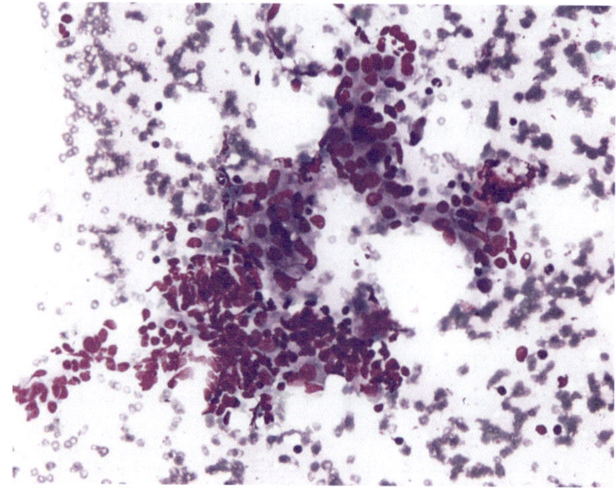

Fig. 10.46 Idiopathic granulomatous mastitis. Cluster of reactive ductal cells (upper right) and inflammatory cells (bottom left) (Diff Quik 20×)

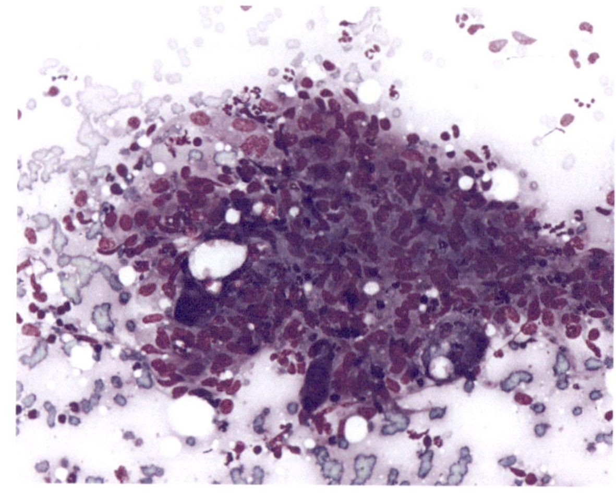

Fig. 10.47 Idiopathic granulomatous mastitis. Non-necrotizing granulomatous inflammation (Diff Quik 20×)

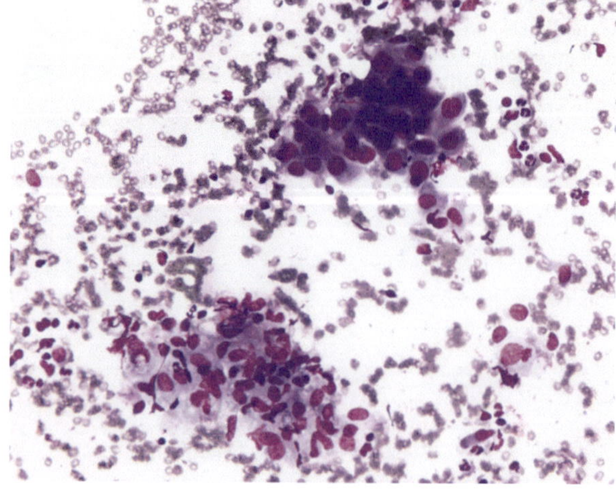

Fig. 10.48 Idiopathic granulomatous mastitis. Cluster of reactive ductal cells (upper) and a granuloma (bottom left) (Diff Quik 20×)

inflammatory infiltrate predominates [120]. With aspiration samples, the lobulocentric distribution of the granulomatous inflammation is not apparent. The cytologic findings are not specific for IGM and overlap with other causes of granulomatous inflammation, such as cystic neutrophilic granulomatous mastitis and granulomatous inflammation due to infectious organisms. Performing special stains, such as AFB and GMS, sending for cultures or performing PCR to detect mycobacteria should be done routinely to exclude infectious etiology. In addition, knowledge of prior trauma or surgical procedures to the breast or history of systemic or autoimmune disorders is required to exclude other causes of granulomatous inflammation [121].

In many parts of the world, the main differential diagnosis of IGM is tuberculous mastitis. Reports have shown that an important finding to differentiate the two disorders on aspiration specimens is the absence of caseous necrosis in IGM [122]. Aspirates of IGM have also been reported to contain abundant neutrophils [117].

Tuberculous Mastitis

Tuberculosis affecting the breast is very rare, accounting for 0.1% of overall breast lesions [123]. Even in parts of the world where tuberculosis is endemic and pulmonary infection rates are high, mammary tuberculosis account for 3% to 4.5% of breast lesions [124]. Breast tuberculosis may be primary when there is no evidence of infection outside the breast, or secondary when there is a known, preexisting lesion in an extra-mammary site [125]. Although breast tuberculosis has been reported in women in a wide age range, the disease typically affects women in child-bearing age [124, 126].

The clinical presentation is variable and may be mistaken as a carcinoma or other forms of mastitis [124]. Three clinical presentations have been described: nodular, disseminated, and sclerosing tuberculosis [127]. In nodular tuberculosis, patients present with a discrete palpable, circumscribed, or ill-defined breast mass associated with erythema and pain. Systemic symptoms may be present, including fever and weight loss. Disseminated tuberculosis occurs when multiple foci coalesce and the disease is more expensive in the breast. In sclerosing tuberculosis, there is diffuse fibrosis with little caseous necrosis [127].

Mammary tuberculosis may have various radiologic presentations [128]. A definitive diagnosis cannot be made on imaging studies, and tissue biopsy is required for a definitive diagnosis [129]. A discrete mass may be seen on mammogram and ultrasound in the nodular form of mammary tuberculosis. The mass may be circumscribed or irregular and be associated with calcifications [128].

FNA samples show epithelioid granulomas in a background of caseous necrosis [[122, 126, 130]) (Figs. 10.49, 10.50 and 10.51). Multinucleated giant cells, a mixed inflammatory infiltrate and granulation tissue may also be seen. In some cases, the only cytologic finding is necrosis. Benign or reactive ductal epithelial cells without evidence of atypia may also be aspirated [130]. Mycobacterial stains have a low

Fig. 10.49 Tuberculous mastitis. Granulomas in a background of necrosis (10× Diff Quik)

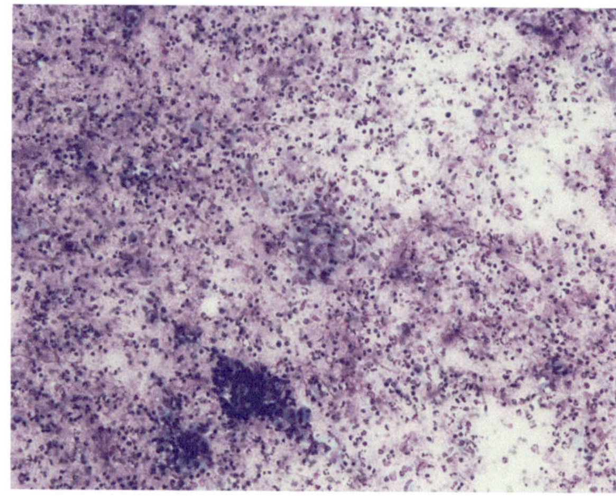

Fig. 10.50 Tuberculous mastitis. Granulomas in a background of necrosis (10× Diff Quik)

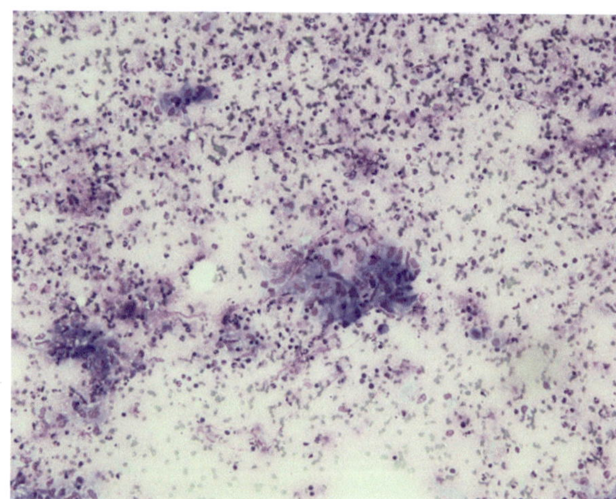

Fig. 10.51 Tuberculous mastitis. Granulomas in a background of necrosis (10× Diff Quik)

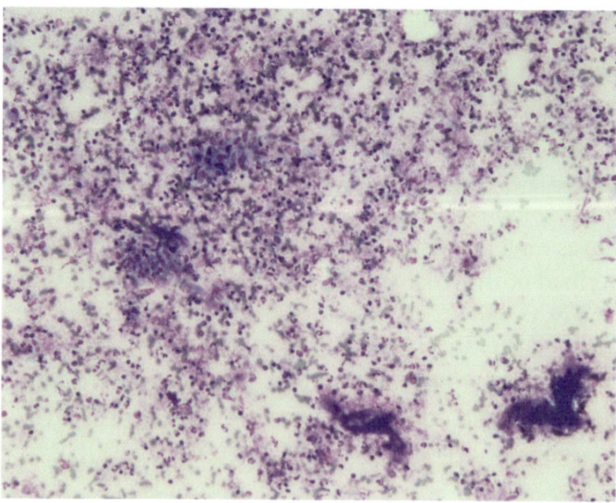

sensitivity for detecting AFB-positive organisms. The percentage of cases identifying acid fast bacilli on smears ranges from 0% to 38.6% [124]. The gold-standard for definitive diagnoses of tuberculous mastitis is mycobacterial culture although results may take up to 10 weeks [131].

The findings of caseous granulomatous inflammation on aspirate samples in areas where tuberculosis is endemic is suggestive of tuberculosis and anti-tuberculosis treatment is initiated as standard practice even if an AFB stain is negative and cultures are pending [131].

Other etiologies for granulomatous mastitis include foreign body reactions, sarcoidosis, fungal and parasitic infections, autoimmune disorders, and idiopathic granulomatous lobular mastitis [122].

Gynecomastia

Gynecomastia is a benign disorder resulting in an increased amount of glandular and stromal tissue of the male breast. The causes of gynecomastia are numerous, but the underlying physiology is an imbalance of the androgen-to-estrogen ratio [132, 133]). This imbalance may be physiologic or may be due to numerous secondary causes. Gynecomastia may occur in the absence of any underlying disorder in three distinct age groups: infancy, puberty, and in men older than 50 years of age. In many patients, gynecomastia is asymptomatic and found only as a subareolar mass on physical exam [134].

Gynecomastia occurring during infancy is transient and is due to the presence of residual maternal estrogen. Adolescent males may also develop self-limiting gynecomastia during puberty, when there is relatively more estrogen production by the testes and peripheral tissues [133]. With time, the amount of androgen production reaches adult levels and in most cases the symptoms of gynecomastia resolve. Persistent gynecomastia into late adolescence and early adulthood occurs in less than 5% of patients [133]. Older men may develop gynecomastia due to decreasing testosterone synthesis and peripheral conversion of androgen to estrogen [133]. It has been estimated that approximately 65% of men between 50 and 80 years of age will have some degree of gynecomastia [132]. In addition to these physiologic causes, there are numerous secondary etiologies of gynecomastia: use of certain medications, including digoxin, antihypertensives, antidepressants, and antiretroviral HIV medications; illicit-drug use; anabolic steroids; chronic illnesses, such as cirrhosis and renal insufficiency; genetic disorders; and primary hypogonadism [132–134]. In up to 25% of cases of gynecomastia, no cause is identified (idiopathic) [132].

Pseudogynecomastia is a disorder in which there an increased amount of adipose tissue in the subareolar region of the breast without an increase in glandular tissue [134]. Aspiration biopsies of pseudogynecomastia will yield fibroadipose tissue with very little or no epithelial cells.

Patients with gynecomastia typically present with a palpable mass behind the nipple/areola that may be unilateral or bilateral. Patients may also complain of pain associated with the mass. On physical exam, the characteristic finding is a rubbery or firm mass in the retroareolar region. Nipple retraction and skin changes are not seen with gynecomastia.

Three patterns of gynecomastia have been described on imaging studies. Early-stage gynecomastia produces a nodular appearance with a subareolar nodular or fan-shaped density on mammography that is hypoechoic on sonogram [135, 136]. Long-standing gynecomastia will show a dendritic pattern with a flame-shaped density radiating outward from the nipple [135, 136]. The dendritic projections represent fibrous tissue extending into the mammary parenchyma from the subareolar region. Gynecomastia associated with long-term exposure to exogenous estrogen will produce a diffuse pattern similar to dense female breast tissue [136].

Several studies indicate that breast FNAs in men constitute a small percentage of overall breast FNAs, approximately 1.5–4% of cases, and the vast majority of breast FNAs in males represent benign lesions, with gynecomastia being the most common diagnosis (Siddiqui 2022; [137, 138]). Gynecomastia is typically a clinical diagnosis, and the indication for fine needle aspiration is to exclude a malignancy and for patient reassurance [134]. FNA also decreases unnecessary surgical biopsies. The sensitivity of male breast FNA ranges from 95% to 100%, while the specificity ranges from 89% to 100% [10, 67, 137, 138].

Aspiration specimens of gynecomastia vary from scant cellularity to hypercellular aspirates depending on the stage of the gynecomastia. In the early, proliferative stage, FNA specimens will yield cellular aspirates with groups of epithelial cells admixed with myoepithelial cells. The groups may appear as flat, monolayered sheets, or have a papillary or cribriform appearance with punched out spaces (Siddiqui 2022). Some aspirates may show a fibroadenomatoid pattern, with large branching sheets of epithelial cells with a staghorn configuration, stromal fragments and bare oval nuclei, reminiscent of a fibroadenoma [67, 139]. Other findings in gynecomastia include apocrine cells, histiocytes, and columnar cells [140] (Figs. 10.52, 10.53, 10.54, 10.55 and 10.56).

While groups of ductal epithelial cells are typically tightly cohesive, some dissociation of epithelial cells may be present [137]. However, dissociated epithelial cells should not be prominent. There may also be epithelial cell atypia characterized by nuclear enlargement, nuclear hyperchromasia, prominent nucleoli, higher nuclear-to-cytoplasmic ratios, and nuclear overlapping. (Siddiqui 2022; [137, 140]). These atypical changes are prominent in the proliferative stage of gynecomastia, and the atypia may be more severe in patients on anabolic steroids or receiving chemotherapy or radiation therapy for non-mammary malignancies [140].

It is important to be aware of the florid proliferative nature of gynecomastia in the early stages and not to overinterpret these findings as atypical or as malignant. The presence of bare oval nuclei and the lack of numerous dissociated epithelial cells should prevent the overinterpretation of gynecomastia. The cytologic features of breast adenocarcinoma in men are similar to those in the female breast. Findings that would favor a diagnosis of adenocarcinoma include a predominant population

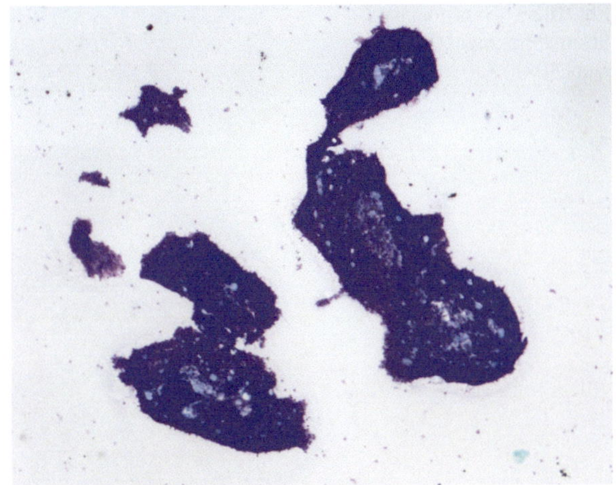

Fig. 10.52 Gynecomastia. Large, branching groups of ductal epithelium and myoepithelial cells. A stromal fragment is present on the left side of the image (Diff Quik 4×)

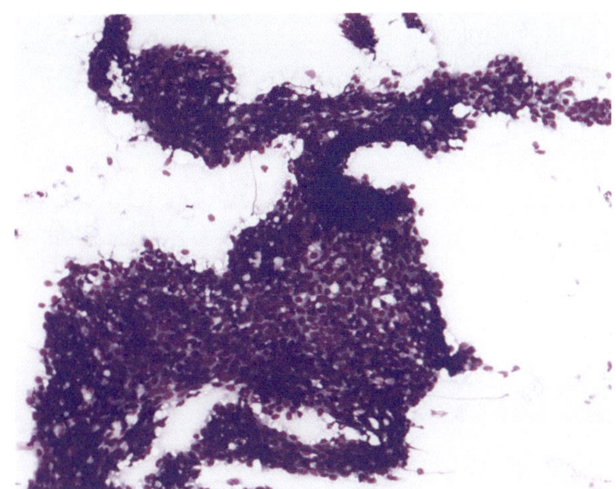

Fig. 10.53 Gynecomastia. Branching group of ductal epithelial cells (Diff Quik 10×)

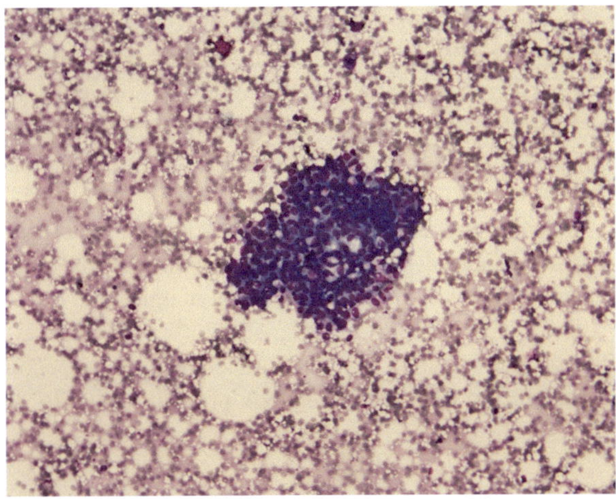

Fig. 10.54 Gynecomastia. Group of benign ductal epithelial cells and myoepithelial cells (Diff Quik 20×)

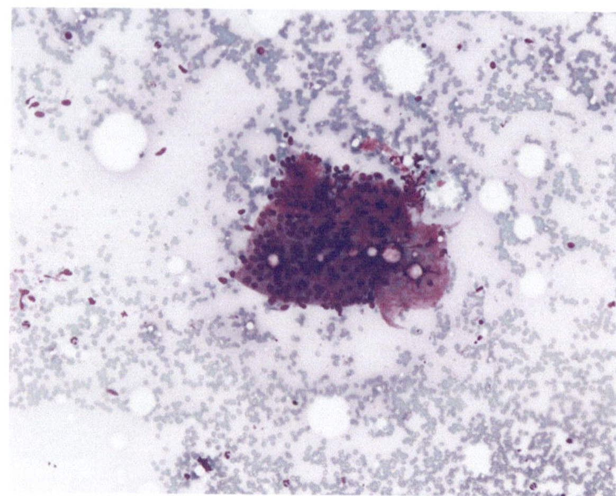

Fig. 10.55 Gynecomastia. Stromal fragment (Diff Quik 10×)

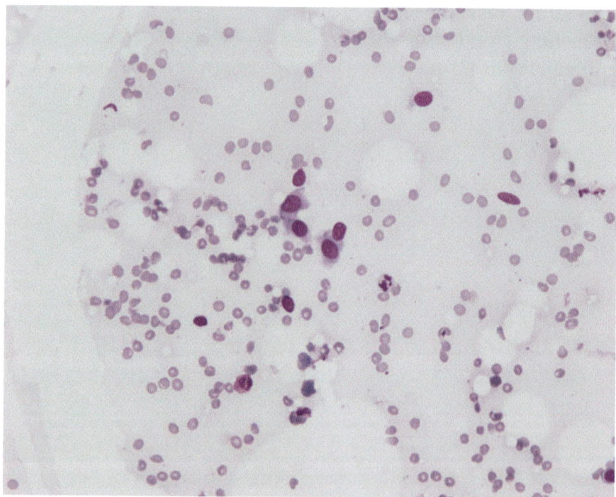

Fig. 10.56 Gynecomastia. Scant dissociated epithelial cells and bar oval nuclei (Diff Quik 20×)

of dissociated epithelial cells with marked nuclear pleomorphism and macronucleoli, intracytoplasmic mucin vacuoles, and absence of myoepithelial cells [141].

Breast tenderness as a result of gynecomastia is typically reported during the early, proliferative phase, and therefore, patients may report pain and discomfort, sometimes severe, during the FNA procedure. This may lead to under-sampling of the mass and to an unsatisfactory diagnosis [141].

Later in the course of gynecomastia, the proliferative changes abate and there will be increased stromal and periductal fibrosis. Aspirations during the inactive, fibrous phase will yield scant groups of epithelial cells and fibrous tissue.

Some studies report an unsatisfactory rate as high as 30%. This may be due to the fibrotic nature during the late or inactive phase gynecomastia or undersampling due to patient not tolerating the FNA procedure due to discomfort during the biopsy [141, 142].

References

Introduction

1. Frable WJ. Fine-needle aspiration biopsy: a review. Hum Pathol. 1983;14(1):9–28.
2. Mathews FS. Aspiration of breast cysts. Ann Surg. 1936;104(2):220–6.
3. Fornage BD, Faroux MJ, Simatos A. Breast masses: US-guided fine-needle aspiration biopsy. Radiology. 1987;162(2):409–14.
4. Tabbara SO, Frost AR, Stoler MH, Sneige N, Sidawy MK. Changing trends in breast fine-needle aspiration: results of the Papanicolaou Society of Cytopathology Survey. Diagn Cytopathol. 2000;22(2):126–30.
5. Li Z, Souers RJ, Tabbara SO, Natale KE, Nguyen LN, Booth CN. Breast fine-needle aspiration practice in 2019: results of a College of American Pathologists National Survey. Arch Pathol Lab Med. 2021;145(7):825–33.
6. Oyama T, Koibuchi Y, McKee G. Core needle biopsy (CNB) as a diagnostic method for breast lesions: comparison with fine needle aspiration cytology (FNA). Breast Cancer. 2004;11(4):339–42.
7. Simsir A, Rapkiewicz A, Cangiarella J. Current utilization of breast FNA in a cytology practice. Diagn Cytopathol. 2009;37(2):140–2.
8. Montezuma D, Malheiros D, Schmitt FC. Breast fine needle aspiration biopsy cytology using the newly proposed IAC Yokohama system for reporting breast cytopathology: the experience of a single institution. Acta Cytol. 2019;15:1–6.
9. Field AS, Raymond WA, Rickard M, Arnold L, Brachtel EF, Chaiwun B, Chen L, Di Bonito L, Kurtycz DFI, Lee AHS, Lim E, Ljung BM, Michelow P, Osamura RY, Pinamonti M, Sauer T, Segara D, Tse G, Vielh P, Chong PY, Schmitt F. The international academy of cytology Yokohama system for reporting breast fine-needle aspiration biopsy cytopathology. Acta Cytol. 2019;63(4):257–73.
10. Hoda RS, Brachtel EF. International academy of cytology Yokohama system for reporting breast fine-needle aspiration biopsy cytopathology: a review of predictive values and risks of malignancy. Acta Cytol. 2019;63(4):292–301. Field AS. Breast FNA biopsy cytology: current problems and the international academy of cytology Yokohama standardized reporting system. Cancer Cytopathol. 2017;125(4):229–30.
11. Field AS, Schmitt F, Vielh P. IAC standardized reporting of breast fine-needle aspiration biopsy cytology. Acta Cytol. 2017;61(1):3–6.
12. Wong S, Rickard M, Earls P, Arnold L, Bako B, Field AS. The international academy of cytology Yokohama system for reporting breast fine needle aspiration biopsy cytopathology: a single institutional retrospective study of the application of the system categories and the impact of rapid onsite evaluation. Acta Cytol. 2019;63(4):280–91.
13. Boler AK, Roy S, Chakraborty A, Bandyopadhyay A. Reproducibility of the "international academy of cytology Yokohama system for reporting breast cytology" - a retrospective analysis of 70 cases. J Cytol. 2022;39(4):159–62.
14. Chauhan V, Pujani M, Agarwal C, Chandoke RK, Raychaudhuri S, Singh K, Sharma N, Khandelwal A, Agarwal A. IAC standardized reporting of breast fine-needle aspiration cytology, Yokohama 2016: a critical appraisal over a 2 year period. Breast Dis. 2019;38(3–4):109–15.
15. Hoda RS, Arpin RN III, Gottumukkala RV, Hughes KS, Ly A, Brachtel EF. Diagnostic value of fine-needle aspiration in male breast lesions. Acta Cytol. 2019a;63(4):319–27.

Fibrocystic Change

16. Masood S. Cytomorphology of fibrocystic change, high-risk proliferative breast disease, and premalignant breast lesions. Clin Lab Med. 2005;25(4):713–31.
17. Hartmann LC, Sellers TA, Frost MH, Lingle WL, Degnim AC, Ghosh K, Vierkant RA, Maloney SD, Pankratz VS, Hillman DW, Suman VJ, Johnson J, Blake C, Tlsty T, Vachon CM, Melton LJ 3rd, Visscher DW. Benign breast disease and the risk of breast cancer. N Engl J Med. 2005;353(3):229–37.
18. Maygarden SJ, Novotny DB, Johnson DE, Frable WJ. Subclassification of benign breast disease by fine needle aspiration cytology. Comparison of cytologic and histologic findings in 265 palpable breast masses. Acta Cytol. 1994;38(2):115–29.
19. Sidawy MK, Tabbara SO, Bryan JA, Poprocky LA, Frost AR. The spectrum of cytologic features in nonproliferative breast lesions. Cancer. 2001;93(2):140–5.
20. Pattari SK, Dey P, Gupta SK, Joshi K. Myoepithelial cells: any role in aspiration cytology smears of breast tumors? Cytojournal. 2008;5:9.
21. Thomas PA, Cangiarella J, Raab SS, Waisman J. Fine needle aspiration biopsy of proliferative breast disease. Mod Pathol. 1995;8(2):130–6.
22. Vetto JT, Pommier RF, Shih RL, Campagna J, Robbins D, Schmidt WA. Breast fine-needle aspirates with scant cellularity are clinically useful. Am J Surg. 2005;189(5):621–5.
23. Zemba-Palko V, Klenn PJ, Saminathan T, Kline TS. Benign breast aspirates: two decades of experience. Arch Pathol Lab Med. 1996;120(11):1056–60.
24. Ventura K, Cangiarella J, Lee I, Moreira A, Waisman J, Simsir A. Aspiration biopsy of mammary lesions with abundant extracellular mucinous material. Review of 43 cases with surgical follow-up. Am J Clin Pathol. 2003;120(2):194–202.
25. Nayar R, De Frias DV, Bourtsos EP, Sutton V, Bedrossian C. Cytologic differential diagnosis of papillary pattern in breast aspirates: correlation with histology. Ann Diagn Pathol. 2001;5(1):34–42.
26. Simsir A, Waisman J, Thorner K, Cangiarella J. Mammary lesions diagnosed as "papillary" by aspiration biopsy: 70 cases with follow-up. Cancer. 2003;99(3):156–65.
27. Cho EY, Oh YL. Fine needle aspiration cytology of sclerosing adenosis of the breast. Acta Cytol. 2001;45(3):353–9.
28. Sreedharanunni S, Das A, Veenu S, Srinivasan R, Singh G. Nodular sclerosing adenosis of breast: a diagnostic pitfall in fine needle aspiration cytology. J Cytol. 2013;30(1):49–51.
29. Lamb J, McGoogan E. Fine needle aspiration cytology of breast in invasive carcinoma of tubular type and in radial scar/complex sclerosing lesions. Cytopathology. 1994;5(1):17–26.
30. Lim JC, Al-Masri H, Salhadar A, Xie HB, Gabram S, Wojcik EM. The significance of the diagnosis of atypia in breast fine-needle aspiration. Diagn Cytopathol. 2004;31(5):285–8.
31. Mulford DK, Dawson AE. Atypia in fine needle aspiration cytology of nonpalpable and palpable mammographically detected breast lesions. Acta Cytol. 1994;38(1):9–17.

Pregnancy-Related Changes

32. Levine PH, Cangiarella J. Cytomorphology of benign breast disease. Clin Lab Med. 2005a;25(4):689–712.
33. Rovera F, Frattini F, Coglitore A, Marelli M, Rausei S, Dionigi G, Boni L, Dionigi R. Breast cancer in pregnancy. Breast J. 2010;16(Suppl 1):S22–5.
34. Vuolo M, Suhrland MJ, Madan R, Oktay MH. Discrepant cytologic and radiographic findings in adjacent galactocele and fibroadenoma: a case report. Acta Cytol. 2009;53(2):211–4.

35. Whang IY, Lee J, Kim KT. Galactocele as a changing axillary lump in a pregnant woman. Arch Gynecol Obstet. 2007;276(4):379–82.
36. Son EJ, Oh KK, Kim EK. Pregnancy-associated breast disease: radiologic features and diagnostic dilemmas. Yonsei Med J. 2006;47(1):34–42.
37. Haliloglu N, Ustuner E, Ozkavukcu E. Breast ultrasound during lactation: benign and malignant lesions. Breast Care (Basel). 2019;14(1):30–4.
38. Langer A, Mohallem M, Berment H, Ferreira F, Gog A, Khalifa D, Nekka I, Chérel P. Breast lumps in pregnant women. Diagn Interv Imaging. 2015;96(10):1077–87.
39. Lee SE, Bae YK. Breast lesions during pregnancy and lactation: a pictorial essay. Ultrasonography. 2020;39(3):298–310.
40. Kieturakis AJ, Wahab RA, Vijapura C, Mahoney MC. Current recommendations for breast imaging of the pregnant and lactating patient. AJR Am J Roentgenol. 2021;216(6):1462–75.
41. Novotny DB, Maygarden SJ, Shermer RW, Frable WJ. Fine needle aspiration of benign and malignant breast masses associated with pregnancy. Acta Cytol. 1991;35(6):676–86.
42. Varshney B, Bharti JN, Saha S, Sharma N. Crystallising galactocele of the breast: a rare cytological diagnosis. BMJ Case Rep. 2021;14(5):e242888.
43. Umasankar P, Lakshmi Priya U, Sideeque A. Crystallizing Galactocele: a rare entity-report of two cases. Diagn Cytopathol. 2018;46(10):873–5.
44. Zaman S, Gupta R, Gupta S. Crystallizing galactocele of the breast masquerading as a malignancy: report of a rare case with cytological diagnosis. Diagn Cytopathol. 2022;50(8):E236–9.
45. Volckmar AL, Leichsenring J, Flechtenmacher C, Pfarr N, Siebolts U, Kirchner M, Budczies J, Bockmayr M, Ridinger K, Lorenz K, Herpel E, Noske A, Weichert W, Klauschen F, Schirmacher P, Penzel R, Endris V, Stenzinger A. Tubular, lactating, and ductal adenomas are devoid of MED12 Exon2 mutations, and ductal adenomas show recurrent mutations in GNAS and the PI3K-AKT pathway. Genes Chromosom Cancer. 2017;56(1):11–7.
46. Chico MJ, Causa Andrieu PI, Wernicke A, Pesce K. Breast lactating adenoma, an example of the utility of the radiological-pathological correlation. Clin Imaging. 2021;71:136–40.
47. Sumkin JH, Perrone AM, Harris KM, Nath ME, Amortegui AJ, Weinstein BJ. Lactating adenoma: US features and literature review. Radiology. 1998;206(1):271–4.

Mammary Duct Ectasia

48. Javadzadeh B, Finley J, Williams HJ. Fine needle aspiration cytology of mammary duct ectasia: report of a case with novel cytologic and immunocytochemical findings. Acta Cytol. 2001;45(6):1027–31.
49. D'Alfonso TM, Ginter PS, Shin SJ. A review of inflammatory processes of the breast with a focus on diagnosis in Core biopsy samples. J Pathol Transl Med. 2015;49(4):279–87.
50. Dillon DA, Lester SC. Lesions of the nipple. Surg Pathol Clin. 2009;2(2):391–412.
51. Moon S, Lim HS, Ki SY. Ultrasound findings of mammary duct ectasia causing bloody nipple discharge in infancy and childhood. J Ultrasound Med. 2019;38(10):2793–8.
52. Chan KW, Lau WY. Duct ectasia in the male breast. Aust N Z J Surg. 1984;54(2):173–6.
53. Hari S, Kumar J, Kumar A, Chumber S. Bilateral severe mammary duct ectasia. Acta Radiol. 2007;48(4):398–400.
54. Lippa N, Hurtevent-Labrot G, Ferron S, Boisserie-Lacroix M. Nipple discharge: the role of imaging. Diagn Interv Imaging. 2015;96(10):1017–32.
55. Samreen N, Madsen LB, Chacko C, Heller SL. Magnetic resonance imaging in the evaluation of pathologic nipple discharge: indications and imaging findings. Br J Radiol. 2021;94(1120):20201013.
56. Ng WK, Kong JH. Significance of squamous cells in fine needle aspiration cytology of the breast. A review of cases in a seven-year period. Acta Cytol. 2003;47(1):27–35.

Fat Necrosis

57. Aqel NM, Howard A, Collier DS. Fat necrosis of the breast: a cytological and clinical study. Breast. 2001;10(4):342–5.
58. Tan PH, Lai LM, Carrington EV, Opaluwa AS, Ravikumar KH, Chetty N, Kaplan V, Kelley CJ, Babu ED. Fat necrosis of the breast--a review. Breast. 2006;15(3):313–8.
59. Pullyblank AM, Davies JD, Basten J, Rayter Z. Fat necrosis of the female breast--Hadfield re-visited. Breast. 2001;10(5):388–91.
60. Agnihotri MA, Kothari KS, Naik LP. Fat necrosis of the breast masquerading as malignancy diagnosed on fine-needle aspiration cytology. J Midlife Health. 2020;11(1):49–50.
61. Nakada H, Inoue M, Furuya K, Watanabe H, Ikegame K, Nakayama Y, Ohmori M, Nakagomi H. Fat necrosis after breast-conserving oncoplastic surgery. Breast Cancer. 2019;26(1):125–30.
62. Saidian L, Lee SJ, Hodges KB, Mahoney MC. Coronary artery bypass graft: an often overlooked cause of breast fat necrosis. Breast J. 2019;25(6):1282–3.
63. Horne CG, Breiner M. Fat necrosis of the breast after coronary artery bypass grafting presenting similarly to inflammatory breast cancer. Cureus. 2022;14(7):e26524.
64. AlQattan AS, Ghulam WZ, Aldaoud N, Algheryafi L, Aleisa N, Aldulaijan FA. Breast fat necrosis secondary to warfarin-induced calciphylaxis, a rare mimicker of breast cancer: a case report and a review of literature. Breast J. 2021;27(3):258–63.
65. Villeirs G, Van Damme S, Heydanus R, Serreyn R, Kunnen M, Mortier M. Heparin-induced thrombocytopenia and fat necrosis of the breast. Eur Radiol. 2000;10(3):527–30.
66. Akyol M, Kayali A, Yildirim N. Traumatic fat necrosis of male breast. Clin Imaging. 2013;37(5):954–6.
67. Siddiqui MT, Zakowski MF, Ashfaq R, Ali SZ. Breast masses in males: multi-institutional experience on fine-needle aspiration. Diagn Cytopathol. 2002a;26(2):87–91.
68. Kerridge WD, Kryvenko ON, Thompson A, Shah BA. Fat necrosis of the breast: a pictorial review of the mammographic, ultrasound, CT, and MRI findings with histopathologic correlation. Radiol Res Pract. 2015;2015:613139.
69. Taboada JL, Stephens TW, Krishnamurthy S, Brandt KR, Whitman GJ. The many faces of fat necrosis in the breast. Am J Roentgenol. 2009;192(3):815–25.
70. Tayyab SJ, Adrada BE, Rauch GM, Yang WT. A pictorial review: multimodality imaging of benign and suspicious features of fat necrosis in the breast. Br J Radiol. 2018;91:20180213.
71. Adejolu M, Huo L, Rohren E, Santiago L, Yang WT. False-positive lesions mimicking breast cancer on FDG PET and PET/CT. Am J Roentgenol. 2012a;198(3):W304.
72. Shabb N, Sneige N, Dekmezian RH. Myospherulosis. Fine needle aspiration cytologic findings in 19 cases. Acta Cytol. 1991;35(2):225–8.
73. Gerhard R, Schmitt FC. Liquid-based cytology in fine-needle aspiration of breast lesions: a review. Acta Cytol. 2014;58(6):533–42.

Silicone Granuloma

74. Majedah S, Alhabshi I, Salim S. Granulomatous reaction secondary to intramammary silicone injection. BMJ Case Rep. 2013;2013:bcr2012007961.
75. Chen TH. Silicone injection granulomas of the breast: treatment by subcutaneous mastectomy and immediate subpectoral breast implant. Br J Plast Surg. 1995;48(2):71–6.
76. van Diest PJ, Beekman WH, Hage JJ. Pathology of silicone leakage from breast implants. J Clin Pathol. 1998;51(7):493–7.
77. Dodd LG, Sneige N, Reece GP, Fornage B. Fine-needle aspiration cytology of silicone granulomas in the augmented breast. Diagn Cytopathol. 1993;9(5):498–502.

78. Mitnick JS, Vazquez MF, Plesser K, Pressman P, Harris MN, Roses DF. Fine needle aspiration biopsy in patients with augmentation prostheses and a palpable mass. Ann Plast Surg. 1993;31(3):241–4.
79. Samreen N, Glazebrook KN, Bhatt A, Venkatesh SK, McMenomy BP, Chandra A, Leng S, Adler KE, McCollough CH. Imaging findings of mammary and systemic silicone deposition secondary to breast implants. Br J Radiol. 2018;91(1089):20180098.
80. Tabatowski K, Elson CE, Johnston WW. Silicone lymphadenopathy in a patient with a mammary prosthesis. Fine needle aspiration cytology, histology and analytical electron microscopy. Acta Cytol. 1990;34(1):10–4.
81. Borghol K, Gallagher G, Skelly BL. Silicone granuloma from ruptured breast implants as a cause of cervical lymphadenopathy. Ann R Coll Surg Engl. 2016;98(7):e118–20.
82. Dragu A, Theegarten D, Bach AD, Polykandriotis E, Arkudas A, Kneser U, Horch RE, Ingianni G. Intrapulmonary and cutaneous siliconomas after silent silicone breast implant failure. Breast J. 2009;15(5):496–9.

Subareolar Abscess

83. Zuska JJ, Crile G Jr, Ayres WW. Fistulas of lactiferous ducts. Am J Surg. 1951;81(3):312–7.
84. Snider HC. Management of Mastitis, abscess, and fistula. Surg Clin North Am. 2022;102(6):1103–16.
85. Meguid MM, Oler A, Numann PJ, Khan S. Pathogenesis-based treatment of recurring subareolar breast abscesses. Surgery. 1995;118(4):775–82.
86. Johnson SP, Kaoutzanis C, Schaub GA. Male Zuska's disease. BMJ Case Rep. 2014;2014:bcr2013201922.
87. Lo G, Dessauvagie B, Sterrett G, Bourke AG. Squamous metaplasia of lactiferous ducts (SMOLD). Clin Radiol. 2012;67(11):e42–6.
88. Ofri A, Dona E, O'Toole S. Squamous metaplasia of lactiferous ducts (SMOLD): an under-recognised entity. BMJ Case Rep. 2020;13(12):e237568.
89. Giess CS, Golshan M, Flaherty K, Birdwell RL. Clinical experience with aspiration of breast abscesses based on size and etiology at an academic medical center. J Clin Ultrasound. 2014;42(9):513–21.
90. Versluijs-Ossewaarde FN, Roumen RM, Goris RJ. Subareolar breast abscesses: characteristics and results of surgical treatment. Breast J. 2005;11(3):179–82.
91. Kasales CJ, Han B, Smith JS Jr, Chetlen AL, Kaneda HJ, Shereef S. Nonpuerperal mastitis and subareolar abscess of the breast. AJR Am J Roentgenol. 2014;202(2):W133–9.
92. Li S, Grant CS, Degnim A, Donohue J. Surgical management of recurrent subareolar breast abscesses: Mayo Clinic experience. Am J Surg. 2006;192(4):528–9.
93. Silverman JF, Raso DS, Elsheikh TM, Lannin D. Fine-needle aspiration cytology of a subareolar abscess of the male breast. Diagn Cytopathol. 1998;18(6):441–4.
94. Silverman JF, Lannin DR, Unverferth M, Norris HT. Fine needle aspiration cytology of subareolar abscess of the breast. Spectrum of cytomorphologic findings and potential diagnostic pitfalls. Acta Cytol. 1986;30(4):413–9.
95. Galblum LI, Oertel YC. Subareolar abscess of the breast: diagnosis by fine-needle aspiration. Am J Clin Pathol. 1983;80(4):496–9.
96. Subramaniam MM, En NM. Subareolar abscess in a male breast: cytological characterisation and distinction from other benign and malignant squamous cell aspirate. Pathology. 2012;44(5):472–4.
97. Rajaram ST, Kini H, Rau AR, Pai RR. Subareolar abscess in the male breast. Diagn Cytopathol. 2008;36(10):766–7.
98. López-Ríos F, Dhimes P, de Agustín PP. Subareolar abscess of the breast in a male. A report of two cases with fine needle aspiration cytology diagnosis. Acta Cytol. 1997;41(6):1819–22.

Lactational Mastitis/Abscess

 99. Cheng L, Reddy V, Solmos G, Watkins L, Cimbaluk D, Bitterman P, Ghai R, Gattuso P. Mastitis, a radiographic, clinical, and histopathologic review. Breast J. 2015;21(4):403–9.
100. Spencer JP. Management of mastitis in breastfeeding women. Am Fam Physician. 2008;78(6):727–31.
101. Berens PD. Breast pain: engorgement, nipple pain, and mastitis. Clin Obstet Gynecol. 2015;58(4):902–14.
102. Marchant DJ. Inflammation of the breast. Obstet Gynecol Clin N Am. 2002;29(1):89–102.
103. Eryilmaz R, Sahin M, Hakan Tekelioglu M, Daldal E. Management of lactational breast abscesses. Breast. 2005;14(5):375–9.
104. Lukassek J, Ignatov A, Faerber J, Costa SD, Eggemann H. Puerperal mastitis in the past decade: results of a single institution analysis. Arch Gynecol Obstet. 2019;300(6):1637–44.
105. Dahlbeck SW, Donnelly JF, Theriault RL. Differentiating inflammatory breast cancer from acute mastitis. Am Fam Physician. 1995;52(3):929–34.
106. Hayes R, Michell M, Nunnerley HB. Acute inflammation of the breast--the role of breast ultrasound in diagnosis and management. Clin Radiol. 1991;44(4):253–6.
107. Tan H, Li R, Peng W, Liu H, Gu Y, Shen X. Radiological and clinical features of adult non-puerperal mastitis. Br J Radiol. 2013;86(1024):20120657.
108. Das DK, Sodhani P, Kashyap V, Parkash S, Pant JN, Bhatnagar P. Inflammatory lesions of the breast: diagnosis by fine needle aspiration. Cytopathology. 1992;3(5):281–9.
109. Nemenqani D, Yaqoob N. Fine needle aspiration cytology of inflammatory breast lesions. J Pak Med Assoc. 2009;59(3):167–70.

Idiopathic Granulomatous Mastitis

110. Nguyen MH, Molland JG, Kennedy S, Gray TJ, Limaye S. Idiopathic granulomatous mastitis: case series and clinical review. Intern Med J. 2021;51(11):1791–7.
111. Benson JR, Dumitru D. Idiopathic granulomatous mastitis: presentation, investigation and management. Future Oncol. 2016;12(11):1381–94.
112. Martinez-Ramos D, Simon-Monterde L, Suelves-Piqueres C, Queralt-Martin R, Granel-Villach L, Laguna-Sastre JM, Nicolau MJ, Escrig-Sos J. Idiopathic granulomatous mastitis: a systematic review of 3060 patients. Breast J. 2019;25(6):1245–50.
113. Wolfrum A, Kümmel S, Theuerkauf I, Pelz E, Reinisch M. Granulomatous mastitis: a therapeutic and diagnostic challenge. Breast Care (Basel). 2018;13(6):413–8.
114. Fazzio RT, Shah SS, Sandhu NP, Glazebrook KN. Idiopathic granulomatous mastitis: imaging update and review. Insights Imaging. 2016;7(4):531–9.
115. Maione C, Palumbo VD, Maffongelli A, Damiano G, Buscemi S, Spinelli G, Fazzotta S, Gulotta E, Buscemi G, Lo Monte AI. Diagnostic techniques and multidisciplinary approach in idiopathic granulomatous mastitis: a revision of the literature. Acta Biomed. 2019;90(1):11–5.
116. Sripathi S, Ayachit A, Bala A, Kadavigere R, Kumar S. Idiopathic granulomatous mastitis: a diagnostic dilemma for the breast radiologist. Insights Imaging. 2016;7(4):523–9.
117. Helal TE, Shash LS, Saad El-Din SA, Saber SM. Idiopathic granulomatous mastitis: Cytologic and histologic study of 65 Egyptian patients. Acta Cytol. 2016;60(5):438–44.
118. Yip CH, Jayaram G, Swain M. The value of cytology in granulomatous mastitis: a report of 16 cases from Malaysia. Aust N Z J Surg. 2000;70(2):103–5.
119. Almobarak AO, Siddig SB, Hassan A, Ahmed MH. Diagnosis of idiopathic granulomatous mastitis in a Sudanese woman. J Microsc Ultrastruct. 2021;10(1):33–5.

120. Gangopadhyay M, De A, Chakrabarti I, Ray S, Giri A, Das R. Idiopathic granulomatous mastitis-utility of fine needle aspiration cytology (FNAC) in preventing unnecessary surgery. J Turk Ger Gynecol Assoc. 2010;11(3):127–30.
121. Kaur AC, Dal H, Müezzinoğlu B, Paksoy N. Idiopathic granulomatous mastitis. Report of a case diagnosed with fine needle aspiration cytology. Acta Cytol. 1999;43(3):481–4.
122. Chandanwale S, Naragude P, Shetty A, Sawadkar M, Raj A, Bhide A, Singh M. Cytomorphological Spectrum of granulomatous mastitis: a study of 33 cases. Eur J Breast Health. 2020a;16(2):146–51.

Tuberculous Mastitis

123. Prathima S, Kalyani R, Parimala S. Primary tubercular mastitis masquerading as malignancy. J Nat Sci Biol Med. 2014;5(1):184–6.
124. Chandanwale SS, Ravishankar R, Garg AA, Ambekar MR. Image-guided fine-needle aspiration cytology or core biopsy - a key to definitive diagnosis of tuberculous mastitis. Int J Mycobacteriol. 2022;11(3):323–5.
125. Sinha RTK, Dey A, Agarwal S. Tuberculous mastitis diagnosed on cytology - case report of a rare entity. J Cytol. 2017;34(3):162–4.
126. Ail DA, Bhayekar P, Joshi A, Pandya N, Nasare A, Lengare P, Narkhede KA. Clinical and cytological Spectrum of granulomatous mastitis and utility of FNAC in picking up tubercular mastitis: an eight-year study. J Clin Diagn Res. 2017;11(3):EC45–9.
127. Shinde SR, Chandawarkar RY, Deshmukh SP. Tuberculosis of the breast masquerading as carcinoma: a study of 100 patients. World J Surg. 1995;19(3):379–81.
128. Sakr AA, Fawzy RK, Fadaly G, Baky MA. Mammographic and sonographic features of tuberculous mastitis. Eur J Radiol. 2004;51(1):54–60.
129. Longman CF, Campion T, Butler B, Suaris TD, Khanam A, Kunst H, Tiberi S, O'Keeffe SA. Imaging features and diagnosis of tuberculosis of the breast. Clin Radiol. 2017;72(3):217–22.
130. Gupta D, Rajwanshi A, Gupta SK, Nijhawan R, Saran RK, Singh R. Fine needle aspiration cytology in the diagnosis of tuberculous mastitis. Acta Cytol. 1999;43(2):191–4.
131. Narayana Reddy RA, Narayana SM, Shariff S. Role of fine-needle aspiration cytology and fluid cytology in extra-pulmonary tuberculosis. Diagn Cytopathol. 2013;41(5):392–8.

Gynecomastia

132. Dickson G. Gynecomastia. Am Fam Physician. 2012;85(7):716–22.
133. Braunstein GD. Clinical practice. Gynecomastia N Engl J Med. 2007;357(12):1229–37.
134. Johnson RE, Murad MH. Gynecomastia: pathophysiology, evaluation, and management. Mayo Clin Proc. 2009;84(11):1010–5.
135. Chau A, Jafarian N, Rosa M. Male breast: clinical and imaging evaluations of benign and malignant entities with histologic correlation. Am J Med. 2016;129(8):776–91.
136. Billa E, Kanakis GA, Goulis DG. Imaging in gynecomastia. Andrology. 2021;9(5):1444–56.
137. Singh R, Anshu SSM, Gangane N. Spectrum of male breast lesions diagnosed by fine needle aspiration cytology: a 5-year experience at a tertiary care rural hospital in Central India. Diagn Cytopathol. 2012;40(2):113–7.
138. Wauters CA, Kooistra BW, de Kievit-van der Heijden IM, Strobbe LJ. Is cytology useful in the diagnostic workup of male breast lesions? A retrospective study over a 16-year period and review of the recent literature. Acta Cytol. 2010;54(3):259–64.

139. Kapila K, Verma K. Cytomorphological spectrum in gynaecomastia: a study of 389 cases. Cytopathology. 2002;13(5):300–8.
140. Amrikachi M, Green LK, Rone R, Ramzy I. Gynecomastia: cytologic features and diagnostic pitfalls in fine needle aspirates. Acta Cytol. 2001;45(6):948–52.
141. Rosa M, Masood S. Cytomorphology of male breast lesions: diagnostic pitfalls and clinical implications. Diagn Cytopathol. 2012;40(2):179–84.
142. MacIntosh RF, Merrimen JL, Barnes PJ. Application of the probabilistic approach to reporting breast fine needle aspiration in males. Acta Cytol. 2008;52(5):530–4.

Chapter 11
Respiratory Tract

Ruhani Sardana and Guoping Cai

Anatomy and Histology of the Low Respiratory System

The lower respiratory tract consists of the larynx, trachea, bronchi, and bronchioalveolar structures. The upper portion of larynx is lined by non-keratinizing squamous epithelium while the lower larynx, trachea, and bronchi are lined by respiratory epithelium. The respiratory epithelium is characteristically pseudostratified, ciliated columnar with admixed goblet cells (Fig. 11.1). Located at the base of the respiratory epithelium are basal or reserved cells. Mucinous and seromucinous glands are present in the subepithelial soft tissue of the tracheal and bronchial wall.

The lung parenchyma is primarily composed of roughly spherical thin-walled alveolar tissue, which is the functional unit of the lung (Fig. 11.2). It is lined by two types of epithelial cells—type I pneumocytes and type II pneumocytes. Type I cells are metabolically inactive, flattened, and with extremely attenuated cytoplasm surfacing approximately 90% of the alveolar wall. Type II cells are plump, cuboidal, and are capable of proliferation especially during chronic inflammation [1]. They synthesize alveolar surfactant that lines the inner alveolar surface to lower the surface tension and prevent pulmonary collapse.

R. Sardana · G. Cai (✉)
Department of Pathology, Yale School of Medicine, New Haven, CT, USA
e-mail: ruhani.sardana@yale.edu; guoping.cai@yale.edu

S. M. Gilani, G. Cai (eds.), *Non-Neoplastic Cytology*,
https://doi.org/10.1007/978-3-031-44289-6_11

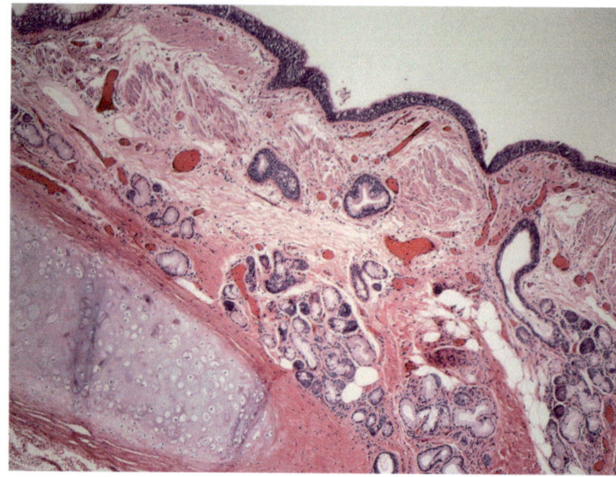

Fig. 11.1 Bronchial wall showing respiratory epithelial lining with subepithelial seromucinous glands (Hematoxylin-eosin stain)

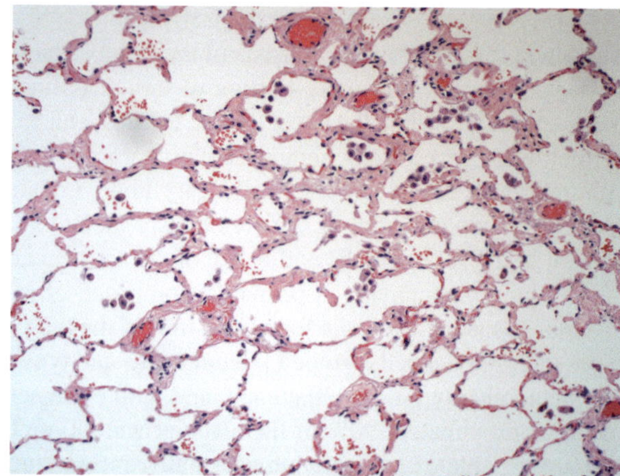

Fig. 11.2 Lung parenchyma showing thin alveolar septa with scattered intra-alveolar macrophages (Hematoxylin-eosin stain)

Specimen Types

The specimens from lower respiratory tract include sputum, bronchial brush, bronchial wash, bronchioalveolar lavage, and fine needle aspiration (Table 11.1).

Sputum

The simplest modality for studying respiratory tract pathology is collection of spontaneously or artificially produced sputum specimen. Patient should be instructed to follow certain precautions like clearing nasal passage and rinsing mouth before

Table 11.1 Sampling techniques for respiratory system disorders

	Method	Adequacy	Advantage	Disadvantage
Sputum	Expectorated spontaneously or induced	Presence of alveolar macrophages	Simple and low cost	Low sensitivity, oral contaminant may mask the findings
Bronchial brush	Direct sampling of bronchial abnormalities under bronchoscope	Whether the findings can explain the lesion of interest. Clinical correlation is required	Relatively simple. Can be combined with biopsy under bronchoscope	Difficult to differentiate reactive changes from dysplastic process and invasive tumor
Bronchial wash	Aspiration of washed saline through bronchoscope	Whether the findings can explain the lesion of interest. Clinical correlation is required	Detect both tumor and infectious lesions from relatively smaller area of lung tissue	Low sensitivity
Bronchioalveolar lavage	Aspiration of large volume of instilled saline through bronchoscope	Presence of alveolar macrophages	Detect mostly infectious lesions from larger area of lung tissue	Low sensitivity for identifying infectious agents
Fine needle aspiration	Direct sampling of the lesion under bronchoscopy or CT-guidance	Whether the findings can explain the lesion of interest. Clinical correlation is required	Direct sampling of the lesion helps to uncover the underlying etiologies	Sampling adequacy is a limiting factor. Rapid on-site evaluation may help improve diagnostic yield Cautious for contaminants such as bronchial cells and mesothelial cells

collecting the specimen, expelling directly into a wide mouth container with fixative and storing in the refrigerator. However, sometimes due to lack of instructions or other constraining factors the material expectorated might not be of diagnostic significance and consist entirely of mouth contents or saliva. Other drawbacks of the modality include contamination from mouth or nasopharynx and relatively low diagnostic yield due to non-productive cough. Sputum can be induced by inhaling heated aerosol of 20% propylene glycol in 10% hypertonic saline or water in salt restricted patients.

Bronchial Brush

The method exploits the utility of flexible bronchoscopes, which aids in the sampling of a visualized mucosal abnormality to confirm and localize occult in situ or early invasive carcinomas. Brushings can be supplemented by tissue biopsy or transbronchial aspiration biopsy. The limitation of the method is that the lesion of interest may not be within the reach of the bronchoscope such as distal peripheral bronchoalveolar region [2].

Bronchial Wash

Bronchial washing is less lesion-directed sampling technique, aiding in the sampling of more peripheral airway lesions, usually small bronchi beyond the reach of bronchoscopy brush. The lesional material is obtained by aspiration of small amount of sterile saline solution applied near the tip of the bronchoscope. Bronchial washing can be used to find tumors as well as infections.

Bronchioalveolar Lavage

Bronchioalveolar lavage was formerly introduced in clinical setting as a therapeutic procedure to remove accumulated secretions blocking the gaseous exchange in the lung. Subsequently, the technique has been widely used for diagnostic purposes particularly in patients with acquired immunodeficiency syndrome (AIDS). Under local anesthesia, the bronchoscope is passed to a secondary or tertiary bronchus and wedged to occlude the lumen. A total of 100–300 mL normal saline is instilled and re-aspirated. The specimen represents the epithelium of the bronchioles beyond the point of occlusion and alveolar contents. It is commonly used to identify various infectious agents—bacteria, fungal, parasitic, and sometimes viral organisms. The modality has replaced open lung biopsy for detection of opportunistic infections such as *Pneumocystis jirovecii pneumonia* [3]. The recent advancement has been detecting rejection and/or infection in post lung transplant patients.

Fine Needle Aspiration

Fine needle aspiration biopsy is an imaging-guided direct sampling of a pulmonary lesion. It can be performed via a percutaneous or transbronchial approach dependent on the location of the lesion. The former is used to sample peripheral lung lesion that might not be within the reach of bronchoscopy, whereas the latter is applied to sample hilar and parahilar lymph nodes, or other near hilar masses which are difficult to access through percutaneous route [4, 5].

Normal Cytology—Cellular Elements

Respiratory Columnar Cells

The normal respiratory epithelium is identified as ciliated columnar cells. They do not desquamate easily, hence are uncommon in exfoliated material and typically seen in specimen obtained by bronchoscopy, bronchial brushing, bronchial wash, and fine needle aspiration. However, respiratory epithelial cells may also originate in the nasal cavity or nasopharynx; therefore, their presence cannot be reliable evidence for sampling of lower respiratory tract.

In brushings, columnar cells can be seen in clusters with cilia better appreciated at periphery, and sometimes even with attached reserve or basal epithelial cells (Fig. 11.3). While cilia may get damaged or lost, prominent linear thickening, the terminal plate or bar, at the luminal end of the epithelial cells is usually retained. The basal end of the cell tapers off representing the site of attachment to the basement membrane. The cytoplasm is lightly basophilic and homogenous, with occasional brown-lipochrome granules in the supranuclear area. The cells have oval-shaped nuclei with fine granular chromatin, and occasionally tiny nucleolus.

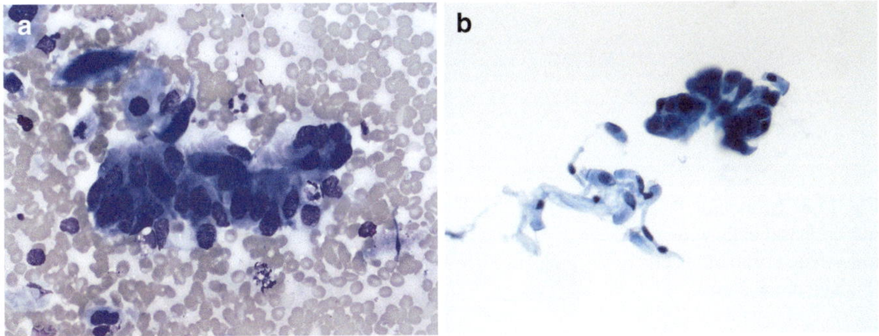

Fig. 11.3 Single and clusters of bronchial epithelial cells with cilia ((**a**) Diff-Quik stain; (**b**) Papanicolaou stain)

Goblet Cells

The mucus producing goblet cells are less predominant than ciliated columnar cells. They are wider than ciliated cells, have a basally placed nucleus with distended supranuclear cytoplasm containing mucinous vacuoles (Fig. 11.4). Goblet cell hyperplasia is seen in asthma and other chronic irritation conditions [6].

Basal or Reserve Cells

The basal or reserve cells form a layer of cells attached to the basement membrane, which are capable of regenerating and proliferating in response to inflammation or injury. These cells are small and have scant cytoplasm (Fig. 11.5). Immunohisto-

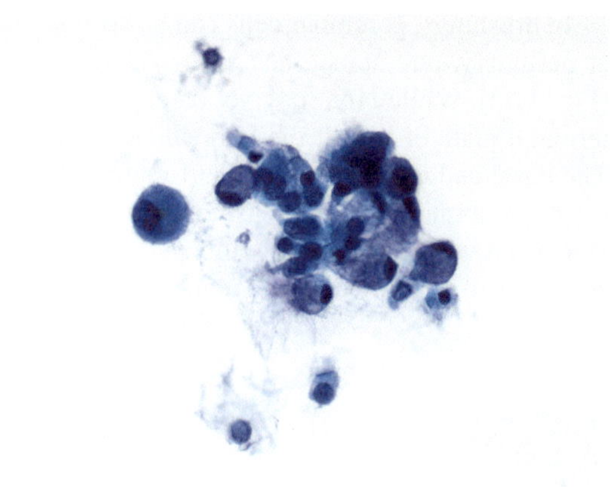

Fig. 11.4 Goblet cells admixed with bronchial epithelial cells (Papanicolaou stain)

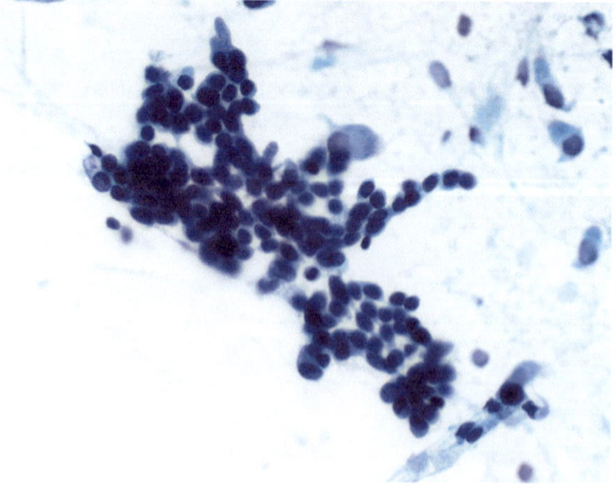

Fig. 11.5 Bronchial reserve/basal cells with a few ciliated bronchial cells (Papanicolaou stain)

chemically, they usually stain positive for p40, which therefore can be used as an internal control when working up subclassification of non-small cell carcinoma.

Squamous Cells

The exfoliated superficial squamous cells predominate the saliva and mostly originate from the superficial and intermediate cells of squamous epithelium. Squamous cells with relatively large but uniform nuclei may be present singly or more often in clusters hinting towards an underlying inflammatory disorder. Squamous cells in the lower respiratory tract likely represent reactive/metaplastic changes. During an inflammatory process, squamous cells may show significant cytologic atypia.

Macrophages

Alveolar macrophage in a cytology sample confirms the origin of the material from pulmonary alveoli. They are the predominant cell type in BAL specimen. They are spherical to oval cells, with amphophilic vacuolated cytoplasm containing variable amounts of brown-black dust particles (dust cells), and round-oval, or kidney-shaped nuclei with fine chromatin (Fig. 11.6). Binucleation can also be seen, also large multinucleated macrophages are not rare. Macrophages may contain other material such as hemosiderin pigments and lipid droplets in case of pulmonary hemorrhage and aspiration pneumonia.

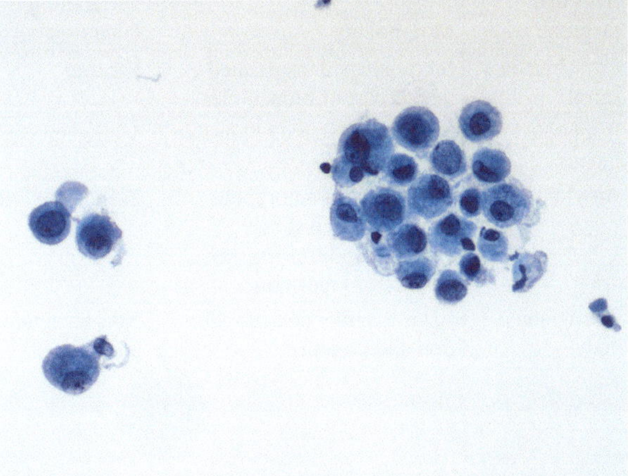

Fig. 11.6 Alveolar macrophages (Papanicolaou stain)

Mesothelial Cells

Mesothelial cells line the serosal surface of the lung. They are not infrequently seen as the contaminant in the percutaneous transthoracic needle biopsy of the peripheral lung lesions. These cells form flat clusters of uniform cells separated by slits or windows.

Non-cellular material (Table 11.2)

Curschmann's Spiral

Casts of inspissated mucus taking the shape of small bronchiolar lumen. It has a coiled appearance with a dark center and translucent periphery (Fig. 11.7). These spirals can be conveniently seen in chronic inflammatory conditions due to excess mucin production.

Inspissated Mucus

Small, dark staining structureless blob, as small as a naked nucleus and can be mistaken for a malignant cell.

Table 11.2 Cytomorphology and diagnostic implications of non-cellular material

Acellular material	Morphology	Differential diagnosis	Diagnostic clue
Curschmann's spiral	Spiral-shaped inspissated mucus cast of bronchioles	Parasite	Non-refractile, stains positive for mucin
Inspissated mucus	Small, dark stained blob-like size of nucleus	Malignant cell	No internal structures
Amyloid	Homogenous-amorphous material which shows apple-green birefringence post Congo red stain	Pseudoamyloid	Pseudoamyloid is fibrillar and does not show birefringence
Ferruginous body	Asbestos fiber coated with iron and protein	Non-ferruginous body	Ferruginous bodies are transparent, segmented bamboo shaped. Non-ferruginous bodies have opaque fibrous core, and may be curved or branched

Fig. 11.7 Curschmann's
spiral (Papanicolaou stain)

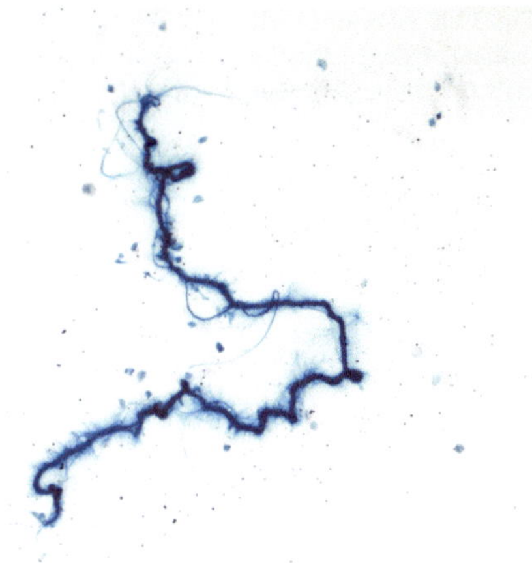

Corpora Amylacea

These are proteinaceous spherical translucent structures with concentric lamination. They are often seen in patients with a history of pulmonary edema, infarction, and chronic bronchitis.

Amyloid and Pseudoamyloid

Amyloid is a homogenous, waxy amorphous material which shows apple-green birefringence under polarized light following Congo red staining. Amyloid deposition in the lung could be diffuse or localized [7]. Localized amyloid deposition, amyloidoma, in the lung parenchyma can present a mass lesion by imaging studies. Pseudoamyloid is fibrillar eosinophilic material with no birefringence which is associated with an underlying light chain deposition disease.

Ferruginous Bodies

Sputum or bronchial samples of patients exposed to asbestos may contain beaded or segmented bamboo-shaped asbestos fibers with knobbed or bulbous ends (Fig. 11.8). These are coated with protein and iron, which lend a golden-yellow hue to the ferruginous body. The presence of asbestos bodies does not necessarily imply asbestos-related disease, moreover, other mineral fibers may have similar appearance.

Fig. 11.8 Asbestos body
with a few degenerated
cells (Papanicolaou stain)

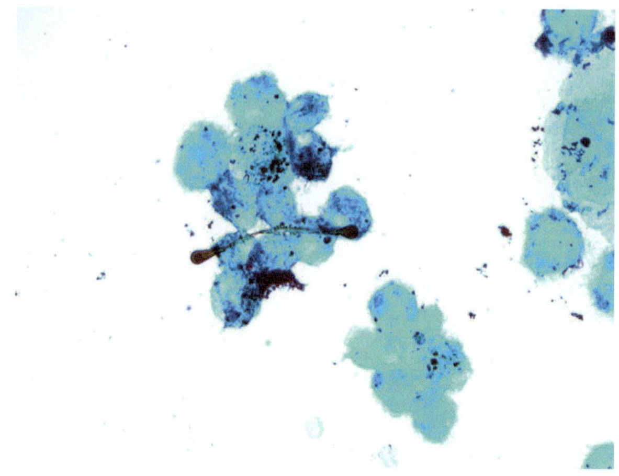

Reactive Cellular changes (Table 11.3)

Reactive Bronchial Cells

As a response to insult, bronchial cells undergo reactive changes including cytomegaly, nuclear enlargement, prominent nucleoli, and multinucleation. Such reactive changes can be observed even after minor trauma like repeated bronchoscopies
or bouts of severe coughing, and in inflammatory processes such as bronchitis, bacterial or viral pneumonia, or tuberculosis.

Ciliocytophthoria

Ciliocytophthoria represents destruction of ciliated bronchial cells mostly due to an
underlying viral pneumonia [8, 9]. The distal ciliated portion of the cells is pinched
off, resulting in anucleated ciliated tufts, and nucleated cytoplasmic remnants.
Nuclear degeneration is a common finding.

Creola Bodies

The chronic inflammatory conditions especially bronchiectasis, triggers papillary
hyperplasia of the respiratory epithelium which sheds spherical or ovoid papillary
clusters of bronchial cells [10]. The surface of this cluster consists of ciliated columnar cells while the core is composed of uniform small basal cells. It is important to

Table 11.3 Reactive cellular changes, differential diagnosis, and diagnostic pitfalls

	Cytomorphology	Differential Diagnosis	Diagnostic Clue
Reactive bronchial cells	Bi- or multinucleation, cytomegaly	Viral infection Adenocarcinoma	Smooth nuclear contours
Creola body	Detached portion of papillary hyperplasia of bronchial epithelium	Adenocarcinoma	Presence of cilia and goblet cells preserved nucleus to cytoplasm ratio
Basal cell hyperplasia	Clusters of small basal cells with hyperchromatic nuclei and scant cytoplasm	Small cell carcinoma	One of the edges is straight, tight clusters, with no nuclear molding
Squamous metaplasia	Clusters of cuboidal or polygonal cells with moderate eosinophilic cytoplasm	Squamous cell carcinoma	Smooth nuclear contour, preserved N:C ratio Some may show a straight edge or terminal plate
Bronchial metaplasia	Columnar epithelial cell accompanying alveolar macrophage in BAL specimen		
Reactive pneumocytes	Cuboidal cells with hyperchromatic nuclei and prominent nucleoli	Adenocarcinoma, atypical adenomatoid hyperplasia	Positive TTF-1 and Napsin A immunostaining

differentiate them from well-differentiated adenocarcinoma by paying attention to the presence of cilia, admixed goblet cells, and relatively maintained nuclear cytoplasmic ratio.

Basal Cell Hyperplasia

The small basal cells situated next to the basement membrane in the respiratory epithelium may undergo an abnormal multiplication to tide over unfavorable environment [11]. Normally, these cells are firmly adhered to the basement membrane hence rarely seen in the sputum. However, they can be seen in specimens obtained through instrumentation causing forceful detachment of the cells. The clusters of small, hyperchromatic cells are tightly packed, and may have a straight edge (Fig. 11.9). It can mimic small cell carcinoma; hence, keen observation is required [12].

Squamous Metaplasia

Respiratory epithelium of the trachea or bronchus can be replaced by squamous epithelium in response to inflammation, infection, or repeat instrumentation. Squamous metaplasia of the bronchial epithelium without atypia must not be considered as a precancerous lesion; however, atypical squamous metaplasia is a potential precursor of bronchogenic squamous cell carcinoma.

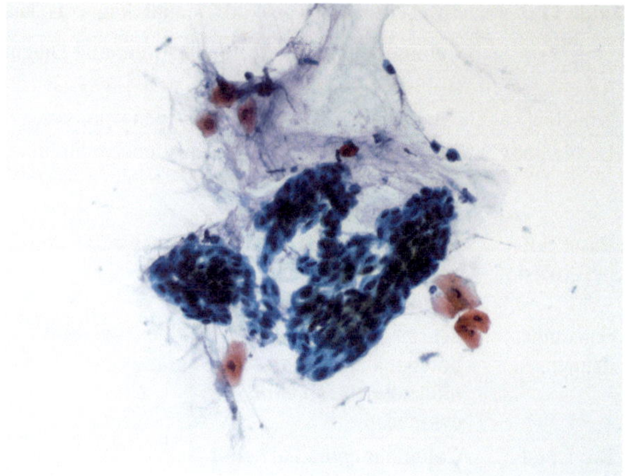

Fig. 11.9 Clusters of predominant reserve/basal cells (Papanicolaou stain)

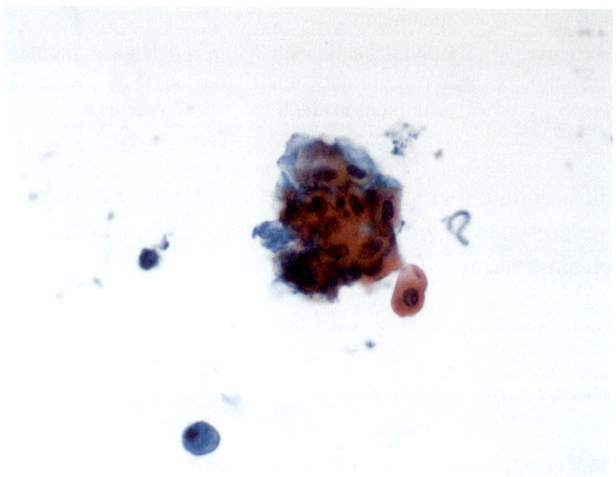

Fig. 11.10 Cluster of metaplastic squamous cells (Papanicolaou stain)

In sputum sample, it is difficult to differentiate the normal squamous cells from metaplastic. In bronchial washings, aspirates, and brush specimens, the metaplastic squamous cells can be well identified, when contamination from upper respiratory tract is excluded. Cytologically, the metaplastic squamous cells are small, adhered to each other in clusters or sheets (Fig. 11.10). They have round to oval nuclei and eosinophilic cytoplasm resembling parabasal cells.

Bronchial Metaplasia of Alveolar Epithelium

The pulmonary alveoli are lined by small cuboidal pneumocytes. In a variety of chronic inflammatory/obstructive processes, the pneumocytes can be replaced by one or more layers of columnar epithelial cells that are in continuity with the surrounding bronchioles. This phenomenon is commonly seen in areas adjacent to

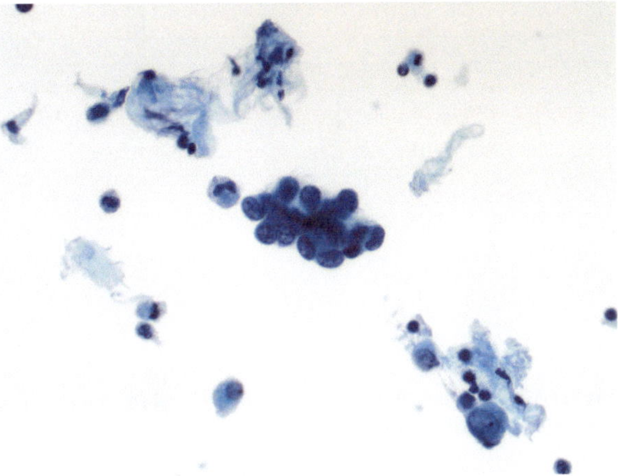

Fig. 11.11 Cluster of reactive pneumocytes with a few macrophages and lymphocytes (Papanicolaou stain)

scars or fibrosis and associated with cystic honeycomb lung changes. In setting of radiological findings suggestive of honeycomb lung changes, the presence of significant numbers of columnar epithelial cells accompanying alveolar macrophages in BAL specimens may suggest alveolar bronchial metaplasia.

Reactive Pneumocytes

Type II pneumocytes are highly reactive cells that respond to various pathologic processes. Reactive pneumocytes present individually or in sheets or rosette-like clusters with fine textured cyanophilic cytoplasm, occasional cytoplasmic vacuoles, and enlarged hyperchromatic nuclei with smooth nuclear contours and single or multiple prominent nucleoli (Fig. 11.11) [12]. The pulmonary diseases that are associated with reactive changes includes chronic pneumonia, viral pneumonitis, pulmonary fibrosis, infarcts, and chemo or radiation therapy.

Bacterial infections (Fig. 11.10)

Tuberculosis

It is caused by acid-fast mycobacterium tuberculosis, characterized by formation of caseating granulomas composed of epithelioid histiocytes, giant cells, and lymphocytes (Fig. 11.12). Epithelioid histiocytes have elongated nuclei and eosinophilic cytoplasm with poorly defined cell borders. Giant cells have multiple nuclei, which may be arranged with a peripheral wreath pattern, known as Langhans' cells [13]. Presence of Langhans' giant cell in cytology material is a non-specific finding and should not be considered as a hallmark feature for tuberculosis diagnosis.

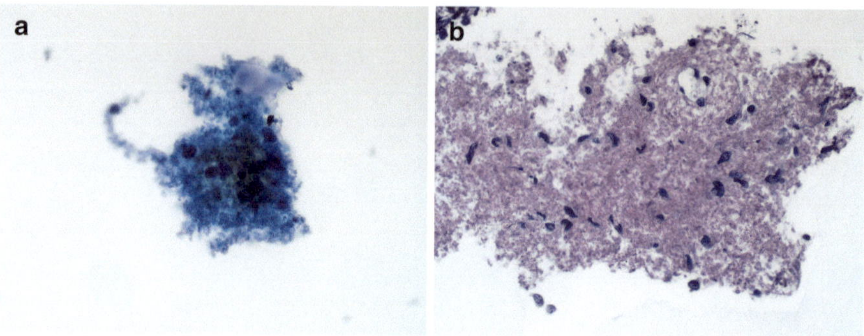

Fig. 11.12 Loose clusters of necrotic debris and scattered histiocytes ((**a**) Papanicolaou stain; (**b**) Hematoxylin-eosin stain)

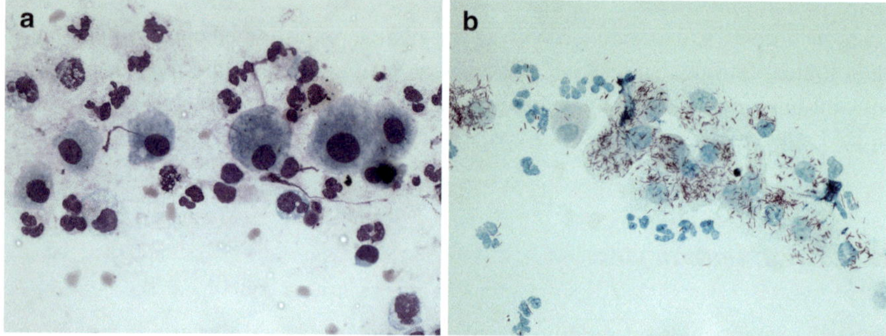

Fig. 11.13 Macrophages with intracytoplasmic negative images ((**a**) Diff-Quik stain) and acid-fast bacilli; ((**b**) Acid-fast bacilli stain)

Granuloma is rarely seen in exfoliative cytology specimens. Direct sampling of the lesions via FNA usually yields granular necrotic debris and a mixture of inflammatory cells. The presence of granuloma-like cluster of spindly epithelioid histiocytes with necrosis is not specific but should raise the possibility of tuberculosis. Mycobacterial organisms (*mycobacteria tuberculosis*) are sparse and difficult to identify even with special stains. Special attention should be given in high-risk patients with AIDS, in whom disease is severe and highly contagious. In such patients, the granulomas are poorly formed, and likely to contain a greater number of atypical mycobacteria (*mycobacterium avium-intracellulare*) (Fig. 11.13).

Actinomycosis

Suppurative infections caused by Gram-positive filamentous bacteria which are mostly saprophytic but can be pathogenic in immune compromised patients. They can commonly present as contaminants in the sputum, with no clinical significance.

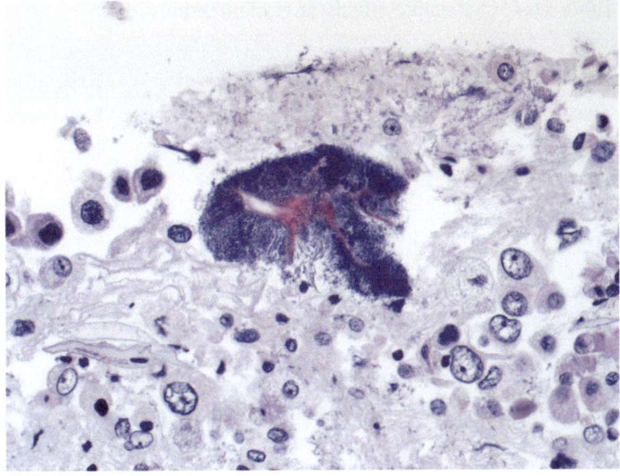

Fig. 11.14 Actinomycin colony with scattered macrophages and lymphocytes (Hematoxylin-eosin stain)

Pulmonary lesions sampled through bronchial brush or bronchial aspirate, usually represent secondary or complicating infections of already damaged or inflamed lung tissue. Actinomyces may produce lung abscesses, which can grow into pleura and chest wall resulting in empyema and fistulous tracts. They present as dense colonies made of hematoxylin-stain tangled filaments that radiate outwards and are more eosinophilic at the periphery (Fig. 11.14), known as sulfur granules [14].

Nocardiosis

Nocardiosis is aerobic branching filamentous bacteria that is Gram positive and resembles actinomyces but does not usually form colonies [15, 16]. Nocardia stains positive with Fite stain.

Viral Infections (Table 11.4)

Herpes Simplex Virus

Herpes infection is more often seen in immunosuppressed patients, which may progress to herpetic pneumonia [17]. Cytology specimen reveals multinucleated cells with moderately enlarged basophilic nuclei of ground glass appearance, or nuclei with margination of chromatin and molding. There are no cytoplasmic inclusions.

Table 11.4 Cytopathic effects of viral infections

Virus	Cytoplasmic Inclusions	Nuclear Inclusions	Giant Cells
Herpes simplex	No	Yes, ground-glass and eosinophilic	Yes
Cytomegalovirus	Yes, eosinophilic, or basophilic with halo	Yes, eosinophilic, or basophilic with large halo	Occasional
Adenovirus	No	Yes, multiple basophilic	No
Respiratory syncytial virus	Multiple basophilic halos	No	Always
Measles	Multiple small eosinophilic	Rare	Always

Cytomegalovirus (CMV)

CMV infection is mostly seen in immunocompromised patients. On cytology, CMV is characterized by significantly enlarged nuclei with large basophilic intranuclear inclusions surrounded by a clear halo. Multiple tiny basophilic cytoplasmic inclusions are sometimes seen. Virus can affect bronchiolar or alveolar epithelial cells, macrophages, and endothelial cells. In equivocal cases, immunocytochemistry, in situ hybridization, or molecular testing can help confirm the diagnosis.

Adenovirus

The cytopathic effects of this virus infection are characterized by enlarged nuclei containing multiple eosinophilic intranuclear inclusions with halos, which can merge into a single basophilic inclusion presenting as a smudge nucleus. The infected bronchial epithelial cells retain their cilia; however, ciliocytophthoria can be seen [18].

Respiratory Syncytial Virus

The infection predominantly occurs in infants or children with immunodeficiency but can also be seen in immunosuppressed adults. The classic finding is the presence of large syncytial groups of cells which contain multiple basophilic inclusions within the degenerated cytoplasm. Multinucleated giant cells with similar cytoplasmic inclusions.

Measles Virus

Measles is a common infection of childhood, usually in a transient nature, but can be complicated in immunocompromised patients. The hallmark feature is the formation of multinucleated giant cells (Warthin-Finkeldey cells) which can have up to

100 nuclei and contain spherical eosinophilic intracytoplasmic and intranuclear inclusions [19]. Also seen are syncytial epithelial giant cells which are formed by coalescence of type II pneumocytes and contain similar inclusions [20].

Viral Mimickers

Small eosinophilic intracytoplasmic inclusions can be seen in desquamated bronchial cells like the inclusions seen in ciliocytophthoria. These inclusions are aggregates of intermediate filaments and represent an underlying degenerative process.

Pulmonary Mycoses (Table 11.5)

Cryptococcus neoformans *(Hominis)*

Commonly seen in immunocompromised patients with leukemia, AIDS, etc. with meningitis being the typical presentation. However, lung is believed to be the site of entry for the fungus, hence early detection helps in preventing an accelerated disseminated form.

Table 11.5 Morphologic characteristics of pulmonary fungi

Fungal organism	Cytomorphologic features	Differential diagnosis
Cryptococcus neoformans	Transparent capsule, narrow based budding	Bronchogenic carcinoma
Blastomyces dermatitidis	Broad based budding, granuloma	Tuberculosis
Coccidioides immitis	Large thick wall spherules with multiple endospores	
Paracoccidioides brasiliensis	Large spore surrounded by buds (Ship's wheel)	
Histoplasma capsulatum	Tiny dot like structures with halo in macrophage	Tuberculosis
Sporothrix schenckii	Multiple, eosinophilic intracytoplasmic yeast in macrophages, non-staining cell wall	Candida albicans Histoplasma capsulatum
Aspergillus	Septate hyphae branching at acute angle. Oxalate crystals sign of *Niger* species	Mucor Tuberculosis
Mucor	Aseptate broad hyphae branching at obtuse angle	Aspergillus
Candida	Pseudohyphae, narrow based budding yeast	Trichophyton
Pneumocystis jirovecii	Uniform spherical or cup-shaped cysts with internal dots	Candida yeast

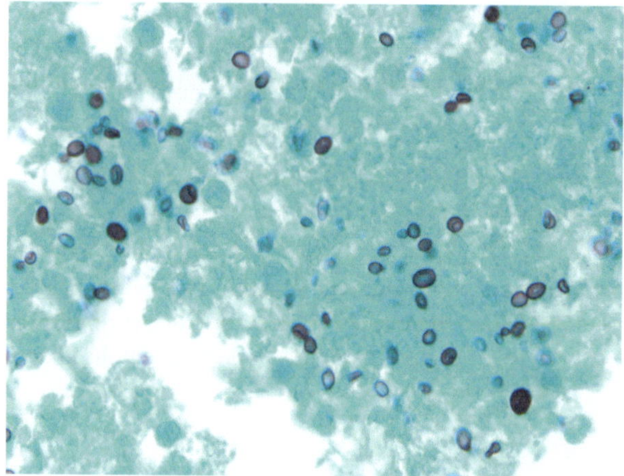

Fig. 11.15 Cryptococcus—pleomorphic organisms with uneven narrow-based budding (Grocott's methenamine silver stain)

The cytology shows spherical, pleomorphic, yeast-form organisms, measuring 6 to 20 mm, and have characteristic uneven narrow-based budding (Fig. 11.15). The organisms have thick sharply demarcated capsule and stain positive with mucicarmine, periodic acid-Schiff (PAS), and Gomori methenamine silver stains [21].

Blastomyces Dermatitidis

Pulmonary blastomycosis manifests as granulomatous lesions which can mimic malignancy. In cytology, the yeast forms of the organisms are spherical, relatively uniform, with broad based budding [22]. The organisms are about 20 mm in size, equal or larger to cryptococcus. *Blastomyces* has a refractile, thick wall but no mucoid capsule, stained by methenamine silver.

Coccidioidomycosis Immitis

The pulmonary form of the disease may show cavitary forms, which can be misdiagnosed as tuberculosis. The cytology shows large spherules with endospores [23], the spherules measure up to 100 mm and the endospores about 20 mm. The spherules can have a crushed appearance (Fig. 11.16).

Fig. 11.16 Coccidioidomycosis—large,
crushed spherules
(Diff-Quik stain)

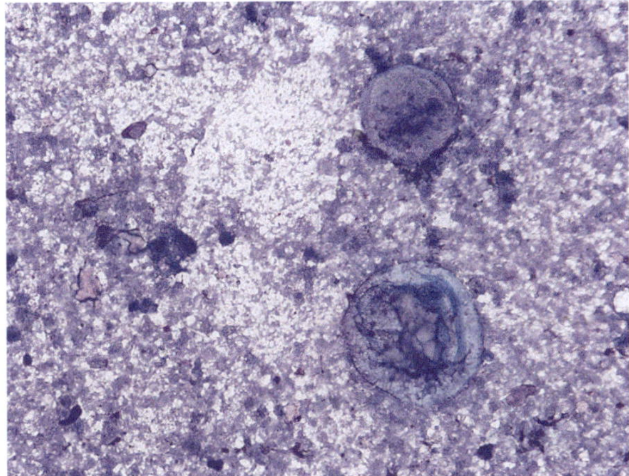

Paracoccidioides Brasiliensis

Paracoccidioidomycosis is characterized by large spores surrounded by multiple peripheral buds (ship's wheel), stained by methenamine silver [24]. The cytology specimens are usually hemorrhagic or purulent with epithelioid and multinucleated giant cells.

Histoplasma Capsulatum

The pulmonary form can mimic tuberculosis and cause sclerosing mediastinitis. The fungal organism fills the cytoplasm of macrophages with tiny dot-like structures with clear halos. The organisms are small with narrow-based budding and measure 2 to 4 mm. They are best seen by silver staining.

Sporothrix Schenckii

Sporotrichosis, caused by thermally dimorphic fungi *Sporothrix schenckii* complex, has become an emerging infection in recent years although pulmonary infection with *S. schenckii* still remains relatively uncommon [25]. The organisms are multiple, small, ovoid, eosinophilic intracytoplasmic yeasts seen within macrophages. Due to the non-staining of the organism wall, a thin halo is seen around. Elongated, budding cigar-shaped forms are also seen which helps to differentiate from histoplasma. This intracellular fungal species should not be confused with extracellular candida.

Aspergillus Species

Aspergillus can present as diffuse pulmonary infection or solitary aspergilloma and mainly infects the immunosuppressed patients [26]. The hyphae branch at 45 (acute angle), helping to differentiate them from *Mucor* species. Rarely calcium oxalate crystals can be seen, suggestive of *Aspergillus niger* species. The cavity wall of aspergilloma can undergo atypical squamous metaplasia, reactive basal epithelial cell hyperplasia, and marked inflammation.

Mucor Species

The family of fungus has strong predisposition towards angioinvasion and causing vascular thrombosis and infarcts. The morphology is characteristic, showing broad, ribbon-like and wavy, aseptate hyphae branching at obtuse angle [27].

Candida Species

Candida presents as pseudohyphae, rarely true hyphae, with narrow neck "teardrop"-shaped budding yeast are documented (Fig. 11.17). It is mostly seen in debilitated patients where it can even become invasive and disseminate. Trichophyton, a common contaminant of oral cavity should be differentiated from candida.

Pneumocystis Jirovecii

Pneumocystis jirovecii pneumonia (PJP) occurs primarily in immunocompromised patients, presenting as diffuse lung lesion on imaging studies. Rapid accurate diagnosis, often achieved by examination of BAL specimens, is crucial for patient

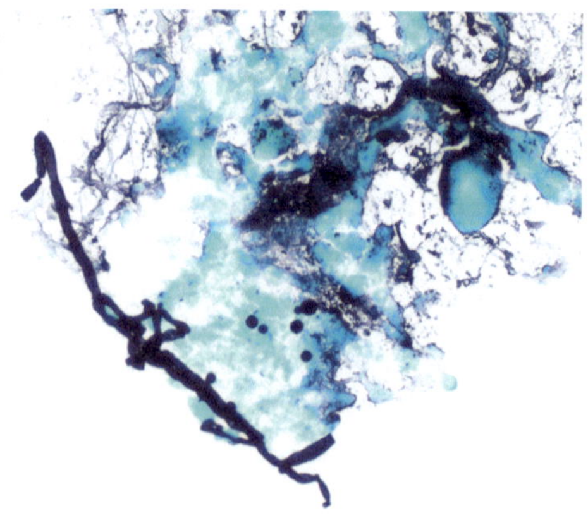

Fig. 11.17 Candida—mixed pseudohyphae and yeast (Grocott's methenamine silver stain)

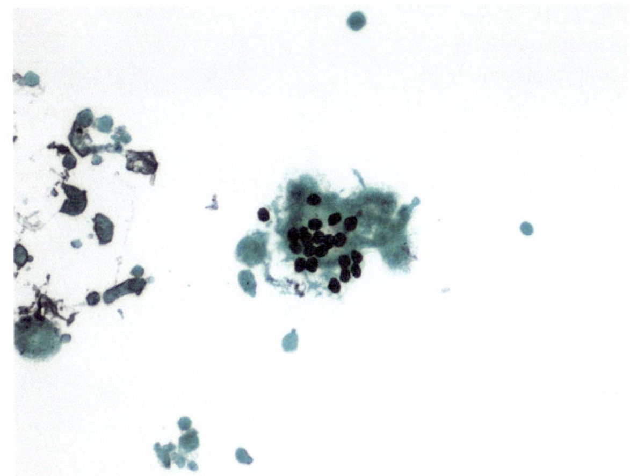

Fig. 11.18 Alveolar cast with pneumocystis jirovecii—uniform spherical organisms (Grocott's methenamine silver stain)

management. Typical findings of BAL specimens include foamy alveolar casts full of microorganisms. The organisms are best revealed by GMS stain, showing relatively uniform 4–6 μm, spherical or cup-shaped cyst structures with 1–2 internal dots (Fig. 11.18).

Other Lung disorders

Lipid Pneumonia

Exogenous lipid pneumonia results from aspiration of oily substance into the lungs. The radiologic appearance can be alarming as localized infiltrate or mass can mimic an underlying carcinoma [28]. The oil gets phagocytized by macrophages which can trigger a granulomatous response. Cytology can yield characteristic features of large macrophages with large cytoplasmic vacuoles or abundant bubbly vacuolated cytoplasm (Fig. 11.19). It is worth differentiating these lipid-rich macrophages from mucus producing cells, the latter tend to have atypia and commonly a single cytoplasmic vacuole.

Endogenous lipid pneumonia represents an underlying destructive process with release of tissue lipid that get phagocytized by macrophages. This is suggestive of involvement of lung by carcinoma, organizing pneumonia, necrotizing granulomatous inflammation, or other chronic inflammation. On cytology, small, finely vacuolated macrophages are seen as opposed to large cytoplasmic vacuoles seen in exogenous pneumonia [29]. Gaucher's disease and side effects of amiodarone should also be considered, while diagnosing lipid pneumonia.

Fig. 11.19 A few
macrophages with
intracytoplasmic lipid
droplets (Oil-Red-O stain)

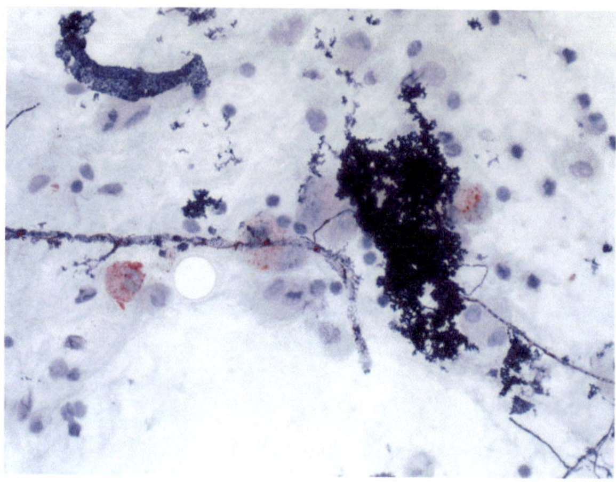

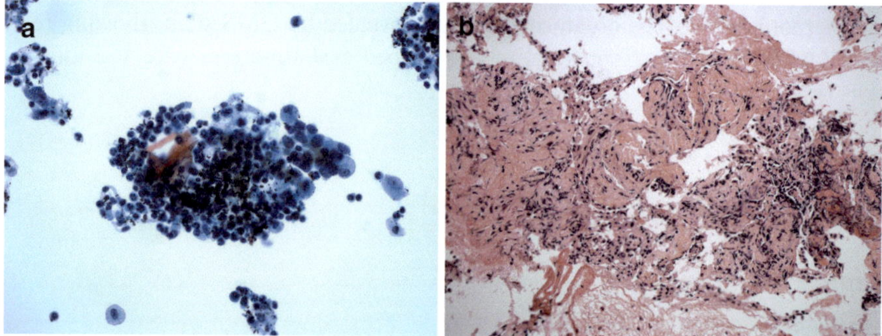

Fig. 11.20 Mixed neutrophils, lymphocytes, and macrophages in BAL specimen ((**a**).
Papanicolaou stain) with current lung biopsy showing inflamed fibrotic lung parenchyma; ((**b**)
Hematoxylin-eosin stain)

Interstitial Pneumonia

It is an umbrella term for disorders of unknown etiology, which have in common
inflammation, progressive fibrosis, and synchronous dilatation of bronchioles forming pseudo-glandular spaces. On cytology marked bronchiolar atypia and pneumo-
cyte hyperplasia can be seen, mimicking adenocarcinoma. The aspirate commonly
shows papillary clusters of bronchiolar and alveolar cells with prominent nucleoli
[30]. BAL of patients with interstitial pneumonia show an increase in macrophages,
lymphocytes, and other inflammatory cells (Fig. 11.20).

Sarcoidosis

This granulomatous disease differs from tuberculosis that does not show caseous necrosis. A characteristic, though not specific feature is laminated crystalline inclusions (Schaumann's bodies) in multinucleated giant cells. Intracytoplasmic asteroid bodies may also be present. A constellation of findings should increase the suspicion of sarcoidosis: tight clusters of epithelioid histiocytes with lymphocytes (Fig. 11.21), alveolar macrophages, and multinucleated giant cells in a relatively clean background. The lymphocytosis in BAL specimen shows an increased ratio of CD4/CD8 with predominance of activated T-cells. In cases with concern for sarcoidosis, a transbronchial FNA of mediastinal lymph node probably has a higher diagnostic yield than percutaneous aspiration; however, final diagnosis requires clinical correlation [31].

Wegener's Granulomatosis

Vasculitis of small and medium size vessels and necrotizing granulomatous inflammation involving upper respiratory tract and lung, where it can mimic cavitating tuberculosis. The diagnosis can be suggested, not confirmed by FNA of lung yielding amorphous or filamentous necrotic tissue, and an inflammatory cellular infiltrate [30, 32]. It is however difficult to diagnose this disease on cytology specimens. The diagnosis is often rendered by a supplementary biopsy and positive anti-neutrophilic cytoplasmic antigen test (cANCA) and ELISA for proteinase 3.

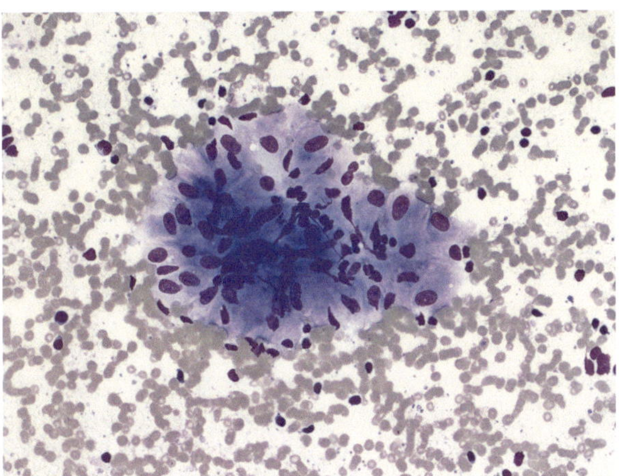

Fig. 11.21 A tight cluster of epithelioid histiocytes and scattered lymphocytes (Diff-Quik stain)

Langerhans Cell Histiocytosis

Pulmonary Langerhans cell histiocytosis is a proliferative, usually clonal, disorder of Langerhans cells, with associated interstitial changes in the lung tissue [33]. The diagnosis may be suspected when a BAL specimen shows more than 4–5% of CD1a positive large mononuclear cells, often with increase eosinophils and Charcot-Leyden crystals [34, 35]. Occasionally, transbronchial or percutaneous aspirate can show CD1a and S-100 positive Langerhans' cells with round to oval, cleaved, or convoluted nuclear contour, fine chromatin, and long cytoplasmic processes.

Rheumatoid Granuloma

Classic manifestation of pulmonary involvement by rheumatoid arthritis is seen in pleural effusion cytology, however, limited cytologic findings can be seen in sputum and bronchoalveolar specimens. Necrobiotic nodules, presented as mass-like lesions, may be subjected to FNA, showing multinucleated giant cells in a necrotic background [36]. The background necrosis on cytology specimen is generally considered to be the representation of the necrotic center of the granuloma.

Alveolar Proteinosis

Acquired autoimmune disorder caused by antibodies targeting surface receptor for granulocyte-macrophage colony stimulating factors, which is expressed on alveolar macrophages [37]. The phospholipid-rich proteinaceous material filling the alveoli is due to the defective clearance by macrophages. BAL specimens demonstrate globules of amorphous or fibrillar PAS-positive casts which is suggestive of the disease in the correct clinical settings [35, 38].

Therapy-Related Changes

Systemic or local therapies such as chemotherapy and radiation can cause significant cellular changes in squamous epithelium, respiratory epithelium, and pneumocytes of the respiratory system. The cellular changes are characterized by cytomegaly, cytoplasmic vacuolization, nuclear enlargement, prominent nucleoli, and occasionally multinucleation (Fig. 11.22). These changes, sometimes quite atypical, may overlap with cytomorphologic features of malignant tumors, raising a concern. It

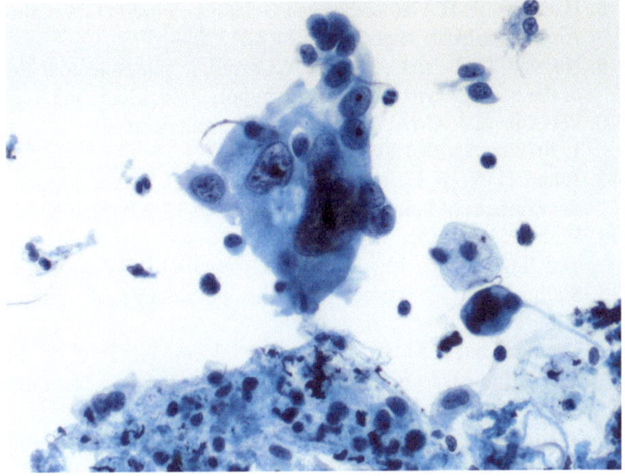

Fig. 11.22 Reactive bronchial cells with enlarged nuclei, multinucleation, and prominent nucleoli (Papanicolaou stain)

should be extremely cautious to interpret cytological atypia in the specimens from patients who receive therapies. The presence of cytoplasmic vacuoles with low nuclear-to-cytoplasmic ratios favors therapy-related atypia over an underlying malignancy.

Acknowledgments None.

Conflict of Interest None.

References

1. Zhao CZ, Fang XC, Wang D, Tang FD, Wang XD. Involvement of type II pneumocytes in the pathogenesis of chronic obstructive pulmonary disease. Respir Med. 2010;104(10):1391–5.
2. Chen CC, Bai CH, Lee KY, Chou YT, Pan ST, Wang YH. Evaluation of the diagnostic accuracy of bronchial brushing cytology in lung cancer: a meta-analysis. Cancer Cytopathol. 2021;129(9):739–49.
3. Bateman M, Oladele R, Kolls JK. Diagnosing pneumocystis jirovecii pneumonia: a review of current methods and novel approaches. Med Mycol. 2020;58(8):1015–28.
4. Ferretti GR, Busser B, de Fraipont F, et al. Adequacy of CT-guided biopsies with histomolecular subtyping of pulmonary adenocarcinomas: influence of ATS/ERS/IASLC guidelines. Lung Cancer. 2013;82(1):69–75.
5. Błach J, Frąk M, Krawczyk P, et al. Observational cross-sectional study of 5279 bronchoscopy results for the practical effectiveness of various biopsy techniques in the diagnosis of lung diseases with particular emphasis on lung cancer. BMJ Open. 2021;11(8):e043820.
6. Samitas K, Carter A, Kariyawasam HH, Xanthou G. Upper and lower airway remodelling mechanisms in asthma, allergic rhinitis and chronic rhinosinusitis: the one airway concept revisited. Allergy. 2018;73(5):993–1002.
7. Khoor A, Colby TV. Amyloidosis of the lung. Arch Pathol Lab Med. 2017;141(2):247–54.

8. Hadziyannis E, Yen-Lieberman B, Hall G, Procop GW. Ciliocytophthoria in clinical virology. Arch Pathol Lab Med. 2000;124(8):1220–3.

9. Nuovo GJ, Magro C, Mikhail A. Cytologic and molecular correlates of SARS-CoV-2 infection of the nasopharynx. Ann Diagn Pathol. 2020;48:151565.

10. Persson C. Creola bodies and pathogenesis of childhood asthma. Eur Respir J. 2022;60(5):2201204.

11. Adam D, Roux-Delrieu J, Luczka E, et al. Cystic fibrosis airway epithelium remodelling: involvement of inflammation. J Pathol. 2015;235(3):408–19.

12. Witt BL, Wallander ML, Layfield LJ, Hirschowitz S. Respiratory cytology in the era of molecular diagnostics: a review. Diagn Cytopathol. 2012;40(6):556–63.

13. Stellmacher F, Perner S. Histopathology of pulmonary tuberculosis. Pathologe. 2021;42(1):71–7.

14. Gómez Mateo Mdel C, Urbano Salcedo A, Toro de Méndez M, Ferrández Izquierdo A. Pulmonary actinomycosis. Fine needle aspiration diagnostic. Investig Clin. 2011;52(4):358–64.

15. Sharma S, Gupta P, Gupta N, Lal A, Behera D, Rajwanshi A. Pulmonary infections in immunocompromised patients: the role of image-guided fine needle aspiration cytology. Cytopathology. 2017;28(1):46–54.

16. Sood R, Tyagi R, Selhi PK, Kaur G, Kaur H, Singh A. Role of FNA and special stains in rapid Cytopathological diagnosis of pulmonary Nocardiosis. Acta Cytol. 2018;62(3):178–82.

17. Clark NM, Lynch JP 3rd, Sayah D, Belperio JA, Fishbein MC, Weigt SS. DNA viral infections complicating lung transplantation. Semin Respir Crit Care Med. 2013;34(3):380–404.

18. Martínez-Girón R, Pantanowitz L. Lower respiratory tract viral infections: diagnostic role of exfoliative cytology. Diagn Cytopathol. 2017;45(7):614–20.

19. Pritt BS, Aubry MC. Histopathology of viral infections of the lung. Semin Diagn Pathol. 2017;34(6):510–7.

20. Fraire AEWB. Viruses and the lung. Springer; 2013.

21. George B, Rivera Rolon MDM, Clement CG. Role of fine-needle aspiration cytology in early diagnosis of fungal infections. Diagn Cytopathol. 2020;48(7):645–51.

22. Montes MA, DiNisco S, Dry S, Galvanek E. Fine needle aspiration cytology of primary isolated splenic Blastomyces dermatitidis. A case report. Acta Cytol. 1998;42(2):396–8.

23. Aly FZ, Millius R, Sobonya R, Aboul-Nasr K, Klein R. Cytologic diagnosis of coccidioidomycosis: Spectrum of findings in southern Arizona patients over a 10 year period. Diagn Cytopathol. 2016;44(3):195–200.

24. de Souza Vianna LM, Pirani Carneiro F, Calvalca Tavares A, Soares Takano GH, Silva Guerra EN, de Melo NS. Cytological diagnosis of paracoccidioidomycosis: a report of four cases. Diagn Cytopathol. 2013;41(4):374–6.

25. Aung AK, Spelman DW, Thompson PJ. Pulmonary Sporotrichosis: an evolving clinical paradigm. Semin Respir Crit Care Med. 2015;36(5):756–66.

26. Singh L, Jain D, Madan K, et al. Pulmonary mycoses diagnosed using exfoliative cytology: infection or colonization? Acta Cytol. 2013;57(6):604–10.

27. Lee FY, Mossad SB, Adal KA. Pulmonary mucormycosis: the last 30 years. Arch Intern Med. 1999;159(12):1301–9.

28. Sung S, Tazelaar HD, Crapanzano JP, Nassar A, Saqi A. Adult exogenous lipoid pneumonia: a rare and underrecognized entity in cytology - a case series. Cytojournal. 2018;15:17.

29. Kim CH, Kim EJ, Lim JK, et al. Comparison of exogenous and endogenous lipoid pneumonia: the relevance to bronchial anthracofibrosis. J Thorac Dis. 2018;10(4):2461–6.

30. Silverman JF. Inflammatory and neoplastic processes of the lung: differential diagnosis and pitfalls in FNA biopsies. Diagn Cytopathol. 1995;13(5):448–62.

31. Crombag LMM, Mooij-Kalverda K, Szlubowski A, et al. EBUS versus EUS-B for diagnosing sarcoidosis: the international sarcoidosis assessment (ISA) randomized clinical trial. Respirology. 2022;27(2):152–60.

32. Kaneishi NK, Howell LP, Russell LA, Vogt PJ, Lie JT. Fine needle aspiration cytology of pulmonary Wegener's granulomatosis with biopsy correlation. A report of three cases. Acta Cytol. 1995;39(6):1094–100.
33. Roden AC, Yi ES. Pulmonary Langerhans cell Histiocytosis: an update from the Pathologists' perspective. Arch Pathol Lab Med. 2016;140(3):230–40.
34. Lommatzsch M, Bratke K, Stoll P, et al. Bronchoalveolar lavage for the diagnosis of pulmonary Langerhans cell histiocytosis. Respir Med. 2016;119:168–74.
35. Costabel U, Guzman J, Bonella F, Oshimo S. Bronchoalveolar lavage in other interstitial lung diseases. Semin Respir Crit Care Med. 2007;28(5):514–24.
36. Filho JS, Soares MF, Wal R, Christmann RB, Liu CB, Schmitt FC. Fine-needle aspiration cytology of pulmonary rheumatoid nodule: case report and review of the major cytologic features. Diagn Cytopathol. 2002;26(3):150–3.
37. Chou CW, Lin FC, Tung SM, Liou RD, Chang SC. Diagnosis of pulmonary alveolar proteinosis: usefulness of papanicolaou-stained smears of bronchoalveolar lavage fluid. Arch Intern Med. 2001;161(4):562–6.
38. Jouneau S, Ménard C, Lederlin M. Pulmonary alveolar proteinosis. Respirology. 2020;25(8):816–26.

Chapter 12
Gastrointestinal Tract

Rita Abi-Raad

Esophagus:

Normal Epithelial Cells [1]

- Smears are composed primarily of superficial and intermediate squamous epithelial cells, often present in large to small sheets, as well as scattered single cells in brushings (Fig. 12.1).

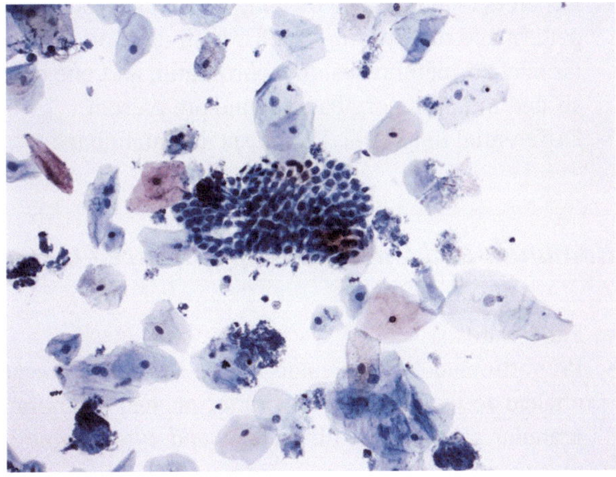

Fig. 12.1 Normal esophageal elements: Squamous epithelial cells with fundic-type glandular epithelial cells in a brushing from the lower end of the esophagus (Papanicolaou stain, x200)

R. Abi-Raad (✉)
Department of Pathology, Yale-New Haven Hospital, New Haven, CT, USA
e-mail: rita.abiraad@yale.edu

© The Author(s), under exclusive license to Springer Nature Switzerland AG 2023
S. M. Gilani, G. Cai (eds.), *Non-Neoplastic Cytology*,
https://doi.org/10.1007/978-3-031-44289-6_12

- Parabasal squamous cells are single cells with round to ovoid contours, dense cyanophilic cytoplasm, and relatively high nuclear to cytoplasmic (N:C) ratio. They are usually absent from esophageal brush but may be encountered as a result of forceful brushing.
- Gastric glandular cells from the gastroesophageal junction may be present (Fig.12.1). They are arranged in monolayer cohesive sheets of mucin-secreting cells with a honeycomb pattern when viewed en face and columnar shape when viewed on edge, with mucin vacuoles, basally located nuclei, delicate and finely granular cytoplasm and round nuclei with smooth nuclear contours.

Contaminants

- From nasopharyngeal tract: single ciliated respiratory columnar cells.
- From the oral cavity: yeast forms.
- Vegetable matter.

Reactive and Reparative Changes [2]

- Caused by mucosal injuries, ulceration, and infections.
- Repair is characterized by cohesive flat sheets of squamous cells with streaming pattern and rare/no single cells, with uniform, mildly enlarged nuclei with regular nuclear membranes, fine chromatin, and one or more nucleoli. Normal mitosis and inflammatory background are present.
- Differential diagnosis: Dysplasia and malignancy.

Radiation and Chemotherapy-Induced Changes [1]

- Parakeratosis.
- Proportionate cellular enlargement and nucleomegaly with retention of normal nuclear to cytoplasm (N:C) ratio, nuclear membranes irregularities, and finely granular chromatin with nuclear and cytoplasmic vacuolization and intracytoplasmic neutrophils.
- Multinucleated cells can be present.

Microorganisms: [2, 3–5]

- Candida:
  - Brushing is more sensitive than tissue biopsies [2, 6, 7].

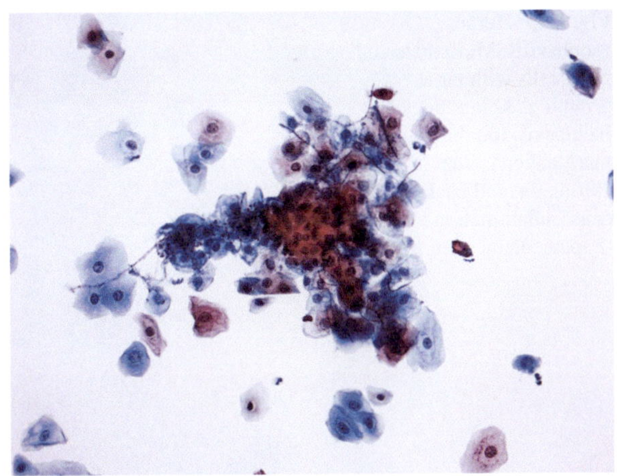

Fig. 12.2 Candida esophagitis. Fungal hyphae embedded within reactive squamous cells (Papanicolaou stain, x200)

- Pseudohyphae with small round budding yeast forms embedded within squamous cells with acute inflammation (Fig.12.2).
  - Reactive squamous cells with intracytoplasmic neutrophils, vacuolization, and mildly enlarged nuclei with perinuclear halos.

- Cytomegalovirus (CMV):

  - Rare enlarged cells with a single owl's eye intranuclear and intracytoplasmic inclusion (single large central dark area surrounded by a zone of pallor and irregular thickened nuclear membrane).
  - Epithelial, stromal, and endothelial cells can be infected.
  - Background reactive epithelial cells, acute inflammation, and granulation tissue.

- Herpes Simplex Virus (HSV):

  - Most frequent viral cause of esophagitis.
  - Rare cells with multinucleation, nuclear molding, characteristic classic intranuclear ground glass inclusion (Cowdry type A), and chromatin margination (3Ms) (Fig. 12.3).
  - Dirty/necrotic background with neutrophilic debris and squamous cells with reactive atypia.

Duplication Cyst [8]

- Paucicellular specimen with scattered epithelial cells.
- Squamous and ciliated cells, inflammatory cells, hemosiderin-laden macrophages, and detached ciliary tufts in a background of proteinaceous material, debris, and crystals.

Fig. 12.3 Herpes esophagitis. Multinucleated giant cells with large ground glass intranuclear inclusions, molding and margination of the chromatin, and background acute inflammation (Papanicolaou stain, x600)

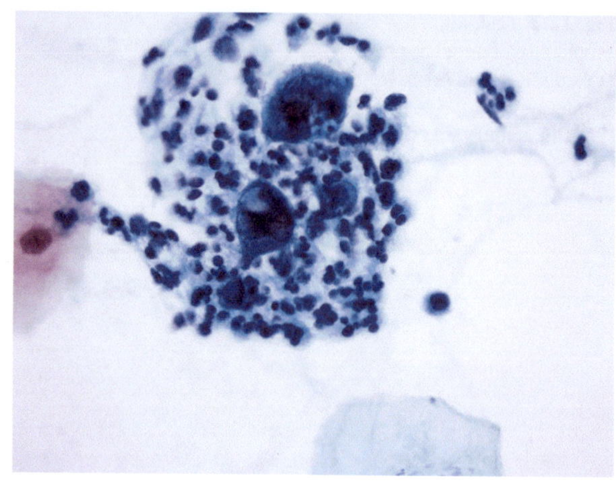

Heterotopic Tissue [9–11]

- Congenital anomaly of the cervical esophagus consisting of heterotopic gastric mucosa (inlet patch).
- Most common histologic type: oxyntic mucosa followed by cardiac and antral mucosa. Pancreatic tissue can rarely be present.
- Inflammation is common.
- Production of acid in the ectopic gastric mucosa predisposes to *Helicobacter Pylori* colonization.

Barrett's Esophagus [1, 2]

- Replacement of the normal esophageal squamous epithelium by metaplastic large flat sheets of cohesive glandular epithelium in a honeycomb appearance.
- Differential diagnosis: cells derived from the gastroesophageal junction when the metaplasia is of the fundic or cardiac type without specialized goblet cells.
- Cytological distinction between Barrett's esophagus and normal gastroesophageal junction glandular epithelium depends on the sampling site.
- The presence of goblet cells, which may be only few, is diagnostic of intestinal metaplasia.

Stomach

Normal Epithelial Cells [1, 2, 5]

- Smears from stomach brushings are composed of surface mucous cells arranged in large tightly cohesive monolayered sheets in a honeycomb pattern and uniformly distributed nuclei, cohesive palisaded rows arranged in a picket-fence

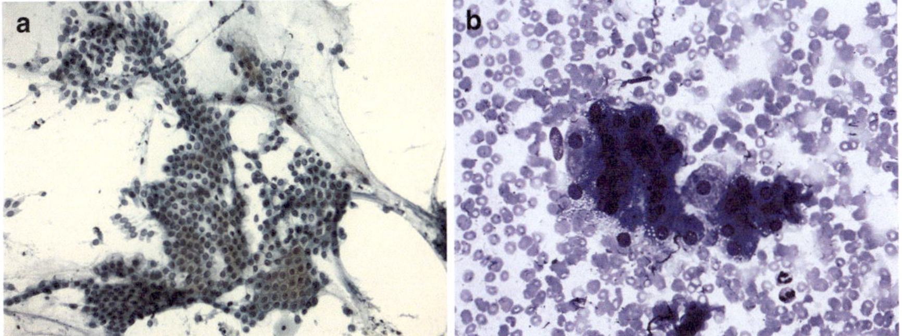

Fig. 12.4 (**a**) Normal gastric mucinous epithelium. Flat sheet arranged in a honeycomb pattern with pale mucinous cytoplasm, well-defined cell borders, and uniform round bland nuclei (Papanicolaou stain, x200). (**b**) Normal gastric elements: Small round chief cells with dark purple blue granules with interspersed large pyramidal parietal cells with granular lavender cytoplasm (Diff-Quik stain, x400)

pattern and single cells with small clear apical vacuoles, oval to elongated basally located nuclei with finely granular chromatin and inconspicuous nucleoli (Fig.12.4a).

- Surface mucous cells contain a moderate amount of pale cytoplasm, which appears pale green on Papanicolaou stain, light blue on Diff-Quik stain, and eosinophilic on hematoxylin-eosin-stained smears.
- Mucous cells from the cardiac and pyloric regions share cytologic similarities with the surface glandular cells and are present in a background of mucus.
- Mucus is red-violet on Diff-Quik and blue-green on Papanicolaou stains.
- Chief and parietal cells may also be seen in samples from the fundus and body of the stomach, present as single cells or arranged in small clusters.
- Chief cells are small round to cuboidal cells with finely granular chromatin and granular green cytoplasm on Papanicolaou stain and coarse basophilic granules on Diff-Quik stain (Fig. 12.4b).
- Parietal cells are characterized by a centrally placed round nucleus with finely granular chromatin and abundant orange granular cytoplasm on Papanicolaou stain and lavender with purple granules on Diff-Quik stain.

Contaminants

- Squamous cells from the oral cavity.
- Columnar respiratory epithelial cells.
- Alveolar histiocytes.
- Vegetable matter and meat fibers.

Heterotopic Tissue [12, 13]

- Pancreatic tissue: composed of acinar tissue, ductal cells, islet cells, or a combination of all types of cells.

Duplication Cyst [14, 15]

- Fluid with gastric, small intestinal and/or respiratory-type epithelium. Pancreatic tissue, cartilage, and ceruminous glands can be present.
- Columnar cells aggregated in small clusters in a palisade configuration or single cells, with long cilia and brush border, oval nuclei with finely dispersed chromatin and small nucleoli.
- Background consists of amorphous debris, crystal formations, lymphocytes, and macrophages.
- The presence of detached ciliary tufts is pathognomonic of a duplication cyst.

Helicobacter Pylori [1, 16, 17]

- Cytology is more sensitive compared to biopsy since brush cytology samples a larger surface and *H. pylori* organisms are scattered throughout the gastric mucosa.
- Curved or spiral rod-shaped bacteria arranged in parallel within strands of mucus.
- The rods are better visualized on Diff-Quik or Wright stain compared to Papanicolaou stain.
- Can be overlooked in mucus.
- Reactive epithelium secondary to gastritis and ulceration.

Atypical Mycobacteria [1]

- Abundant macrophages with vacuolated cytoplasm.
- Reactive epithelial cells.

Reactive and Reparative Changes

- Associated with gastritis or ulcers.
- Cohesive monolayered sheets and clusters with only rare single cells with enlarged nuclei with smooth nuclear borders and homogeneous prominent nucleoli.

- Differential diagnosis: normal gastric glandular epithelium (foveolar epithelium in cohesive flat sheets in honeycomb arrangement with uniform nuclei) and intestinal adenocarcinoma (discohesive cells, coarse chromatin, irregular nuclei and nuclear membrane, prominent nucleoli).

Gastritis

- Tightly cohesive two-dimensional sheets of glandular cells with preserved polarity and occasional single cells with enlarged cells with enlarged nuclei, preserved N:C ratio, regular nuclear membrane, and prominent nucleoli.
- Inflammatory background with neutrophils and lymphocytes, degenerated and necrotic cellular debris.
- Giant cells and granulomas are present in granulomatous gastritis.

Ulcer

- Cohesive sheets of glandular cells with enlarged nuclei, preserved N:C ratio, regular nuclear membrane, and prominent nucleoli.
- Inflammatory background with neutrophils.

Differential diagnosis between reactive/reparative epithelium and malignant neoplasms.

	Malignant neoplasms	Reactive/reparative changes
Cellularity	High	Low—moderate
Architecture	Three-dimensional clusters, crowding/overlapping, loosely cohesive groups, abundant single cells	Cohesive flat uniform sheets with streaming, rare single cells
Background	Necrosis	Clean or inflammatory
N:C ratio	High	Not increased
Cytologic atypia	Markedly pleomorphic cells	Mild to moderate
Nuclear enlargement	Present	Present
Nucleoli	Prominent	Prominent
Nuclear membrane	Irregular	Smooth
Chromatin	Coarse	Fine

Small intestine [1, 4]

Cytology

Normal Epithelial Cells

- Cytologic specimens are often obtained from the duodenum.
- Commonly seen as contaminants in FNA samples from the pancreatic head and bile duct brushings.
- Cohesive sheets, small clusters, rows, and single cells.
- Honeycomb sheets of absorptive enterocytes and interspersed circular clear goblet cells in a starry sky or "Swiss cheese" pattern. When lying on their edge, the enterocytes reveal their columnar shape, with low N:C ratio, basally located nuclei and accentuated luminal border, and scattered goblet cells with a basally located crescent shape nucleus and a vacuole of mucus distending the apical cytoplasm (Fig.12.5).
- On Papanicolaou stain, the cytoplasm appears blue-green, granular and finely vacuolated. The nuclei are round with regular nuclear membrane and an inconspicuous nucleolus.
- FNA shows smooth muscle cells consisting of spindle-shaped cells with blunt ended nuclei.

Contaminants

- Columnar cells from the bile and pancreatic ducts.
- Squamous cells from the esophagus.

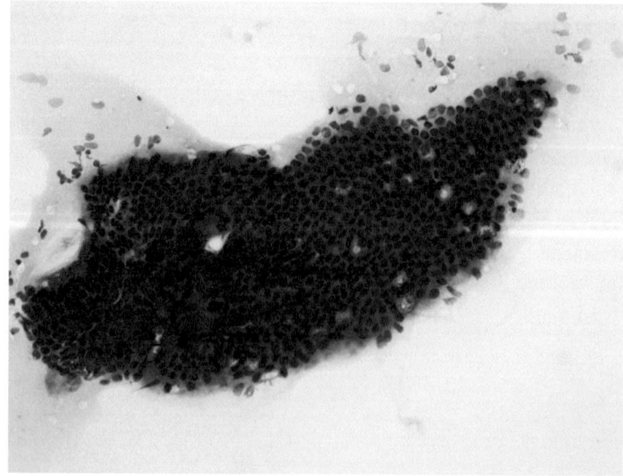

Fig. 12.5 Normal duodenal epithelium. Cohesive sheet of benign enterocytes arranged a honeycomb pattern with interspersed clear goblet cells in a "swiss cheese" pattern and a brush border at the edge (Papanicolaou stain, x200)

Reactive and Reparative Changes

- Cohesive monolayered sheets of cells with mild nuclear enlargement, smooth nuclear membrane, evenly dispersed chromatin, multiple prominent uniform nucleoli, and increased mitosis.
- Dense or vacuolated cytoplasm.
- Background is inflammatory.

Common Pathogens

- Giardia:

  - Identified in duodenal brushing specimens, better visualized on Diff-Quik stain.
  - The trophozoites measure 12–15 μm in maximum dimension and have a characteristic pear-shaped configuration with a rounded anterior end with two symmetrically placed nuclei, one on each side of the midline, and a tapered posterior end.

- Cryptosporidium:

  - Causes diarrhea in normal or immunocompromised individuals.
  - Round basophilic intracytoplasmic protozoa, measures 1–4 μm in diameter, better visualized on Diff-Quik smears.
  - Develops in the brush border of intestinal cells, may be dispersed in the background where they may be confused with platelets or yeast in brushing specimens.

- CMV:

  - Common infection in immunocompromised patients.
  - Characteristic cellular inclusions in glandular, stromal, and endothelial cells.
  - Nucleomegaly and cytomegaly, with large basophilic inclusions within the nucleus and occasional cytoplasmic inclusions.

- Mycobacteria:

  - Atypical mycobacterial infections (MAC) are more commonly encountered in immunocompromised patients.
  - Smears show granulomas, necrotic debris, lymphocytes, and foamy striated histiocytes (pseudo-Gaucher cells).
  - Negative images of MAC organisms can be seen on Diff-Quik stain.
  - The diagnosis can be confirmed with Ziehl-Neelsen and AFB stains.

Large Intestine: [1]

Cytology

Normal Epithelial Cells

- The role of cytology in large bowel disease is limited.
- The colonic epithelium also shows a honeycomb sheet of absorptive and goblet cells with sharply defined external edges and peripherally arranged columnar cells with evenly distributed and basally located round nuclei with regular nuclear membrane and an inconspicuous nucleolus.
- Washings may be composed predominantly of single cells, sometimes with degenerative changes.
- Background mucin is pale blue on Diff-Quik and light cyanophilic on Papanicolaou stain.
- Polymorphous lymphocytes are occasionally present.
- Smooth muscle cells from the muscularis propria and serosal mesothelial cells are occasionally present.

Reactive and Reparative Changes

- Brushings of hyperplastic polyps show similar cytomorphologic features compared to normal colonic epithelium with increased number of goblet cells.
- Reactive epithelial cells maintain their polarity within cohesive sheets, with mildly enlarged nuclei with fine chromatin, nucleoli, and mild nuclear irregular nuclear membrane.
- Inflammatory cells can be present in acute and chronic colitis.

Inflammatory Bowel Disease

- Cytology is a potential adjunct to biopsies, is particularly helpful in strictures and allows for the examination in larger mucosal surface area, highly sensitive in detecting dysplasia and malignancy.
- Mucosal brushings show cohesive aggregates of enlarged glandular epithelial cells displaying enlarged nuclei with smooth nuclear membrane, fine chromatin, and macronucleoli.
- Granulomas can be present in patients with Crohn's disease, abundant neutrophils are present in active inflammatory bowel disease.

- Differential diagnosis: malignancy and dysplasia, small aggregates with loss of normal polarity, crowding and overlapping, larger nuclei with high N:C ratio, irregular nuclear membrane, coarsely granular chromatin, and prominent nucleoli. Single cells are present.

Abscess

- Abundant acute inflammation.
- Cohesive sheets of epithelial cells with enlarged nuclei, smooth nuclear membrane, fine chromatin, and macronucleoli.

Endometriosis

- FNA is useful for the diagnosis of endometriosis.
- Tightly cohesive, three-dimensional groups of small glandular cells, stromal cells with elongated nuclei, and hemosiderin-laden macrophages.

Polyps

- Slender elongated columnar cells arranged in small clusters and single cells with long thin nuclei with fine granular chromatin and nucleoli.

Lymph Node

- The presence of GI tract mucosal fragments in EUS-FNA specimens of lymph nodes can be misinterpreted as metastatic carcinoma.
- The sampling technique, location of the lymph node, and clinical history are helpful in discerning contaminant from metastasis.
- Flat sheets of uniform cells favor gastrointestinal contaminants.

References

1. Patonay E, Geisinger K, Bergman S. Alimentary tract (esophagus, stomach, small intestine, colon, rectum, anus, biliary tract). In: Comprehensive cytopathology. 4th ed. London: Saunders; 2015.
2. Sheaff MT, Singh N. The gastrointestinal system, including the biliary tract, pancreas and liver. In: Cytopathology. London: Springer; 2013.

3. Amaro R, Poniecka A, Goldberg R. Herpes esophagitis. Gastrointest Endosc. 2000;51(1):68.
4. Juric-Sekhar G, Upton M, Swanson P, Westerhoff M. Cytomegalovirus (CMV) in gastrointestinal mucosal biopsies: should a pathologist perform CMV immunohistochemistry if the clinician requests it? Hum Pathol. 2017;60:11–5.
5. Jhala N, Jhala D. Gastrointestinal tract cytology: advancing horizons. Adv Anat Pathol. 2003;10(5):261–77.
6. Geisinger KR. Endoscopic biopsies and cytologic brushings of the esophagus are diagnostically complimentary. Am J Clin Pathol. 1995;103(3):295–9.
7. Wang H, Jonasson J, Ducatman B. Brushing cytology of the upper gastrointestinal tract. Obsolete or not ? Acta Cytol. 1991;35(2):195–8.
8. Eloubeidi M, Cohn M, Cerfolio R, Chhieng D, Jhala N, Jhala D, Eltoum I. Endoscopic ultrasound-guided fine-needle aspiration in the diagnosis of foregut duplication cysts: the value of demonstrating detached ciliary tufts in cyst fluid. Cancer Cytopathol. 2004;102(4):253–8.
9. Tang P, McKinley M, Sporrer M, Kahn E, Inlet patch. Prevalence, histologic type, and association with esophagitis, Barrett esophagus, and antritis. Arch Pathol Lab Med. 2004;128:444–7.
10. Ciocalteu A, Popa P, Ionesu M, Gheonea D. Issues and controversies in esophageal inlet patch. World J Gastroenterol. 2019;25(30):4061–73.
11. Shamoon D, Sostre V, Patel V, Volfson A. A case of heterotopic pancreatic tissue discovered in the distal esophagus. Case Rep Gastrointest Med. 2020;2020:4695184.
12. Yang L, Zhang H, Zhang X, Sun Y, Cao Z, Su Q. Synchronous occurrence of carcinoid, signet-ring cell carcinoma and heterotopic pancreatic tissue in stomach: a case report and literature review. World J Gastroenterol. 2006;12(44):7216–20.
13. Strutynska-Karpinska M, Nienartowicz M, Markowska-Woyciechowska A, Budrewicz-Czapska K. Heterotopic pancreas in the stomach (type II according to Heinrich) – literature review and case report. Pol Przegl Chir. 2011;83(3):171–4.
14. Ponder T, Collins B. Fine needle aspiration biopsy of gastric duplication cysts with endoscopic ultrasound guidance. Acta Cytol. 2003;47:571–4.
15. Napolitano V, Pezzullo A, Zeppa P, Schettino P, D'Armineto M, Palazzo A, Della Pietra C, Napolitano S, Conzo G. Foregut duplication of the stomach diagnosed by endoscopic ultrasound guided fine-needle aspiration cytology: case report and literature review. World J Surg Oncol. 2013;11:33.
16. Mendoza ML, Martin-Rabadan P, Carrion I, Morillas JD, Lopez-Alonso G, Diaz-Rubio M. Helicobacter pylori infection. Rapid diagnosis with brush cytology. Acta Cytol. 1993;37(2):181–5.
17. Mostaghni A, Afard M, Eghbali S, Kumar P. Evaluation of brushing cytology in the diagnosis of helicobacter pylori gastritis. Acta Cytol. 2008;52(5):597–601.

Chapter 13
Pancreas

Xi Wang and Guoping Cai

Anatomy and Histology of the Pancreas

The pancreas is a hammer-shaped organ located deeply in the retroperitoneum. It is divided into four grossly indistinct regions: the head, neck, body, and tail. The pancreatic head, including a blunt extension portion known as the uncinate process, is adjacent to the proximal duodenum. The neck is a short, constricted area anterior to the mesenteric vessels. The body is the midportion of the pancreas resting on the aorta. The tail flattens out as it approaches the spleen. The anterior surface of pancreas is covered by peritoneum, especially at the body and tail regions.

The pancreas has exocrine and endocrine components. The exocrine pancreas is composed of lobules made up of numerous acini, separated by the fibrous septa (Fig. 13.1). Digestive enzymes secreted from the acini drain into the duodenum by the delicate ductal system, which is lined by flattened ductal epithelium. The endocrine component accounts for a very minor portion of pancreatic tissue and consists mostly of Islets of Langerhans cells. The islet cells are small polyhedral cells with amphophilic cytoplasm. Depending on the hormones produced, the islet cells may be classified as insulin-producing β cells, glucagon-producing α cells, somatostatin-producing δ cells, and pancreatic polypeptide-producing (PP) cells, which can be identified by immunohistochemistry or electron microscopy [1, 2].

X. Wang · G. Cai (✉)
Department of Pathology, Yale School of Medicine, New Haven, CT, USA
e-mail: xi.d.wang@yale.edu; guoping.cai@yale.edu

Fig. 13.1 Histopathology
of the pancreas
(hematoxylin-eosin stain)

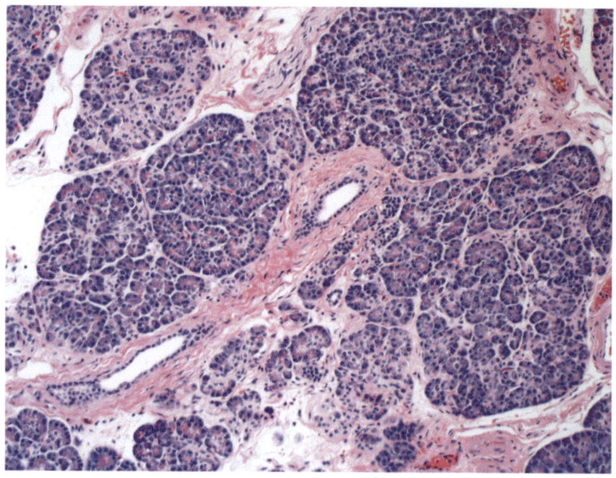

Sampling Methods

Cytological assessment is an important modality in the diagnosis of the pancreatic lesion given its complex anatomy. Traditionally, various methods are available to collect cytologic samples from the pancreas, including duodenal lavage, endoscopic cytologic sampling via the common bile duct, using ultrasound or retrograde pancreatography or pancreatic juice collection [3]. With the advent of endoscopic ultrasound-guided find needle aspiration (EUS-FNA), diagnostic FNA has become the procedure of choice for establishing the diagnosis of pancreatic lesions. EUS-FNA provides real-time visualization of the needle tip, better visualization of small lesions than CT, and can identify local invasion or metastases, thus allowing simultaneous diagnosis and staging [4]. It is well known with excellent specificity (around 100% in nearly all studies), variable sensitivity (60–96%), and rare complications (<0.5%) [5, 6]. Whenever possible, rapid on-site evaluation (ROSE) should be performed to reduce the chance of adequate sampling, especially during the evaluation for solid mass [3].

Normal Pancreas Cytology

Adequacy: The entire slide should be quickly scanned at low magnification to assess preservation and cellularity. The sample adequacy depends on the nature of the sampled lesion [7]. There is no requirement for a specific number of cells to be evaluated. The cells of pancreatic origin include acinar cells, ductal cells, and islet cells (Table 13.1).

Acinar cells: Acinar cells are the predominant cell type found in FNA from normal pancreatic tissue. They are usually arranged in small cohesive clusters or acini,

Table 13.1 Cytomorphologic features of pancreatic cells

	Acinar cells	Ductal epithelial cells	Islet cells
Arrangement	Clusters or acini, grape-like, few stripped nuclei and isolated cells	Flat cohesive, monolayer sheet, honeycomb	Large or small aggregates, in ribbons or as single cells
Cytoplasm	Abundant granular, may have fine red granules, small vacuoles	Relatively abundant, may contain vacuoles	Scant granular
Nuclei	Round	Round to slightly oval	Round to oval
Nuclear contour	Smooth	Smooth	Smooth
Chromatin	Fine granular	Fine granular	Speckled, salt and pepper
Nucleoli	Distinct	Inconspicuous	Inconspicuous

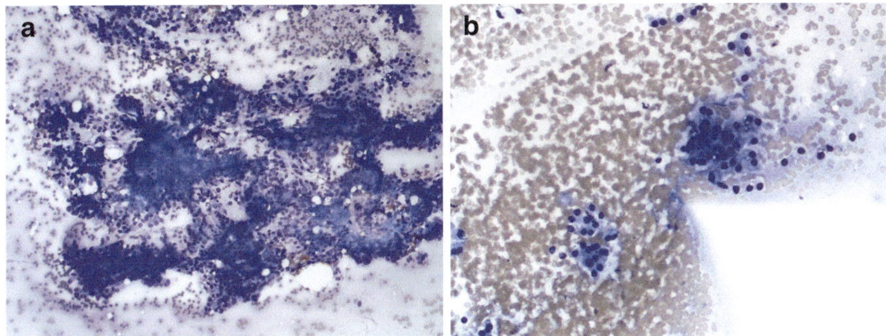

Fig. 13.2 Cytomorphology of pancreatic acinar cells. (**a**) Acinar cells in sheets and clusters; (**b**) acinar cells with acinar pattern (Diff-Quik stain)

lobulated groups, or less frequently as single cells (Fig. 13.2). The nuclei are round, relatively uniform, and often eccentrically located, with smooth nuclear contours and small but distinct nucleoli. Strapped naked nuclei are frequently seen. The chromatin is finely granular and evenly distributed. The cytoplasm is relatively abundant, which may contain small vacuoles and appear fine granular.

Ductal epithelial cells: The ductal cells are often seen as monolayered sheets of uniform cuboidal cells with centrally placed small round nuclei. The cell borders are often well defined, and the cytoplasm is transparent, giving the appearance of "honeycomb" pattern (Fig. 13.3). The nuclei have smooth contours, evenly distributed fine chromatin, and inconspicuous nucleoli. Occasionally, large areas of the ductal epithelium form thick, multilayered sheets with overlapping nuclei, raising a concern for malignancy. Close examination of the edges will reveal the above-mentioned normal cytologic features.

Islet cells: Islet cells less likely to be seen in the cytological samples of the pancreas. In the case of sclerosing cholangitis and atrophic pancreas, loose, spherical, or oval aggregates of islet cells may be present. Like other endocrine cells, islet cells have round to oval nuclei, granular "salt and pepper" like chromatin, small nucleoli, and ill-defined cell borders.

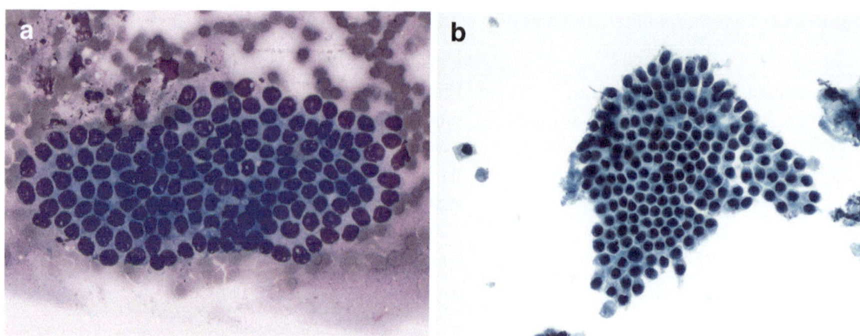

Fig. 13.3 Cytomorphology of pancreatic ductal cells. Uniform epithelial cells arranged in flat sheet. (**a**) Diff-Quik stain; (**b**) papanicolaou stain

Table 13.2 Common contaminants and their mimics

Cell type	Approach	Cytomorphology	Mimics
Gastric epithelial cells	Endoscopic transgastric (lesions in the body and tail)	Sheets of bland appearing cells with mucinous cytoplasm (foveolar cells)	Low-grade mucinous neoplasm
Gastric parietal cells and chief cells	Endoscopic transgastric (lesions in the body and tail)	In small clusters, or singly with granular cytoplasm (parietal cells)	Neuroendocrine cells
Intestinal epithelial cells	Endoscopic transduodenal (lesions in the head and uncinate)	Nonmucinous epithelium in large sheets, admixed with goblet cells, "starry sky" appearance. Intraepithelial lymphocytes are sprinkled among enterocytes "sesame seeds"	Epithelial neoplasm
Hepatocytes	Percutaneous	Polygonal cells with granular cytoplasm, prominent nucleoli, intranuclear inclusions, lipofuscin granules, and bile pigment	Oncocytic neoplasm
Mesothelial cells	Percutaneous	Flat sheets with intercellular windows	–
Splenic tissue	Percutaneous (lesions in the tail)	Predominantly lymphocytes in a vascular background	Neuroendocrine tumors; intraparenchymal lymph node

Possible cells from other organs/contaminants: Other cells may be aspirated as the needle passes through adjacent organs. Examples include gastric and intestinal epithelial cells, hepatocytes, and mesothelial cells [8] (Table 13.2). Both duodenal and gastric epithelial cells are ever-present contaminants in the EUS-FNA specimens. Like pancreatic ductal cells, they also appear as flat, monolayer sheets with honeycomb pattern. The sheet of duodenal cells is intermixed with occasional goblet cells, given a "starry sky" appearance (Fig. 13.4). Intraepithelial lymphocytes are also seen sprinkled among the enterocytes. Surface gastric foveolar cells have mucinous cytoplasm (Fig. 13.5). Other cells of gastric epithelium including chief cells and parietal cells may also be present. Hepatocytes have modest amount of granular cytoplasm and round nuclei with prominent nucleoli and occasional intranuclear inclusions. Cytoplasmic lipofuscin granules and bile pigments are frequently seen. The mesothelial cells have round to oval nuclei containing finely granular chromatin. Intercellular spaces or "windows" are characteristic features. Reactive mesothelial cells contain large distinct nucleoli, which must be distinguished from malignancy. Benign splenic tissue may be also seen on the smear for pancreatic tail lesion [9].

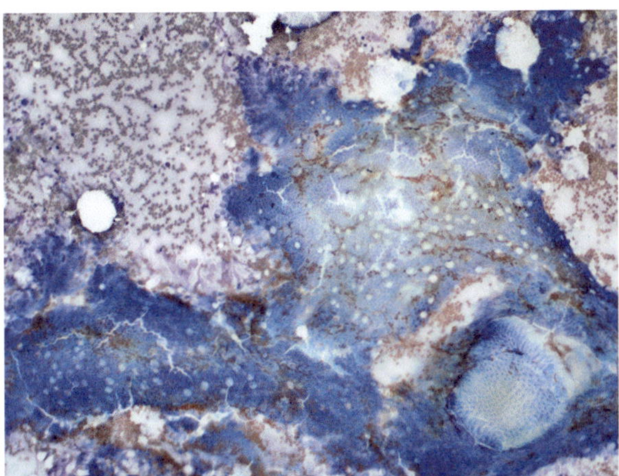

Fig. 13.4 Cytomorphology of duodenal epithelial contaminant (Diff-Quik stain)

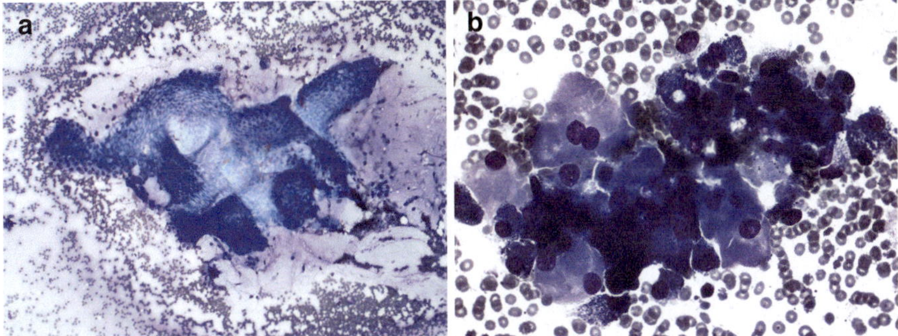

Fig. 13.5 Cytomorphology of gastric epithelial contaminant. (**a**) Foveolar epithelial cells; (**b**) mixed parietal cells and chief cells (Diff-Quik stain)

Reactive Changes

Acute Pancreatitis

The injury to the pancreatic parenchyma will result in the destruction by the digestive enzymes, leading to autodigestion of the pancreas and surrounding tissues. In
the United States, acute pancreatitis is most often caused by alcohol use, followed
by biliary stones, trauma, and medications and genetic factors. Classic clinical presentations, combined with lab findings including elevated white blood cell count,
high amylase and lipase levels, often render the clinical diagnosis of acute pancreatitis. Radiologically, it seldom appears as a mass lesion. Thus, acute pancreatitis is
rarely encountered in FNA specimens. When present, benign ducts and acinar cells
admixed with fat necrosis and inflammation components are expected.

Chronic Pancreatitis

Chronic pancreatitis is a common but yet challenging diagnosis by cytology. Patients
often have recurrent abdominal pain, with or without elevated serum amylase and
lipase. There may be bile duct obstruction and jaundice, mimicking the presentation
of pancreatic carcinoma. Chronic pancreatitis usually forms fibrosis, which appears
as a mass like lesion on imaging. Therefore, FNA is a commonly used diagnostic
method to rule out malignancy in such scenarios.

Histologically, chronic pancreatitis is characterized by fibrosis, atrophy and
dropout of acini, and variable dilation of pancreatic ducts. Islets of Langerhans are
embedded in the sclerotic tissue, which may be readily visible and appear enlarged
than normal. The dilated ductal epithelium may show hyperplasia with reactive
atypia, and even squamous metaplasia. Inflammatory cells such as lymphocytes and
plasma cells infiltrate into the stroma. Ductal dilation and intraluminal protein plugs
and calcifications are often seen in alcoholic chronic pancreatitis. In the end stage
of the disease, the ducts may be distorted by diffuse fibrosis, with or without mucinous metaplasia.

Reactive atypia associated with chronic pancreatitis should be distinguished
from well-differentiated ductal adenocarcinoma (Tables 13.3 and 13.4). Overall,
there is low cellularity in pancreatitis comparing with ductal adenocarcinoma. At
low power view, the cytological specimens of chronic pancreatitis show clusters of
ducal cells, acinar cells, and mixed inflammation (Fig. 13.6). The inflammatory
cells include neutrophils (early stage), histiocytes, lymphocytes, and plasma cells.
Relatively clean background may be seen in the late stage of chronic pancreatitis.

Characteristic features for ductal adenocarcinoma include an uneven distribution
of ductal cell clusters (drunken honeycomb) (Fig. 13.7). Isolated single abnormal
cells are also seen. The cytological atypia include irregular nuclear contours and

Table 13.3 Cytomorphologic features of chronic pancreatitis and well-differentiated adenocarcinoma

	Chronic pancreatitis	Well-differentiated adenocarcinoma
Cellularity	Low to modest	Modest to high
Cell type	Mixed ductal and acinar cells	Predominantly ductal cells
Configuration of ductal cell clusters	Honeycomb	Drunk honeycomb
Single ductal cells	Minimal	Present
Nuclear size	Enlarged	Enlarged
Anisonucleosis	Absent	Present
Nuclear crowding and overlapping	Absent	Present
Nuclear contour	Smooth	Irregular
Nucleoli	Present	Present
Background	Mixed inflammation	Clear or scattered inflammation

Table 13.4 Cytomorphologic features of common reactive conditions

Conditions	Cytomorphologic features
Acute pancreatitis	• Rarely seen in FNA samples • Benign ducts and acinar cells, fat necrosis, and inflammatory cells

Chronic pancreatitis	• Background inflammation, fat necrosis, calcific debris
	• Pancreatic elements with mild atypia:
	  – Monolayered sheets with few/rare isolated single cells
	  – Smooth nuclear membranes
	  – Low N/C ratio
	  – Mild anisonucleosis
	  – Occasional mitoses

Autoimmune pancreatitis	• Cellularly stromal fragments • Inflammatory cells including plasma cells admixed with reactive epithelial cells
Groove pancreatitis	• Spindled stromal cells, sometimes with atypia, foamy cells, and granular debris • Brunner glands can be seen
Ectopic splenic tissue	• Small lymphocytes in clusters admixed with other hematopoietic cells in a background of traversing vessels • CD8 highlighted endothelial cells of splenic sinus
Nesidioblastosis	• Neuroendocrine cells with positive insulin immunostaining

anisonucleosis. Prominent nucleoli and nuclear enlargement are common in both benign reactive and malignant conditions. Ductal carcinoma and chronic pancreatitis may co-exist, adding an additional layer of difficulty for diagnosis. A high threshold for malignancy is needed for diagnosis of malignancy in the presence of significant inflammation.

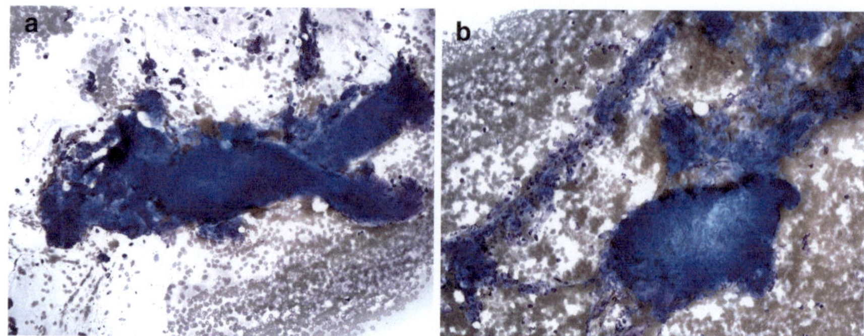

Fig. 13.6 Cytomorphology of chronic pancreatitis. (**a**) Mixed epithelial cells and stromal fragments; (**b**) stromal fragments with crushed lymphocytes (Diff-Quik stain)

Fig. 13.7 Cytomorphology of well-differentiated ductal adenocarcinoma (Papanicolaou stain)

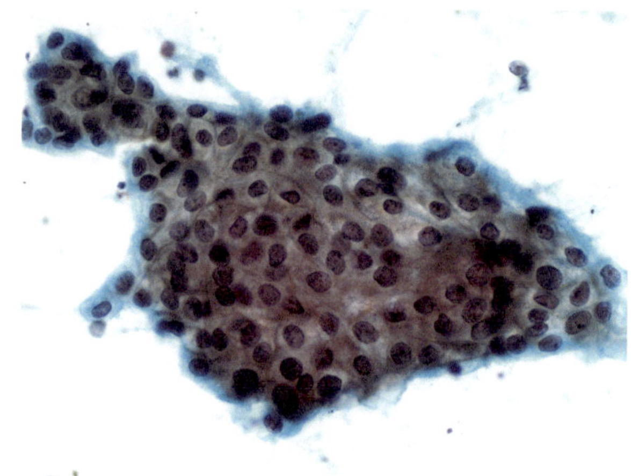

Autoimmune Pancreatitis (AIP)

AIP is a chronic inflammatory syndrome defined by clinical laboratory and pathologic criteria. Type 1 AIP is a systemic disease characterized by storiform-type fibrosis, obliterative phlebitis, and increased IgG4-positive plasma cells. Type 2 API is a pancreas-specific disorder with characteristic granulocytic epithelial lesions and occasional IgG-4 positive plasma cells [10]. It is well known that cytologic diagnosis is quite challenging given its overlapping clinical and imaging features with nonspecific chronic pancreatitis and ductal adenocarcinoma.

One of the diagnostic challenges is the cytologic atypia seen in autoimmune pancreatitis. At least 50% of cases showed varying degree of atypia, including severe atypia, as reported in the literature [10–12]. The presence of cellular stromal fragments and inflammatory cells admixed with epithelial cells may suggest the

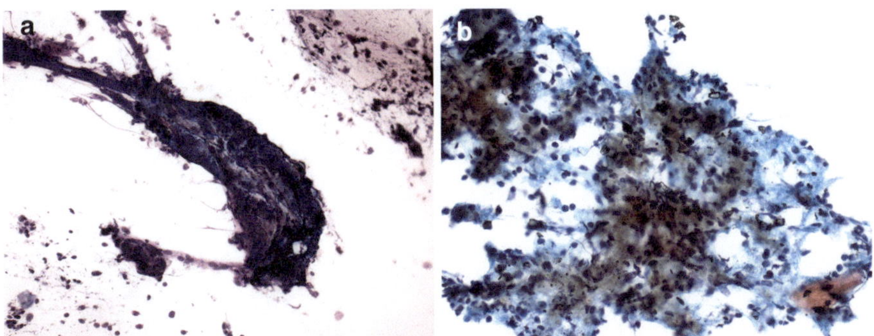

Fig. 13.8 Cytomorphology of autoimmune pancreatitis. (**a**) Stromal fragment with crushed lymphocytes, Diff-Quik stain; (**b**) loosely cohesive clusters of epithelial cells with crushed lymphocytes, Papanicolaou stain

diagnosis (Fig. 13.8). In addition, plasma cells can be rare and difficult to find in cytology samples although critical in the histological diagnosis. *KRAS* mutation may help with the differential diagnosis as it is more commonly associated with malignancy [11] although further studies are needed. Nevertheless, since the clinical management of AIP and adenocarcinoma differs significantly, it is important to keep AIP in the differential diagnosis, especially in cases with absence of classic malignant cytomorphology.

Groove Pancreatitis/Paraduodenal Pancreatitis

Groove pancreatitis, or paraduodenal pancreatitis, is an uncommon form of recurrent pancreatitis involving the "groove" region—the area between duodenum, the head of pancreas, and the common bile duct. This is an underrecognized entity often occurs in middle-aged men with alcohol use history [13]. Groove pancreatitis can cause duodenal wall fibrosis, inflammatory stroma, and duodenal wall/grove cysts mimicking mucinous cysts or pseudocysts [5]. There is limited knowledge regarding the cytopathologic features of groove pancreatitis, which are highly variable. The most common reported findings include spindled stromal cells, sometimes with atypia suggesting a spindle cell neoplasm, foamy cells, and granular debris [14]. When there forms paraduodenal wall cyst, it contains cystic contents such as debris and amorphous proteinaceous material. Bland epithelial cells with abundant foamy cytoplasm consistent with Brunner glands can also be seen [15]. Occasional mitotic figures with background necrotic debris are appreciated, leading to the suspicion for a neoplasm [13]. Florid spindle cell proliferation may also mimic gastrointestinal stromal tumor or a vascular neoplasm. Combination of clinical history, imaging studies, serology and cytologic features help leading to the suspicion for groove pancreatitis.

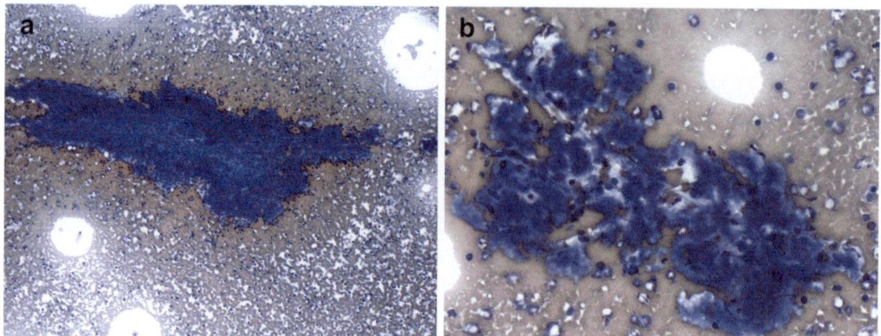

Fig. 13.9 Cytomorphology of accessary spleen. (**a**) Large lymphoid aggregate with dispersed lymphocytes; (**b**) large platelet aggregates (Diff- Quik stain)

Ectopic Splenic Tissue

Ectopic splenic tissue includes accessory spleen, a congenital anomaly, and splenosis, an acquired deposition of splenic tissue by autoimplantation after abdominal surgery or trauma. Both are not rare occurrences in the pancreas, easily mimicking a pancreatic neoplasm especially neuroendocrine tumor. The diagnosis should be considered when there are clusters of predominantly small lymphocytes admixed with other hematopoietic cells in a background of traversing small vessels [16]. Large platelet aggregates are frequently present (Fig. 13.9). The most helpful feature in the diagnosis of ectopic splenic tissue is the use of CD8 immunohistochemical staining in the cell block, which highlights the endothelial cells of the splenic sinus [17].

Nesidioblastosis

Nesidioblastosis is a heterogenous disease presented as persistent hyperinsulinemic hypoglycemia of infancy and rarely in adults. It is characterized by islet cell proliferation, thus mimicking pancreatic neuroendocrine tumor [18, 19]. Rare reports on cytologic features of nesidioblastosis showed neuroendocrine cells with positive immunostaining for insulin [20].

Cystic Lesions

The cystic lesions of the pancreas represent a broad-spectrum of entities including neoplastic and nonneoplastic. They are quite common but diagnostically challenging due to the sparse cellularity. Neoplastic cysts include mucinous (intraductal papillary mucinous neoplasms, IPMN and mucinous cystic neoplasms, MCN) and

Table 13.5 Characteristics of nonneoplastic cystic lesions in the pancreas

Entities	Cytomorphologic features	Cyst fluid analysis
Pseudocyst	• Degenerative debris, abundant inflammatory cells, histiocytes, sometimes yellow pigment and crystals • No epithelial components	High amylase (>250 U/L), often in thousands; low CEA
Retention cyst	• Nonciliated simple cuboidal or columnar epithelium which may contain mucin	
Squamoid cyst	• Squamous epithelium with eosinophilic cytoplasm may contain mucin	High CEA and amylase [24]
Lymphoepithelial cyst	• Squamous cells, squamous and amorphous debris, lymphocytes, macrophages, and cholesterol crystals	May have high CEA and amylase
Cystic lymphangioma	• Nonspecific findings including scattered lymphocytes and histocytes in the background of proteinaceous material • If applicable, CD31 and D2-40 highlight endothelial cells	High triglycerides Chylous appearance [25]
Dermoid cyst	• Benign mature squamous cells, inflammation, and keratin debris • Adnexal tissue in the cystic wall	
Epidermoid cyst of the accessory spleen	• Benign mature squamous cells, inflammation, keratin debris • Accessory splenic components	High CEA and CA19-9 reported [29, 31]
Duplication cyst/ ciliated foregut cyst	• Ciliated epithelial cells, mucinous material, histiocytes and amorphous proteinaceous debris • Duplication cyst has muscle layers	
ADPKD-associated cyst	• Simple epithelial cyst: small flat bland epithelial cells in a honey-comb pattern	
VHL-associated cyst	• Serous lining cyst, similar to serous cystadenoma	*VHL* gene mutation detected

nonmunicous cysts (serous cystadenomas, SCA, solid pseudopapillary tumors, cystic pancreatic neuroendocrine tumors, and other rare cystic malignancy). Nonneoplastic cysts include pseudocysts, lymphoepithelial cysts, retention cysts, cystic lymphangioma, and other congenital cysts. Here we will be focusing on the cytologic features and differential diagnosis for nonneoplastic cysts (Table 13.5).

Pseudocyst

As the most common nonneoplastic cystic lesion, pancreatic pseudocysts usually occur after acute or chronic pancreatitis. The diagnosis is often based on the patient's clinical history and imaging findings. Cytologically, it composed of degenerative debris, abundant inflammatory cells, histiocytes, and sometimes yellow pigment

Fig. 13.10 Cytomorphology of pancreatic pseudocyst (Diff-Quik stain)

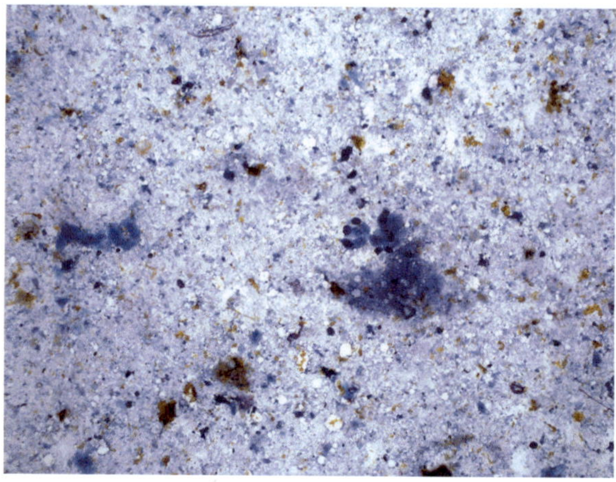

and crystals (Fig. 13.10) [21]. Pseudocysts have no epithelial lining by definition; thus, the presence of epithelial cells should raise a concern for a cystic neoplasm rather than pseudocysts. Pseudocysts should have high level of amylase (often in thousands) while low concentration of CEA, which is helpful for differentiation from IPMN and MCN [22].

Retention Cyst/Squamoid Cyst

Retention cysts are small (0.5–1.0 cm) cysts commonly associated with pancreatic duct obstruction or narrowing with upstream pancreatic duct dilation [21]. They are lined by nonciliated simple cuboidal or columnar epithelium which may contain mucin. A mucin-containing retention cyst should be differentiated from other neoplastic mucinous cysts, which often have intramural nodules or a solid component. Squamoid cyst is a distinct type of retention cyst lined by squamous epithelium, resulting from unilocular cystic dilatation of pancreatic ducts due to obstruction [23, 24].

Lymphoepithelial Cyst (LEC)

Pancreatic LECs are uncommon cysts that are similar to branchial cleft cysts in the neck, occurring predominantly in middle-aged men. Histologically, they are characterized by stratified squamous epithelium surrounded by dense lymphoid tissue with lymphoid follicles. On FNA aspirate, they typically contain squamous cells, squamous and amorphous debris, lymphocytes, macrophages, and cholesterol crystals. LECs may contain elevated CEA and amylase, leading to potential confusion with mucinous neoplasms. Occasionally, mucus cells and the sebaceous differentiation are present, which should be differentiated from dermoid cysts.

Cystic Lymphangioma

Cystic lymphangiomas are congenital malformations of the lymphatic system resulted from the blockage of lymphatic flow leading to the development of lymphangiectasias. Pancreatic cystic lymphangiomas are rare indolent findings, tending to occur more commonly in women. The aspirate cyst fluid is usually chylous, serous, or serosanguineous [25]. High triglyceride contents, if present, can help confirm the diagnosis. FNA usually shows nonspecific findings such as scattered lymphocytes and histocytes in the background of proteinaceous material. Immunostains of endothelial markers CD31 and D2-40, if performed on the cell block, could highlight the cystic lining [21].

Dermoid Cyst

Dermoid cyst, also called cystic teratoma, is a rare benign lesion in the pancreas [26]. Cytomorphologic features include benign mature squamous cells, inflammation, and abundant keratin debris. Adnexal tissues are present within the cystic wall, which distinguishes dermoid cyst from epidermoid cyst. Mucicarmine stains may be helpful to rule out mucinous lesions.

Epidermoid Cyst of Accessory Spleen

An epidermoid cyst arising within an intrapancreatic accessory spleen is an extremely rare entity, the majority of which were reported from Asia [27–29]. The histogenesis is thought to be mesothelial cells from the spleen parenchyma form an inclusion cyst with subsequent squamous metaplasia [30]. While the detection of solid components associated with an accessory spleen might be the diagnostic clue, only a few cases were diagnosed preoperatively. In addition, cases with abnormally high CA19-9 and CEA have been reported [29, 31], making it difficult to distinguish from malignant tumors. Nevertheless, it is helpful to keep this entity in mind when a cystic lesion encountered especially in the pancreatic tail.

Duplication Cyst/Ciliated Foregut Cyst

Enteric duplication cysts are very rare congenital malformations of the foregut that can be found in the head of pancreas. The cytomorphologic features include a mix of epithelial cells, mucinous material, histiocytes, and amorphous proteinaceous debris. The epithelial lining can be squamous, columnar, gastric, or normal intestinal and is often ciliated [21]. On histological examination, duplication cysts contain layers of smooth muscle cells, recapitulating those of normal gut. Those without muscle cells should be designated as ciliated foregut cyst (CFC) [32]. The differential diagnosis includes bronchogenic cysts which contain cartilage and respiratory glands [33].

Others

Solitary cysts occur in patients with autosomal dominant polycystic kidney disease (ADPKD). Although the lesions are not often biopsied, FNA can help rule out other cystic lesions or malignancy in those patients. FNA aspirate has a simple epithelial cyst appearance, consisting of small flat group of uniform epithelial cells in a honeycomb pattern [34]. The pancreatic cysts seen in the patients with von Hippel-Lindau disease are similar to findings of serous cystadenomas, with serous lining cells with distinct cytoplasmic borders. Instead of forming a distinct lesion, VHL-associated cysts are often distributed irregularly. *VHL* gene mutations are detected in those lesions [35].

Ancillary Testing

As mentioned above, a number of ancillary tests have been utilized to help with the diagnosis of pancreatic cystic neoplasms. The cystic fluid biochemical analysis, including CEA and amylase levels, is one of the most important ones to help differentiate between mucinous and nonmucinous cysts [36, 37]. Of note, the cutoff value may differ among institutions and vary for different assays, which should be validated.

CEA: So far, the most accurate tumor markers for mucinous cysts remains CEA [38, 39]. It has been well known that high level of CEA is typically associated with cystic carcinomas and mucinous cysts [39]. While the generally accepted cutoff value is >192 ng/mL (accuracy of 79%), studies have shown the level >800 ng/mL are highly predicative for mucinous neoplasms (specificity of 98%). In contrast, a very low CEA level <5 ng/mL strongly suggests a serous cystadenoma or a pseudocyst (specificity of 95%) [38].

Amylase: This pancreatic enzyme levels are often used to distinguish between pseudocysts and neoplastic cyst [40]. Pseudocysts consistently contain elevated levels of amylase, typically in thousand units per liter.

Background Features

Necrotic background is one of the most common background features for pancreatic malignancy [41]; thus, nonneoplastic debris should be differentiated from tumor necrosis. Tumor necrosis associated with pancreatic ductal adenocarcinoma can be either diffuse or focal, associated with slightly atypical or evidently malignant cells [42]. As necrosis can be also seen in nonneoplastic conditions such as pancreatitis or cystic degeneration [43], investigating the presence and frequency of atypical and malignant cells is critical.

Mucinous background is one of the diagnostic findings for mucinous neoplasms such as IPMNs, MCNs, and colloid carcinomas. Therefore, it is important to avoid misinterpretation for mucinous background in the presence of gastric contamination. Gastroduodenal mucin seems to be watery or colloid-like, while neoplastic mucins are thicker [44]. In addition, conventional smear is superior than liquid-based cytology for the evaluation of mucinous background. Nevertheless, it is challenging to distinguish different types of mucins, the cytologic features should be interpretate in combination of the clinical context and imaging findings. For example, in the right clinical setting, abundant thick mucin alone may suggest the diagnosis of mucinous neoplasm [21]. On the other hand, scant thin mucin seen with low-grade mucinous epithelium is indistinguishable from that of normal gastric epithelium.

Acknowledgments None.

Conflict of Interest None.

References

1. Herzberg AJ, Raso DS, Silverman JF. Color atlas of normal cytology. New York: Churchill Livingstone; 1999.
2. Koss LG, Melamed MR. Koss' diagnostic cytology and its histopathologic bases. 5th ed. Philadelphia: Lippincott Williams & Wilkins; 2006.
3. Pitman MB, Layfield LJ. Guidelines for pancreaticobiliary cytology from the Papanicolaou Society of Cytopathology: a review. Cancer Cytopathol. 2014;122(6):399–411.
4. Erickson RA, Garza AA. Impact of endoscopic ultrasound on the management and outcome of pancreatic carcinoma. Am J Gastroenterol. 2000;95(9):2248–54.
5. Reid MD. Cytologic assessment of cystic/intraductal lesions of the pancreatobiliary tract. Arch Pathol Lab Med. 2022;146(3):280–97.

6. Ylagan LR, et al. Endoscopic ultrasound guided fine-needle aspiration cytology of pancreatic carcinoma: a 3-year experience and review of the literature. Cancer. 2002;96(6):362–9.

7. Conrad R, et al. Cytopathology of the pancreatobiliary tract—the agony, and sometimes, the ease of it. J Gastrointest Oncol. 2013;4(2):210–9.

8. Pitman MB, et al. Standardized terminology and nomenclature for pancreatobiliary cytology: the Papanicolaou Society of Cytopathology Guidelines. Cytojournal. 2014;11(Suppl 1):3.

9. Cibas ES, Ducatman BS. Cytology: diagnostic principles and clinical correlates. 5th ed. Philadelphia: Saunders/Elsevier; 2019.

10. Deshpande V, et al. Endoscopic ultrasound guided fine needle aspiration biopsy of autoimmune pancreatitis: diagnostic criteria and pitfalls. Am J Surg Pathol. 2005;29(11):1464–71.

11. Cai G, et al. Endoscopic ultrasound-guided fine-needle aspiration biopsy of autoimmune pancreatitis: diagnostic clues and pitfalls. J Am Soc Cytopathol. 2015;4(4):211–7.

12. Thangaiah JJ, et al. Revisiting the cytologic features of autoimmune pancreatitis: an institutional experience. Cancer Cytopathol. 2023;131(4):234–44.

13. DeSouza K, Nodit L. Groove pancreatitis: a brief review of a diagnostic challenge. Arch Pathol Lab Med. 2015;139(3):417–21.

14. Chute DJ, Stelow EB. Fine-needle aspiration features of paraduodenal pancreatitis (groove pancreatitis): a report of three cases. Diagn Cytopathol. 2012;40(12):1116–21.

15. Brosens LA, et al. EUS-guided FNA cytology diagnosis of paraduodenal pancreatitis (groove pancreatitis) with numerous giant cells: conservative management allowed by cytological and radiological correlation. Cytopathology. 2015;26(2):122–5.

16. Tatsas AD, et al. Fine-needle aspiration of intrapancreatic accessory spleen: cytomorphologic features and differential diagnosis. Cancer Cytopathol. 2012;120(4):261–8.

17. Saunders TA, Miller TR, Khanafshar E. Intrapancreatic accessory spleen: utilization of fine needle aspiration for diagnosis of a potential mimic of a pancreatic neoplasm. J Gastrointest Oncol. 2016;7(Suppl 1):S62–5.

18. Hong R, Choi DY, Lim SC. Hyperinsulinemic hypoglycemia due to diffuse nesidioblastosis in adults: a case report. World J Gastroenterol. 2008;14(1):140–2.

19. Bergeron JP, et al. Endoscopic ultrasound-guided pancreatic fine-needle aspiration: potential pitfalls in one institution's experience of 1212 procedures. Cancer Cytopathol. 2015;123(2):98–107.

20. Catton JA, et al. Diffuse nesidioblastosis causing hyperinsulinemic hypoglycemia: the importance of pancreatic sampling on EUS. Gastrointest Endosc. 2008;68(3):571–2; discussion 572.

21. Abdelkader A, et al. Cystic lesions of the pancreas: differential diagnosis and cytologic-histologic correlation. Arch Pathol Lab Med. 2020;144(1):47–61.

22. Brugge WR. Diagnosis and management of cystic lesions of the pancreas. J Gastrointest Oncol. 2015;6(4):375–88.

23. Park JI. Squamoid cyst of pancreatic ducts: a case report. Ann Hepatobiliary Pancreat Surg. 2021;25(2):293–8.

24. Hanson JA, Salem RR, Mitchell KA. Squamoid cyst of pancreatic ducts: a case series describing novel immunohistochemistry, cytology, and quantitative cyst fluid chemistry. Arch Pathol Lab Med. 2014;138(2):270–3.

25. Carvalho D, et al. Cystic pancreatic lymphangioma—diagnostic role of endoscopic ultrasound. GE Port J Gastroenterol. 2016;23(5):254–8.

26. Lee SE, et al. Dermoid cyst of the pancreas: a rare cystic neoplasm. Int J Surg Case Rep. 2015;17:72–4.

27. Kato S, et al. Epidermoid cyst in an intrapancreatic accessory spleen: case report and literature review of the preoperative imaging findings. Intern Med. 2016;55(23):3445–52.

28. Matsumoto K, Kato H, Okada H. Epidermoid cyst in an intrapancreatic accessory spleen diagnosed by typical radiographic images and endoscopic ultrasound fine-needle aspiration findings with contrast agent. Clin Gastroenterol Hepatol. 2018;16(2):e13–4.

29. Lo CH, et al. Epidermoid cyst in an intrapancreatic accessory spleen with abnormally high CEA level in cyst fluid: a case report. Autops Case Rep. 2022;12:e2021369.

30. Burrig KF. Epithelial (true) splenic cysts. Pathogenesis of the mesothelial and so-called epidermoid cyst of the spleen. Am J Surg Pathol. 1988;12(4):275–81.
31. Takagi C, et al. Epidermoid cyst within an intrapancreatic accessory spleen exhibiting abrupt changes in serum carbohydrate antigen 19-9 level: a case report. Surg Case Rep. 2020;6(1):133.
32. Dua KS, et al. Ciliated foregut cyst of the pancreas: preoperative diagnosis using endoscopic ultrasound guided fine needle aspiration cytology—a case report with a review of the literature. Cytojournal. 2009;6:22.
33. Huang H, Solanki MH, Giorgadze T. Cytomorphology of ciliated foregut cyst of the pancreas. Diagn Cytopathol. 2019;47(4):347–50.
34. Silverman JF, Prichard J, Regueiro MD. Fine needle aspiration cytology of a pancreatic cyst in a patient with autosomal dominant polycystic kidney disease. A case report. Acta Cytol. 2001;45(3):415–9.
35. Volkan Adsay N. Cystic lesions of the pancreas. Mod Pathol. 2007;20(Suppl 1):S71–93.
36. Martin AK, Zhou Z. Endoscopic ultrasound-guided fine-needle aspiration for the diagnosis of pancreatic cysts by combined cytopathology and cystic content analysis. World J Gastrointest Endosc. 2015;7(15):1157–69.
37. Talar-Wojnarowska R, et al. Pancreatic cyst fluid analysis for differential diagnosis between benign and malignant lesions. Oncol Lett. 2013;5(2):613–6.
38. van der Waaij LA, van Dullemen HM, Porte RJ. Cyst fluid analysis in the differential diagnosis of pancreatic cystic lesions: a pooled analysis. Gastrointest Endosc. 2005;62(3):383–9.
39. Hammel P, et al. Preoperative cyst fluid analysis is useful for the differential diagnosis of cystic lesions of the pancreas. Gastroenterology. 1995;108(4):1230–5.
40. Pitman MB, et al. Pancreatic cysts: preoperative diagnosis and clinical management. Cancer Cytopathol. 2010;118(1):1–13.
41. Hirabayashi K, Saika T, Nakamura N. Background features in the cytology of pancreatic neoplasms. DEN Open. 2022;2(1):e105.
42. Mitsuhashi T, et al. Endoscopic ultrasound-guided fine needle aspiration of the pancreas: cytomorphological evaluation with emphasis on adequacy assessment, diagnostic criteria and contamination from the gastrointestinal tract. Cytopathology. 2006;17(1):34–41.
43. Rau B, et al. Role of ultrasonographically guided fine-needle aspiration cytology in the diagnosis of infected pancreatic necrosis. Br J Surg. 1998;85(2):179–84.
44. Geramizadeh B, et al. Intraductal papillary mucinous neoplasm of the pancreas: cytomorphology, imaging, molecular profile, and prognosis. Cytopathology. 2021;32(4):397–406.

Chapter 14
Liver and Biliary Tract

Xi Wang and Guoping Cai

The Liver

Anatomy and Histology of the Liver

The liver is a wedge-shaped intra-abdominal organ beneath the diaphragm. It is enveloped by peritoneal reflections except an area on the posterior surface. The liver is divided by deep grooves into two large lobes, the left and right lobes, and two small lobes, the caudate and quadrate lobes [1]. The dual blood supply of the liver includes the portal vein and hepatic artery, which enter the liver at the porta hepatis. Venous blood drains via the left and right hepatic veins, eventually into the inferior vena cava [2].

Histologically, the liver consists of hexagonal lobules, with the central vein in the center and hepatocytes radiating outwards (Fig. 14.1). Three to six portal tracts are located at the periphery of the lobules, composing of the portal vein, the hepatic arterioles, bile ducts, and ductules and lymphatic vessels invested by connective tissue.

A more generally accepted classification is the acinar units defined by Rappaport, based on the circulatory flow in the liver. This three-dimensional, spherical shaped compound acinus is subdivided into zones 1, 2, 3 with decreasing oxygenation and increasing susceptibility to injury. Zone 1 surrounds the portal tract; zone 3 lines the acinar periphery; while zone 2 is positioned between zone 1 and 3. Blood flows from the terminal portal vein and hepatic arteriole, through the sinusoids into the terminal hepatic venules at the periphery of the acinus.

X. Wang · G. Cai (✉)
Department of Pathology, Yale School of Medicine, New Haven, CT, USA
e-mail: xi.d.wang@yale.edu; guoping.cai@yale.edu

S. M. Gilani, G. Cai (eds.), *Non-Neoplastic Cytology*,
https://doi.org/10.1007/978-3-031-44289-6_14

247

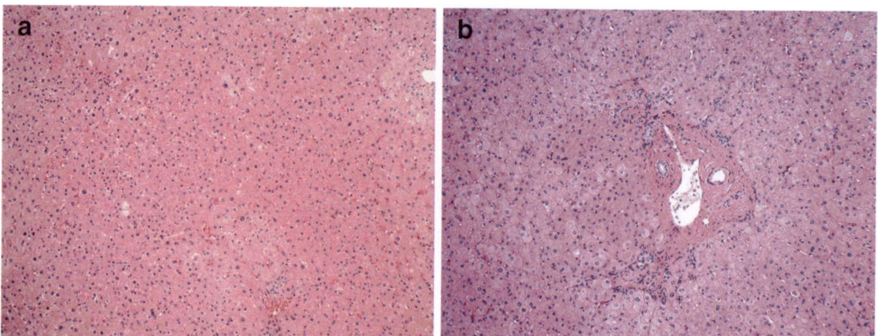

Fig. 14.1 Histopathology of the liver. (**a**) Hexagonal lobule of the liver parenchyma (Hematoxylin-eosin stain). (**b**) Liver parenchyma around the portal tract (Hematoxylin-eosin stain)

Sampling Methods

The diagnosis of liver mass is generally accomplished by fine needle aspiration (FNA) and core needle biopsy, whether percutaneously with guidance by computed tomography (CT), ultrasonography, magnetic resonance imaging (MRI), or more recently with the aid of endoscopic ultrasonography (EUS) [3–7]. The large core needle biopsy is usually reserved for diffuse liver disease including hepatitis and cirrhosis, with at least six complete portal tracts to be adequate for evaluation [8]. The sensitivity and specificity of FNA in the liver lesions have been well established, with an overall accuracy above 90% [3, 5, 6, 9, 10]. EUS-FNA has also been used for the diagnosis of tumors at the hilum of the liver, especially cholangiocarcinoma [11, 12].

Normal Cytology

Hepatocytes and bile duct cells are common components of the liver aspirate, and occasionally in aspirates of adjacent organs including the pancreas, right kidney, right adrenal gland, etc. Other cell types, such as sinusoidal endothelial cells, Kupffer cells, and mesothelial cells from the peritoneal reflection can also be seen. Gastrointestinal epithelial cells are commonly seen as contaminants in the EUS-FNA specimens.

Normal and reactive hepatocytes are the largest cells found in the liver aspirates. They are flat polygonal with well-demarcated cellular contours, sometimes with clean, thin linear spaces between adjacent hepatocytes as bile canaliculi. Isolated cells, thin ribbons (trabeculae), or large tissue fragments can be present [8]. Hepatocytes usually contain one or two round central to eccentric nuclei and granular foamy cytoplasm (Fig. 14.2). The nuclei have a smooth membrane, evenly distributed granular chromatin, and one to two distinct nucleoli. The nucleoli stain

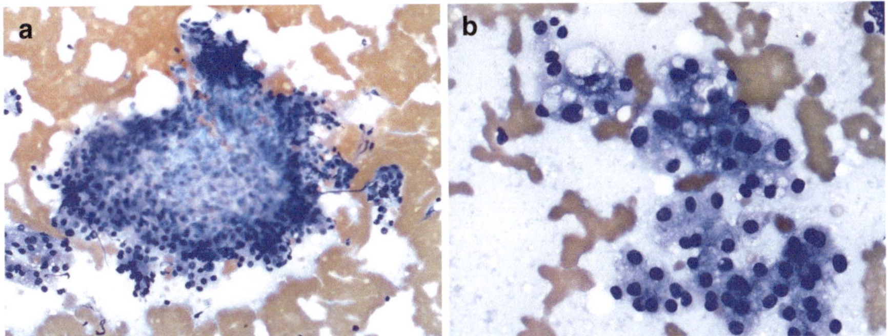

Fig. 14.2 Benign hepatocytes. (**a**) Cohesive cluster of hepatocytes (Diff-Quik stain). (**b**) Loosely cohesive cluster of hepatocytes with granular cytoplasm, intracytoplasmic vacuoles, and round nuclei (Diff-Quik stain)

deep red in Diff-Quik stains and blue with Papanicolaou staining [2]. Binucleation and mild anisonucleosis is normal, especially in older individuals with increased polyploid DNA content, and should be distinguished from malignancy. Stripped naked nuclei can be seen in normal liver FNA and are not exclusive to hepatocellular carcinoma. Intranuclear pseudoinclusions are not uncommon. Reactive hepatocytes may show variations in size and some degree of pleomorphism; however, a low nucleocytoplasmic (N/C) ratio should be maintained.

Pigments in hepatocytes Hepatocytes have abundant granular cytoplasm containing pigments (Table 14.1 and Fig. 14.3).

- **Lipofuscin** is a very common fine nonrefractile pigment which appears golden with Papanicolaou stains and green-brown with Diff-Quik stains. It is composed of tertiary lysosomes that accumulate as end products of intracellular digestion, thus commonly seen in older individuals. Lipofuscin can be stained with acid-fast stain (Fite stain) without clinical significance; however, it may be confused with other pathologic pigments [13].
- **Hemosiderin** is relatively uncommon coarse refractile pigment which appears yellow-brown with Papanicolaou staining and blue-green in Diff-Quik stains. It can be confirmed by iron staining such as Prussian blue. The presence of hemosiderin may indicate iron overload that leading to cirrhosis. When present in large quantities, disorders of iron metabolism such as hemochromatosis or hemosiderosis should be considered. Hemosiderin can also be seen in Kupffer cells.
- **Bile pigment** is nonrefractile pigment stains green to greenish-brown in Papanicolaou staining, and dark blue in Diff-Quik staining. It is only produced by hepatocytes and often observed in intercellular bile canaliculi. Accumulation of bile in benign hepatocytes is associated with hepatitis and obstructive jaundice. On the other hand, bile in the cytoplasm of malignant cells is diagnostic of HCC [13].

Table 14.1 Cytoplasmic pigments of normal/reactive hepatocytes

Pigments	Characteristics	Papanicolaou staining	Diff-Quik staining	Special stains	Significance
Lipofuscin	Fine nonrefractile	Golden	Green-brown	Acid fast (Fite)	Normal; end product of intracellular digestion (aging)
Hemosiderin	Coarse refractile	Yellow-brown	Blue-green	Iron stain (Prussian blue)	Iron deposition, may be seen in iron overload conditions (hemochromatosis, hemosiderosis, etc.)
Bile	Nonrefractile	Green-brown	Dark blue		• Normal in benign hepatocytes: accumulation may be associated with hepatitis or jaundice • In malignant hepatocytes: diagnostic for HCC
Copper	Coarse nonrefractile	Green-brown		Copper stain	Copper metabolism disorders (Wilson's disease, PBC, etc.)
Melanin	Nonrefractile	Brown	Blue		Metastatic melanoma

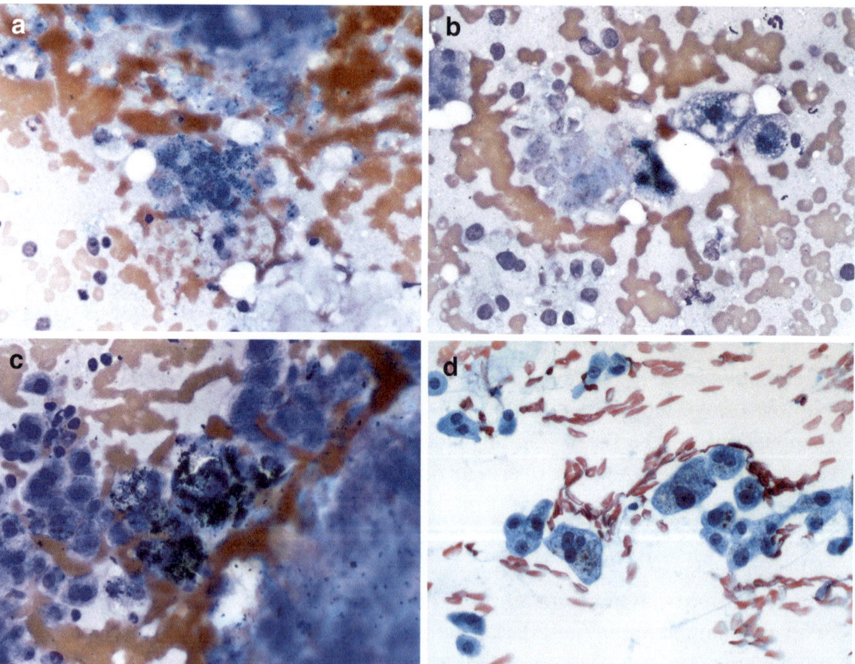

Fig. 14.3 Pigments in hepatocytes. (**a, b**) Bile pigments in hepatocytes (Diff-Quik stain). (**c, d**) Hemosiderin pigments in hepatocytes (**c** Diff-Quik stain; **d** Papanicolaou stain)

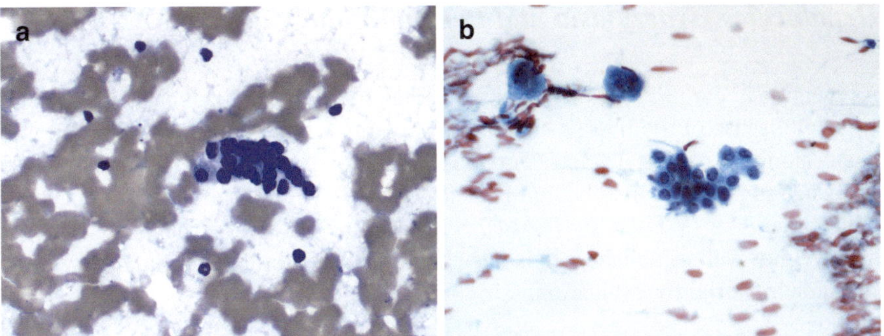

Fig. 14.4 Benign bile ductal epithelial cells (**a** Diff-Quik stain; **b** Papanicolaou stain)

- **Copper** is a coarse, green-brown pigment seen in the cytoplasm of hepatocytes in the patients with copper metabolism disorders, such as Wilson's disease, primary biliary cirrhosis (PBC), and other chronic cholestatic disease. Copper special stains highlight the pigments.
- **Melanin** is usually associated with melanoma metastasized to the liver. It stains brown in Papanicolaou staining and blue in Diff-Quik staining. It may also be phagocytized by Kupffer cells.

Bile duct cells are less frequently encountered in the liver FNA. The epithelial cells of the interlobular bile ducts, smaller ducts in portal tracts, are cuboidal shaped cells smaller than hepatocytes. The cells have round nuclei with smooth contours, evenly distributed chromatin, inconspicuous nucleoli, and scant cytoplasm (Fig. 14.4). They are often arranged in flat sheets and clusters. In contrast, the intralobular bile ducts have tall columnar epithelium, usually arranged in a palisaded, picket fence-like configuration. The cells have basally located nuclei and a moderate amount of cytoplasm on the luminal side. Sometimes they are arranged in sheets with evenly distributed nuclei, while the columnar epithelium can be appreciated at the edges.

Sinusoidal endothelial cells have elongated spindle-shaped nuclei with fine chromatin and relatively scant cytoplasm. The tips can be blunt or pointed. **Kupffer cells** often have a bean-shaped nucleus and stellate cytoplasmic projections. Occasionally, **mesothelial cells** from the peritoneal reflections can be found in liver aspirate. They have ovoid nuclei with very fine chromatin, tiny nucleoli, are often arranged in flat sheets with intercellular spaces (windows). The sheets are sometimes folded. Single mesothelial cells can also be seen.

Hepatocytes Hyperplasia and Regeneration

As mentioned earlier, FNA is of limited value regarding the diagnosis of diffuse or medical disease of the liver, which usually requires tissue biopsies to include adequate numbers of portal tracts. For most FNAs of the liver, the main diagnostic challenge is to distinguish benign liver lesions from well-differentiated hepatocellular carcinoma (WD-HCC) [8, 14]. Standardized criteria for hepatocyte atypia have yet not well established, thus one should be careful to diagnose HCC without sufficient material for evaluation.

Focal nodular hyperplasia (FNH) and hepatocellular adenoma (HCA) Both FNH and HCA are benign hepatic lesions often occur in non-cirrhotic livers of young women, with the latter strongly associated with oral contraceptive pills (OCPs). FNH is often an incidental finding on imaging while HCA are mostly symptomatic, with symptoms ranging from abdominal pain to circulatory collapse in the setting of acute rupture or hemorrhage. On imaging, FNH most commonly presents as a well-demarcated solitary mass with a characteristic central scar, which can be diagnosed alone without tissue diagnosis. MRI has been reported to have high sensitivity and specificity for the diagnosis of HCA, thus tissue sampling is only needed when imaging findings are not typical [15].

Histologically, FNH is characterized by a central fibrotic tissue containing abnormally thick-walled vessels and ductular reaction admixed with inflammatory cells. By immunohistochemistry, FNH demonstrates classic "map-like" pattern by glutamine synthetase (GS) staining. HCA is composed of bland hepatocytes with absence of central veins and portal triads [16].

Cytologically, both lesions comprise bland appearing hepatocytes forming loosely cohesive sheets and clusters (Fig. 14.5) [17]. For FNH, bile duct epithelium and stromal fragments may be present while HCA usually contains hepatocytes only [17–19]. Reactive atypia can be seen, such as increased number of binucleated cells, hyperchromasia, anisocytosis, and coarse chromatin; however, the low nuclear to cytoplasmic (N/C) ratio should be maintained [20]. Hemorrhage and necrosis may be seen in HCA.

Differentiating HCA from well-differentiated HCC can be challenging due to the morphologic overlap, especially on small biopsies (Table 14.2). One helpful diagnostic clue for HCC is the presence of either basketing-endothelial cells wrap around hepatocytes, or traversing capillaries through groups of hepatocytes, both of which are rarely seen in benign lesions (Fig. 14.6). Another feature that favors WD-HCC is the presence of prominent "cherry red" nucleoli and acinar formation [17]. Ancillary studies may be helpful if there are cell blocks available. A reticulin stain can highlight the intact reticulin network in HCA while outline the thickened trabeculae that seen in HCC. CD34 highlights arterialization of sinusoids which are typically seen in HCC. Not uncommonly, some HCAs may not be distinguishable from WD-HCC on aspirates or small biopsies, which may be reported as "well-differentiated hepatocytic neoplasm/lesion" or hepatocytic neoplasm of uncertain potential (HUMP) [21, 22].

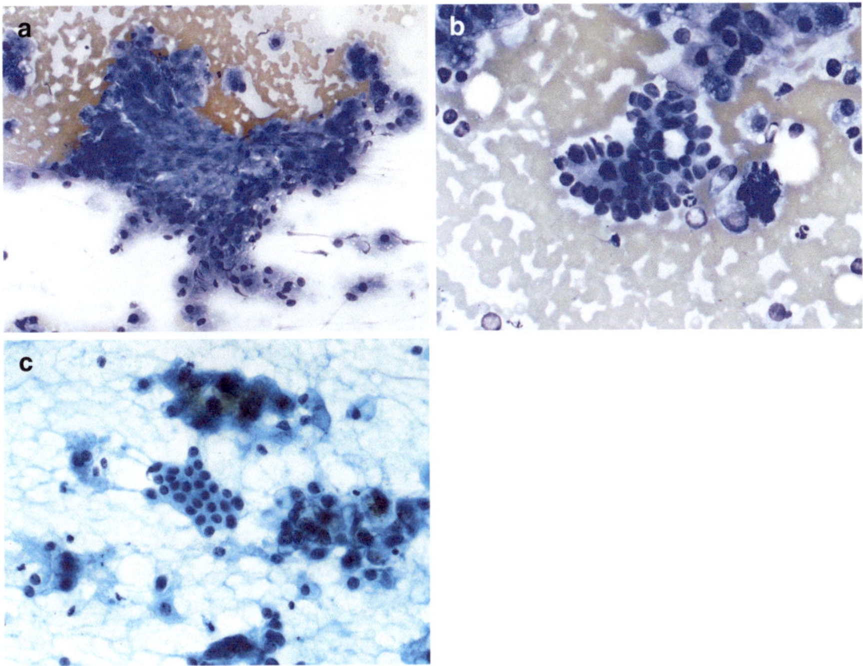

Fig. 14.5 Focal nodular hyperplasia. (**a**) Cluster of benign-appearing hepatocytes (Diff-Quik stain). (**b, c**) Mixed reactive hepatocytes and bile duct epithelial cells (**b** Diff-Quik stain; **c** Papanicolaou stain)

Table 14.2 Cytomorphologic features of benign hepatic disorders and well-differentiated hepatocellular carcinoma

	Cytomorphologic features	IHC
Focal nodular hyperplasia	• Benign hepatocytes in sheets or clusters • Bile duct epithelium or stromal fragment (fibrotic) may be present • Reactive atypia	• "Map like" pattern on glutamine synthetase staining
Hepatocellular adenoma	• Benign hepatocytes in sheets or clusters • Hepatocytes only, no bile duct epithelium • Reactive atypia	• Depending on the subtypes of HCA: L-FABP, SSA/CRP, b-catenin, GS [16]
Cirrhosis	• Hyperplastic hepatocytes • Ductal epithelium may be present • Reactive atypia	
WD-HCC	• Hypercellular smears • Thickened cords (>2 cells thick) of cohesive malignant hepatocytes: high N/C ratio, large nucleus with prominent nucleolus, intranuclear pseudoinclusions • Endothelial wrapping • Transgressing vessels • Pseudoacini containing bile • Atypical large naked nuclei • Bile duct epithelial cells, if present, are few and apart	• CD34 highlights sinusoidal capillarization • CK19 demonstrates absence of ductular reaction • HepPar1, ARG-1 (arginase-1), polyclonal carcinoembryonic antigen (pCEA), etc. [26]

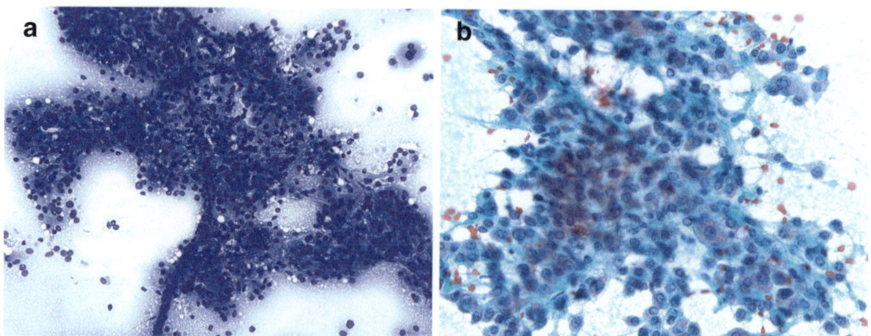

Fig. 14.6 Well-differentiated hepatocellular carcinoma: clusters of hepatocytes with prominent transgressing blood vessels (**a** Diff-Quik stain; **b** Papanicolaou stain)

Cirrhosis

Cirrhosis is an irreversible process at the end stage of alcoholic liver disease, chronic viral hepatitis, or other diseases. Excessive growth of connective tissue led to the disruption of the normal liver architecture, resulting in the fibrous bands separating regenerative nodules. These sometimes may mimic malignancy on imaging. Given that cirrhotic patients are at increased risks for developing hepatocellular carcinoma, it is critical to differentiate cirrhosis from HCC.

Cytologically, cirrhotic liver is similar to that of normal liver (Fig. 14.7). Aspirates show hyperplastic hepatocytes, bile ductal epithelium, endothelial cells, and Kupffer cells, along with features of regeneration and repair [23]. Reactive atypia including increased N/C ratio, variable nuclear size, coarse chromatin, prominent nucleoli, and binucleation can be seen. Again, it can be challenging to differentiate a "dysplastic nodule" and HCC on cytology alone. The presence of bile ductular epithelium usually indicates parenchymal-stromal interface restoration, which favor benign lesion [23].

Cystic Lesions of the Liver (Table 14.3 and Fig. 14.8)

Echinococcal Cyst (Hydatid Cyst)

Human cystic echinococcosis, or hydatid cyst disease is caused by the larval form of *Echinococcus granulosus*. Dogs are the definitive hosts while sheep are the major intermediate host. Although Hippocrates have recognized hydatid disease more than 2000 years ago, hydatid cyst remains endemic in sheep-raising areas including countries bordering the Mediterranean and Baltic seas, in Africa, Australia and New Zealand [24]. The most common infected site is the liver, followed by the lung, the brain, and other viscera.

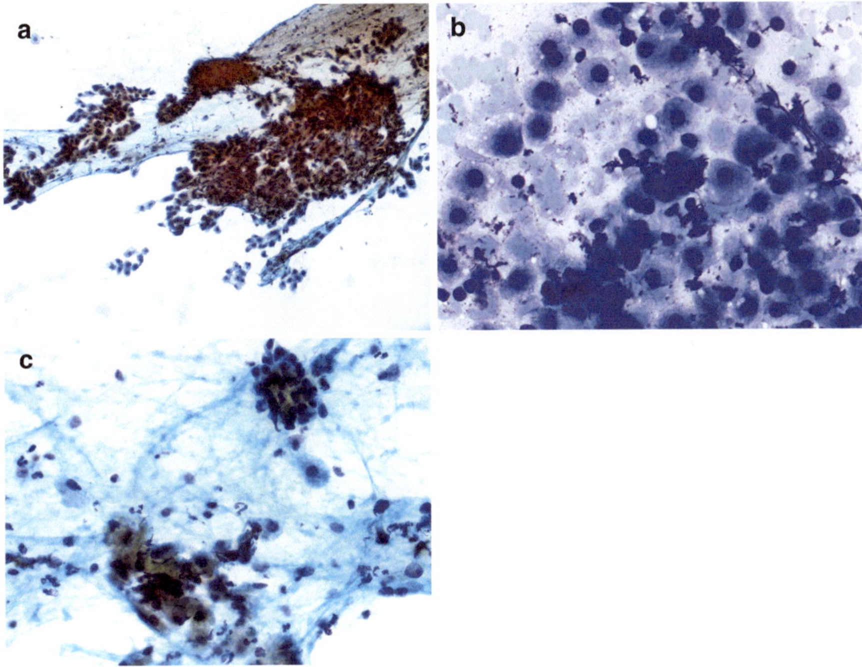

Fig. 14.7 Cirrhosis. (**a**) Loosely cohesive clusters of hepatocytes and scant fibrous tissue (Papanicolaou stain). (**b**) Reactive hepatocytes (Diff-Quik stain). (**c**) Mixed hepatocytes, bile duct epithelial cells and inflammatory cells (Papanicolaou stain)

Table 14.3 Cytomorphologic features of cystic lesions in the liver

	Etiology	Cytology
Infectious cysts		
Echinococcal cyst	*Echinococcus granulosus*	• Laminated acellular membrane with striations • Hooklets and scolices
Amebic liver abscess	*Entamoeba histolytica*	• Necrotic debris with little inflammation • Amebic trophozoites resembling histiocytes • Round nucleus • Peripheral chromatin • Phagocytosis of RBCs in the cytoplasm
Noninfectious cysts		
Simple cysts		• Cuboidal or columnar epithelium like bile duct epithelium • Macrophages
Polycystic liver disease	Mutations in *PRKCSH* and *SEC63* (*isolated*); *or PKD1* and *PKD2* (*associated with ADPKD*)	• Similar to simple cysts: bile duct epithelium and histiocytes

(continued)

Table 14.3 (continued)

	Etiology	Cytology
Liver pseudocysts	Rare complications of acute pancreatitis	• Nonspecific: inflammation and debris • No epithelial lining
Caroli disease	Mutations in *PKHD1 gene* (*associated with ARPKD*)	• Cystic components • Papillary structure and epithelial atypia may be present
Ciliated hepatic foregut cyst		• Ciliated pseudostratified epithelial cells are diagnostic

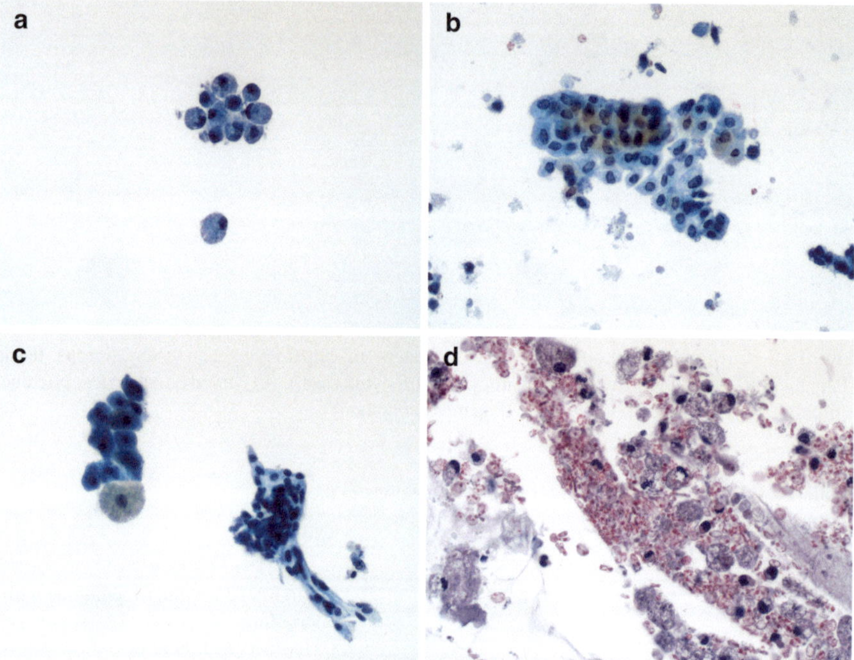

Fig. 14.8 Cystic liver disorders. (**a**) Scattered histocytes (Papanicolaou stain). (**b**) Benign-appearing epithelial cells with scattered histiocytes in a biliary cyst (Papanicolaou stain). (**c**) Mixed hepatocytes, cystic lining cells, and rare histiocytes (Papanicolaou stain). (**d**) Mixed mucinphages and histiocytes in a mucinous cystic neoplasm (Hematoxylin-eosin stain)

Historically, percutaneous aspiration of the hydatid cyst has been contraindicated due to the risk of leakage of cystic contents, leading to anaphylaxis and seeding of the peritoneum. Recently, many health care centers adopted the strategy of pre- and postoperative chemotherapy with albendazole or mebendazole, combined with percutaneous aspiration of hepatic hydatid cysts with great clinical efficacy and safety [24]. Cytologically, fragments of the laminated acellular membrane with striations are diagnostic for echinococcal cyst. Hooklets insets and scolices can be seen. Scolices stain positive for PAS/GMS while hooklets stain positive for Ziehl-Neelsen (acid-fast) stain and appear intensely red under fluorescence [25].

Amebic Liver Abscess

An amebic liver abscess is caused by *Entamoeba histolytica*, most commonly from food and water contaminated with feces containing *Entamoeba* cysts. Oral and anal sex are also possible routes of transmission. It is relatively uncommon in North America and often affect immigrants or travelers from endemic region. Although imaging is often helpful to diagnose liver abscesses, it is sometimes challenging to differentiate between liver abscesses and tumor with central necrosis. Another important differential diagnosis is a pyogenic abscess, which requires different treatment [27].

Cytologically, the smear usually shows necrotic material with few inflammatory cells and *E. histolytica* trophozoites [28]. Amebic trophozoites must be distinguished from histiocytes. They contain round nucleus, peripheral chromatin, and characteristic phagocytosis of erythrocytes in the cytoplasm.

Noninfectious Cysts

Non-parasitic liver cysts affect 5–10% of the population with an increased incidence with age [29]. Most patients with liver cysts are asymptomatic, however occasionally they are found incidentally on imaging. There might be a need to distinguish a simple cyst from other cystic lesions such as hydatid cysts or cystic neoplasm [30].

Simple cysts are solitary or multiple, believed to arise from the abnormal development of intrahepatic bile ducts in utero. The aspirated fluid is clear and straw-colored. The smear is nonspecific, with a few cuboidal or columnar epithelium resembling bile duct epithelium [31, 32]. Macrophages can be seen.

Polycystic liver disease (PCLD) is usually associated with Autosomal Dominant Polycystic Kidney Disease (ADPKD), due to the mutations of *PKD1* and *PKD2* genes. Isolated PCLD has also been discovered, which is an autosomal dominant condition caused by germline mutations of the *PRKCSH* and *SEC63* genes [33]. Microscopically, they have similar appearance with simple cysts, consisting of bile duct epithelium and histiocytes.

Ciliated hepatic foregut cyst (CHFC) is an extremely rare congenital cyst lined by ciliated epithelium, similar to bronchogenic cyst in mediastinum [13]. While they appear similar to simple cysts on imaging, it is critical to recognize this entity as they have risk of progressing to malignancy [34]. Cytologically, proteinaceous/serous fluid contents with few epithelial cells and histiocytes. The ciliated pseudostratified epithelial cells, if present, are diagnostic [13].

Liver pseudocysts are a very rare complication associated with acute pancreatitis, usually acute alcoholic pancreatitis. The radiographic findings of the pseudocyst full of debris could mimic neoplasm, and this differential diagnosis can be easily overlooked given its rarity [35]. Cytologically, no lining epithelium or malignant cells are present. Inflammatory cells, histiocytes, and necrosis are the main findings.

Caroli disease is a developmental anomaly characterized by multiple segmental cystic or saccular dilatations of intrahepatic bile ducts. Caroli syndrome consists of Caroli disease and congenital hepatic fibrosis, characterized by bland portal fibrosis, interlobular bile ducts proliferation with preserved normal lobular structure [36]. It is an autosomal recessive disease due to mutations in *PKHD1*, the gene linked to autosomal recessive polycystic kidney disease (ARPKD), thus associated with renal involvement in up to 60% of patients [36]. Aspirates of Caroli case are rarely reported in the literatures. Papillary folding of biliary epithelium are seen in histology and epithelial dysplasia may also be present [37].

Other Infectious Diseases

Pyogenic abscesses may be complications of cholangitis, septicemia, appendicitis, trauma, or they may have no clear predisposing causes. They are often polymicrobial and the most common organisms identified in US patients include *Streptococcus* species and *E. coli* [38]. Other Gram-negative bacteria such as *Klebsiella pneumonia* has also been increasingly reported [39]. Cytologically, pyogenic abscesses have to be distinguished from amebic abscess. Unlikely the latter which contains few neutrophils, pyogenic abscesses contain neutrophilic heavy inflammatory exudate with nuclear debris. Bacteria are often visible. Necrotic and reactive hepatocytes may also be present [40]. Keep in mind that inflammatory cells may obscure the presence of malignancy, thus careful examination for tumor cells are warranted as always.

Fungal infections of the liver often occur in patients with malignancy, especially hematooncologic patients, or in transplanted patients [41]. The most common causes are *Candida* spp. others such as Aspergillus, Mucormycosis, Cryptococcus, *Pneumocystic jirovecii* have been reported [41]. Most of the lesions need early diagnosis so that highly effective antimicrobial can be administrated. Identifying the fungal organisms is the key to render the diagnosis. For example, aspergillus is usually thin, slender with septation and acute angle branching. Mucormycosis consists of the broad fungus with wide angle branching and no septate [42]. Spherical yeasts surrounded by a clear halo (mucoid capsule) is characteristic for Cryptococcus [43].

Penicillium marneffei is an opportunistic pathogen often associated with HIV infection. Cytology shows aggregates of macrophages engorged with yeast-like organisms. The organisms are spherical or oval shaped with an eccentric or central dot and occasional septum [25, 44].

Granulomas

Granulomas in the liver can be caused by a variety of disorders, such as sarcoidosis, tuberculosis, drugs, neoplasms, and other hepatobiliary disorders such as primary biliary cirrhosis. Like granulomas seen in other organs, they consist of epithelioid histiocytes in a background of chronic inflammation. Necrosis may or may not be present [13].

The Biliary Tract

Anatomy and Histology of the Biliary Tract

The extrahepatic biliary tract serves as conduits for the flow of bile from the liver to the duodenum. The left and right hepatic ducts emerge from the liver and join to form the common hepatic duct. The cystic duct emerging from the gallbladder then joins the common hepatic duct, forming the common bile duct. The relationship between the common bile duct and pancreatic duct (duct of Wirsung) is variable at the major papilla of the duodenum. In majority of the cases, they join to form the common channel (sometimes forming the ampulla of Vater) [1, 2].

Histologically, the bile duct is lined by a single layer of tall columnar cells surrounded by connective tissue. Scattered goblet cells may be present in the epithelium. The wall structure varies depending on the anatomic location of the bile duct. The epithelium invaginates into the stroma, forming sacculi of Beale. Small lobular mucous glands surround those saccules, known as periductal glands. At the papilla, accessory pancreatic ducts and mucous glands may be seen in the wall of the common bile duct.

Normal Cytology

Endoscopic retrograde cholangiopancreatography (ERCP) has been widely used for the diagnosis and treatment of biliary tract disease. Samples can be obtained through biliary drainage or fine needle aspiration for exfoliated cells or brushed [45]. Post-brushing biliary lavage fluid may also be obtained to help increasing diagnostic yield.

Benign bile duct epithelium is usually arranged in sheets or clusters, composing of a monolayer of monomorphic cohesive cells. The cells possess small, round to oval nuclei evenly distributed throughout the sheet. The chromatin is finely granular. Nucleoli are inconspicuous. There might be scant cytoplasm when cells are

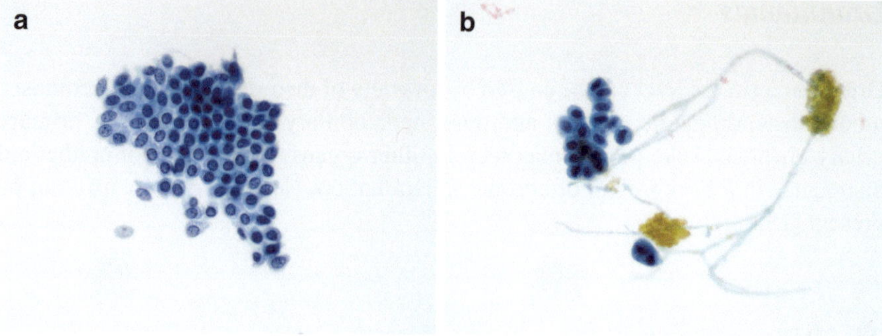

Fig. 14.9 Benign bile duct epithelium and bile. (**a**) Benign ductal epithelial cells arranged in a honeycomb pattern (Papanicolaou stain). (**b**) Benign-appearing bile duct epithelial cells and bile pigments (Papanicolaou stain)

viewed *en face* [2]. However, the abundant cytoplasm should be appreciated at edge, along with the columnar shape of epithelium. Goblet cells with clear cytoplasmic vacuoles, may be scattered throughout the sheet, especially in the distal common bile duct. The background may contain bile, which appears green-yellow in both Diff-Quik and Papanicolaou stains (Fig. 14.9).

The nuclear details may sometimes be obscured by the degenerative changes in the bile fluid. However, the nuclear-to-cytoplasmic (N/C) ratio should be maintained. The monolayered arrangement of cells and uniformed sized nuclei are still evident.

Reactive Conditions

Stricture

Bile duct brushing cytology is an important tool in the evaluation of biliary stricture, which can be caused by neoplastic or inflammatory processes. Patients may have symptoms suspicious for malignancy, while the obtaining endoscopic biopsies can be challenging due to the location. However, the sensitivity of this technique is suboptimal, with the diagnostic yield ranging from 30% to 80% in different studies [46, 47]. On the other hand, biliary tract cytology is challenging for cytopathologists, who should be aware of diagnostic pitfalls and try to differentiate benign reactive ductal epithelium from malignancy, if possible.

Many cytological criteria have been proposed for biliary samples [48–51]. In general, the reactive ductal epithelium has relatively low cellularity comparing with malignant processes such as that seen in cholangiocarcinoma. They are occasionally arranged in papillary clusters with slight nuclear overlapping. However, the N/C ratio should be low (Fig. 14.10). In comparison, dysplastic epithelium usually

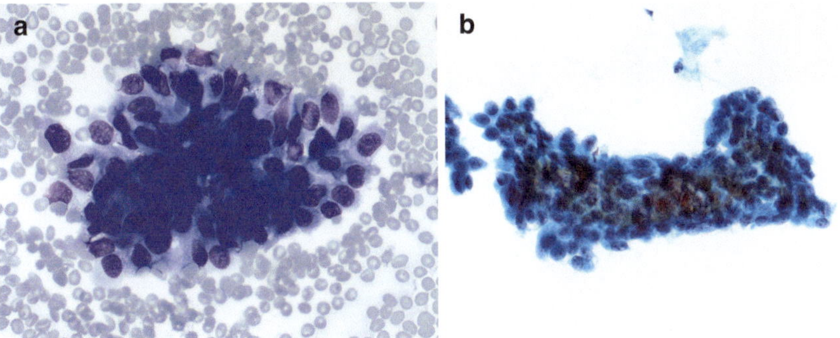

Fig. 14.10 Cholelithiasis-related reactive changes. Ductal epithelial cells show enlarged nuclei with nuclear overlapping and hyperchromasia (**a** Diff-Quik stain; **b** Papanicolaou stain)

demonstrates an increased N/C ratio, and the malignant bile duce epithelium have high N/C ratio. Anisonucleosis, defined as a size variation of at least four times between the largest and smallest nuclei within a cell cluster, if present, favors malignancy. Chromatin changes such as clear chromatin, coarse chromatin, or hyperchromatism are usually seen in malignant processes. The presence of inflammatory cells and degradation of cellular changes (in comparison to the distinct two population in malignancy) are also helpful features for non-malignancy [52]. Recent multivariate study showed that the presence of a single malignant cell has 100% specificity for diagnosing malignancy. In addition, three-dimensional (3D) clusters, anisonucleosis, and N/C ratio >0.5 together could constitute a 100% specific criterion [50].

Primary Sclerosing Cholangitis (PSC)

PSC is a chronic progressive liver disease characterized by inflammation and fibrosis leading to multifocal biliary strictures. It is closely related to inflammatory bowel disease (IBD), with an increased risk for developing malignancy such as cholangiocarcinoma and colorectal cancer [53, 54]. While almost half of the patients will develop dominant biliary strictures [55], it is difficult to distinguish the benign and malignant stenosis on imaging due to the fibrosis. As a result, bile duct brushing cytology under ERCP are commonly used to examine the stenosis and screen for cholangiocarcinoma in patients with PSC.

Although many studies have shown the high specificity but low sensitivity of brush cytology [46, 47, 52, 56, 57], differentiating benign reactive atypia from high-grade dysplasia and cholangiocarcinoma remain challenging in daily practice [58]. There are no well-established objective criteria. In general, a high threshold for malignancy should be warranted in cases of PSC because of the associated reactive changes (Fig. 14.11). Multivariate regression analysis has identified many cytologic features for the diagnosis of cholangiocarcinoma (Table 14.4). The presence of at least three criteria is usually recommended for a definitive diagnosis [49, 59].

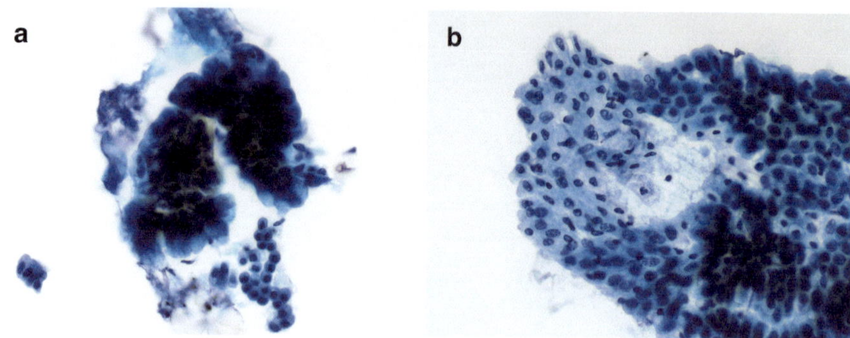

Fig. 14.11 Primary sclerosing cholangitis. Ductal epithelial cells show intracytoplasmic vacuoles, nuclear enlargement, and nuclear streaming (**a**, **b** Papanicolaou stain)

Table 14.4 General cytomorphologic features of benign and malignant bile duct epithelium

Features		Benign reactive	Malignant
Important	3D clusters	Rare	Present
	Two distinct population	No. Gradation of cellular change	Yes
	Nuclear pleomorphism	No	Yes
	Anisonucleosis (1:4)	Absent	Present
	N/C ratio	Relatively low	High
	Chromatin	Evenly distributed	Clear, coarse, or hyperchromatism
	Single malignant cell	Absent	Present
	Additional helpful features	Background inflammation	Necrosis and mitoses; bloody background
Less helpful	Prominent nucleoli	Can be present	Present
	Cellularity	Relatively low	Usually high

Table 14.5 Ancillary testing in biliary brush cytology in primary sclerosing cholangitis

	Utility and interpretation	References
Immunostaining	TP53, KRAS, S100P, pVHL, IMP3, maspin	[60, 61, 67]
Fluorescence in situ hybridization (FISH)	Strong association between polysomy and pancreatobiliary malignancy	[48, 56]
Next-generation sequencing	**CCA**: *TP53, KRAS, GNAS, PIK3CA, ERBB2, SMAD4, APC* **PSC**: *KRAS, GNAS*	[62–64]

Increasing numbers of studies have also been performed to investigate the incorporation of less subjective methods such as ancillary testing in the diagnosis for biliary cytology (Table 14.5). Immunocytochemistry, FISH and next-generation

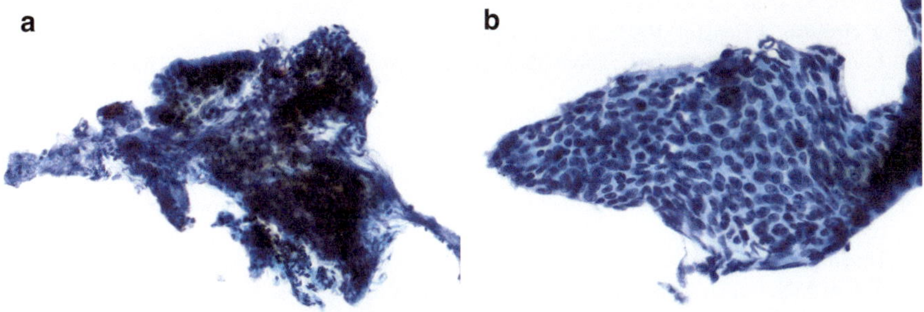

Fig. 14.12 Stent-associated reactive changes. (**a**) Cluster of ductal epithelial cells with mixed inflammatory cells (Papanicolaou stain). (**b**) Ductal epithelial cells with nuclear enlargement, hyperchromasia, and nuclear streaming (Papanicolaou stain)

sequencing have been explored with certain increase in sensitivity and specificity, especially the latter two [48, 51, 56, 60–64]. More further studies are needed to validate their application in common practice.

Stenting

Another challenging condition in biliary cytology is the biliary stent-related changes. In patients with a biliary stricture, ERCP-guided cytology brushing is often followed by placement of a stent, which is a common therapeutic modality [65]. As a result, repeat biliary brush cytology after the stent placement is not uncommon. As described earlier, similar diagnostic exercises should be practiced ruling in/out malignancy. Among all the cytomorphologic features, five of them have been identified critical to differentiate stent-related alterations versus carcinoma. Atypical single cells, two populations, anisonucleosis favored malignancy while distinct cell borders and acute inflammation favored benign (Fig. 14.12) [65, 66].

Acknowledgments None.

Conflict of Interest None.

References

1. Mills SE. Histology for pathologists. 5th ed. Lippincott Williams & Wilkins (LWW); 2019.
2. Herzberg AJ, Raso DS, Silverman JF. Color atlas of normal cytology. New York: Churchill Livingstone; 1999.

3. Borzio M, et al. The evaluation of fine-needle procedures for the diagnosis of focal liver lesions in cirrhosis. J Hepatol. 1994;20(1):117–21.
4. Longchampt E, Patriarche C, Fabre M. Accuracy of cytology vs. microbiopsy for the diagnosis of well-differentiated hepatocellular carcinoma and macroregenerative nodule. Definition of standardized criteria from a study of 100 cases. Acta Cytol. 2000;44(4):515–23.
5. DeWitt J, et al. Endoscopic ultrasound-guided fine needle aspiration cytology of solid liver lesions: a large single-center experience. Am J Gastroenterol. 2003;98(9):1976–81.
6. Guo Z, et al. Radiologically guided percutaneous fine-needle aspiration biopsy of the liver: retrospective study of 119 cases evaluating diagnostic effectiveness and clinical complications. Diagn Cytopathol. 2002;26(5):283–9.
7. Yousaf MN, Cai G, Aslanian HR. EUS evaluation of liver lesions. VideoGIE. 2018;3(1):31–3.
8. Cibas ES, Ducatman BS. Cytology: diagnostic principles and clinical correlates. 5th ed. Philadelphia: Saunders/Elsevier; 2019.
9. Laiq Z, Bishop JA, Ali SZ. Liver lesions in children and adolescents: cytopathologic analysis and clinical correlates in 44 cases. Diagn Cytopathol. 2012;40(7):586–91.
10. Chen QW, et al. Effectiveness and complications of ultrasound guided fine needle aspiration for primary liver cancer in a Chinese population with serum alpha-fetoprotein levels </=200 ng/ml—a study based on 4,312 patients. PLoS One. 2014;9(8):e101536.
11. Fritscher-Ravens A, et al. EUS-guided fine-needle aspiration cytodiagnosis of hilar cholangio-carcinoma: a case series. Gastrointest Endosc. 2000;52(4):534–40.
12. Mohamadnejad M, et al. Role of EUS for preoperative evaluation of cholangiocarcinoma: a large single-center experience. Gastrointest Endosc. 2011;73(1):71–8.
13. Koss LG, Melamed MR. Koss' diagnostic cytology and its histopathologic bases. 5th ed. Philadelphia: Lippincott Williams & Wilkins; 2006.
14. Shyu S, Ali SZ. Significance of hepatocyte atypia in liver fine needle aspiration. Diagn Cytopathol. 2022;50(4):186–95.
15. European Association for the Study of the Liver. EASL Clinical Practice Guidelines on the management of benign liver tumours. J Hepatol. 2016;65(2):386–98.
16. Wang X, Zhang X. Hepatocellular adenoma: where are we now? World J Gastroenterol. 2022;28(14):1384–93.
17. Chhieng DC. Fine needle aspiration biopsy of liver—an update. World J Surg Oncol. 2004;2:5.
18. Ruschenburg I, Droese M. Fine needle aspiration cytology of focal nodular hyperplasia of the liver. Acta Cytol. 1989;33(6):857–60.
19. Erozan YS, Tatsas A. Cytopathology of liver, biliary tract, kidney and adrenal gland. New York: Springer; 2015.
20. Bottles K, Cohen MB. An approach to fine-needle aspiration biopsy diagnosis of hepatic masses. Diagn Cytopathol. 1991;7(2):204–10.
21. Bedossa P, et al. Well-differentiated hepatocellular neoplasm of uncertain malignant potential: proposal for a new diagnostic category. Hum Pathol. 2014;45(3):658–60.
22. Vyas M, Jain D. A practical diagnostic approach to hepatic masses. Indian J Pathol Microbiol. 2018;61(1):2–17.
23. Wee A. Fine-needle aspiration biopsy of hepatocellular carcinoma and related hepatocellular nodular lesions in cirrhosis: controversies, challenges, and expectations. Pathol Res Int. 2011;2011:587936.
24. Smego RA Jr, et al. Percutaneous aspiration-injection-reaspiration drainage plus albendazole or mebendazole for hepatic cystic echinococcosis: a meta-analysis. Clin Infect Dis. 2003;37(8):1073–83.
25. Park J-W, et al. Differential diagnosis in cytopathology. 3rd ed. Cambridge: Cambridge University Press; 2021.
26. Agarwal A, et al. Hepatocyte paraffin-1, CD10, and CD34 immunostaining as a diagnostic aid in cytologic diagnosis of hepatic cancer. J Cancer Res Ther. 2022;18(Suppl):S434–8.
27. Nattakom S, et al. Amebic liver abscesses masquerading as pyemic abscesses. Clin Infect Dis. 2001;33(12):E145–7.

28. Mokhtari M, Kumar PV. Amebic liver abscess: fine needle aspiration diagnosis. Acta Cytol. 2014;58(3):225–8.
29. Gall TM, et al. Surgical management and longterm follow-up of non-parasitic hepatic cysts. HPB (Oxford). 2009;11(3):235–41.
30. Macutkiewicz C, et al. Complications arising in simple and polycystic liver cysts. World J Hepatol. 2012;4(12):406–11.
31. DeMay RM. Practical principles of cytopathology. Chicago: American Society of Clinical Pathologists; 1999.
32. Shi G, et al. A case of a giant cyst in the left lobe of the liver successfully treated with endoscopic ultrasound-guided fine needle aspiration (with video). Endosc Ultrasound. 2017;6(5):343–6.
33. Cnossen WR, Drenth JP. Polycystic liver disease: an overview of pathogenesis, clinical manifestations and management. Orphanet J Rare Dis. 2014;9:69.
34. Wilson JM, et al. Ciliated hepatic cyst leading to squamous cell carcinoma of the liver—a case report and review of the literature. Int J Surg Case Rep. 2013;4(11):972–5.
35. Casado D, et al. Multiple intrahepatic pseudocysts in acute pancreatitis. World J Gastroenterol. 2007;13(34):4655–7.
36. Yonem O, Bayraktar Y. Clinical characteristics of Caroli's syndrome. World J Gastroenterol. 2007;13(13):1934–7.
37. Fozard JB, Wyatt JI, Hall RI. Epithelial dysplasia in Caroli's disease. Gut. 1989;30(8):1150–3.
38. Meddings L, et al. A population-based study of pyogenic liver abscesses in the United States: incidence, mortality, and temporal trends. Am J Gastroenterol. 2010;105(1):117–24.
39. Tsai FC, et al. Pyogenic liver abscess as endemic disease, Taiwan. Emerg Infect Dis. 2008;14(10):1592–600.
40. Wee A, et al. Aspiration cytology of liver abscesses. With an emphasis on diagnostic pitfalls. Acta Cytol. 1995;39(3):453–62.
41. Fiore M, et al. Liver fungal infections: an overview of the etiology and epidemiology in patients affected or not affected by oncohematologic malignancies. Infect Drug Resist. 2018;11:177–86.
42. Gochhait D, et al. Spectrum of fungal and parasitic infections on fine needle aspiration cytology. Diagn Cytopathol. 2015;43(6):450–5.
43. George B, Rivera Rolon MDM, Clement CG. Role of fine-needle aspiration cytology in early diagnosis of fungal infections. Diagn Cytopathol. 2020;48(7):645–51.
44. Jan IS, et al. Cytological diagnosis of Penicillium marneffei infection. J Formos Med Assoc. 2008;107(6):443–7.
45. Sugimoto S, et al. Diagnosis of bile duct cancer by bile cytology: usefulness of post-brushing biliary lavage fluid. Endosc Int Open. 2015;3(4):E323–8.
46. Mahmoudi N, et al. Biliary brush cytology: factors associated with positive yields on biliary brush cytology. World J Gastroenterol. 2008;14(4):569–73.
47. Volmar KE, et al. Pancreatic and bile duct brushing cytology in 1000 cases: review of findings and comparison of preparation methods. Cancer. 2006;108(4):231–8.
48. Barr Fritcher EG, et al. Identification of malignant cytologic criteria in pancreatobiliary brushings with corresponding positive fluorescence in situ hybridization results. Am J Clin Pathol. 2011;136(3):442–9.
49. Avadhani V, et al. Cytologic predictors of malignancy in bile duct brushings: a multi-reviewer analysis of 60 cases. Mod Pathol. 2017;30(9):1273–86.
50. Giovannini D, et al. Biliary cytology: a diagnostic tree for adenocarcinoma based on a cohort of 135 patients with endoscopic retrograde cholangiopancreatography for stenosis of the extrahepatic bile duct. Cancer Cytopathol. 2022;130(6):433–42.
51. Salomao M, et al. Strategies for improving diagnostic accuracy of biliary strictures. Cancer Cytopathol. 2015;123(4):244–52.
52. Mantoo S. Bile duct brush cytology—challenges, limitations and ancillary studies. J Virol Curr Res. 2017;2(1):555578.

53. Karlsen TH, et al. Primary sclerosing cholangitis—a comprehensive review. J Hepatol. 2017;67(6):1298–323.
54. Dyson JK, et al. Primary sclerosing cholangitis. Lancet. 2018;391(10139):2547–59.
55. Chapman MH, et al. Cholangiocarcinoma and dominant strictures in patients with primary sclerosing cholangitis: a 25-year single-centre experience. Eur J Gastroenterol Hepatol. 2012;24(9):1051–8.
56. Barr Fritcher EG, et al. Primary sclerosing cholangitis with equivocal cytology: fluorescence in situ hybridization and serum CA 19-9 predict risk of malignancy. Cancer Cytopathol. 2013;121(12):708–17.
57. Vannas MJ, et al. Value of brush cytology for optimal timing of liver transplantation in primary sclerosing cholangitis. Liver Int. 2017;37(5):735–42.
58. Layfield LJ, Cramer H. Primary sclerosing cholangitis as a cause of false positive bile duct brushing cytology: report of two cases. Diagn Cytopathol. 2005;32(2):119–24.
59. International Academy of Cytology—International Agency for Research on Cancer—World Health Organization Joint Editorial Board. WHO reporting system for pancreaticobiliary cytopathology, IAC-IARC-WHO cytopathology reporting systems series, vol. 2. 1st ed. Lyon, France: International Agency for Research on Cancer; 2022. https://publications.iarc.fr/621.
60. Levy M, et al. S100P, von Hippel-Lindau gene product, and IMP3 serve as a useful immunohistochemical panel in the diagnosis of adenocarcinoma on endoscopic bile duct biopsy. Hum Pathol. 2010;41(9):1210–9.
61. Chen L, et al. Diagnostic value of maspin in distinguishing adenocarcinoma from benign biliary epithelium on endoscopic bile duct biopsy. Hum Pathol. 2015;46(11):1647–54.
62. Dudley JC, et al. Next-generation sequencing and fluorescence in situ hybridization have comparable performance characteristics in the analysis of pancreaticobiliary brushings for malignancy. J Mol Diagn. 2016;18(1):124–30.
63. Singhi AD, et al. Integrating next-generation sequencing to endoscopic retrograde cholangiopancreatography (ERCP)-obtained biliary specimens improves the detection and management of patients with malignant bile duct strictures. Gut. 2020;69(1):52–61.
64. Kamp E, et al. Next-generation sequencing mutation analysis on biliary brush cytology for differentiation of benign and malignant strictures in primary sclerosing cholangitis. Gastrointest Endosc. 2023;97(3):456–465.e6.
65. Heath JE, Goicochea LB, Staats PN. Biliary stent-related alterations can be distinguished from adenocarcinoma on bile duct brushings using a limited number of cytologic features. J Am Soc Cytopathol. 2015;4(5):282–9.
66. Goyal A, et al. Cytologic diagnosis of adenocarcinoma on bile duct brushings in the presence of stent associated changes: a retrospective analysis. Diagn Cytopathol. 2018;46(10):826–32.
67. Ponsioen CY, et al. Value of brush cytology for dominant strictures in primary sclerosing cholangitis. Endoscopy. 1999;31(4):305–9.

Chapter 15
Kidney and Adrenal Gland

Khairya Fatouh and Syed M. Gilani

The normal kidney comprises a cortex and medulla, where the cortex's structural unit consists of glomeruli, proximal tubules, distal tubules, and a portion of collecting ducts. Medulla mainly contains loops of Henle and collecting ducts. The functional unit is the kidney's nephron, composed of glomerulus and associated renal tubules.

Normal Morphology

Glomeruli are compact, cellular, and globular structures surrounded by rich capillary meshwork. Proximal convoluted tubule cells are usually arranged in sheets of flat cells with small bland nuclei and abundant granular cytoplasm (Figs. 15.1 and 15.2). The presence of these cells may raise a differential diagnosis of oncocytic lesion but later has more defined cell borders. Distal tubular cells are less eosinophilic; nuclei are located towards the central lumen and lack brush borders.

Proximal tubular cells are positive for cytokeratin AE1/AE3, CD10, RCC (apical cell membrane), and Pax-8. Distal tubular cells are positive for cytokeratin AE1/AE3, pax-8(+), and kidney-specific cadherin (Ksp)-cadherin, but negative for CD10 and RCC stains [1–4]. Pax-2 staining can be focally seen in distal tubules and rarely in proximal tubules.

K. Fatouh
St. John Hospital and Medical Center, Detroit, MI, USA
e-mail: khairya.fatouh@ascension.org

S. M. Gilani (✉)
Department of Pathology, Albany Medical Center, Albany Medical College,
Albany, NY, USA
e-mail: gilanis@amc.edu

S. M. Gilani, G. Cai (eds.), *Non-Neoplastic Cytology*,
https://doi.org/10.1007/978-3-031-44289-6_15

Fig. 15.1 Renal tubular
cells with abundant
granular cytoplasm
(Diff-Quik stain ×200)

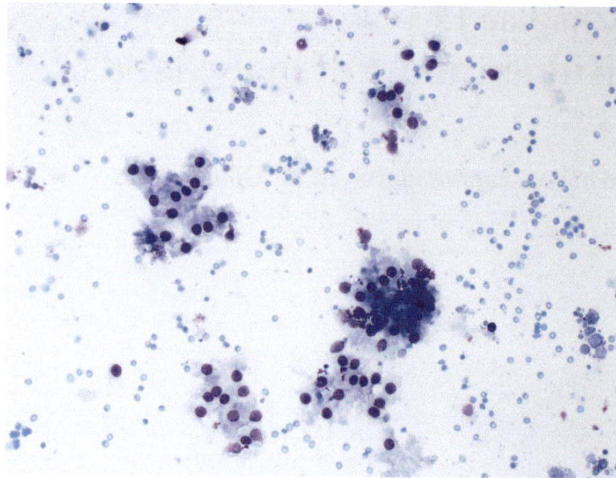

Fig. 15.2 Renal tubular
cells with abundant
granular cytoplasm
(Papanicolaou stain ×400)

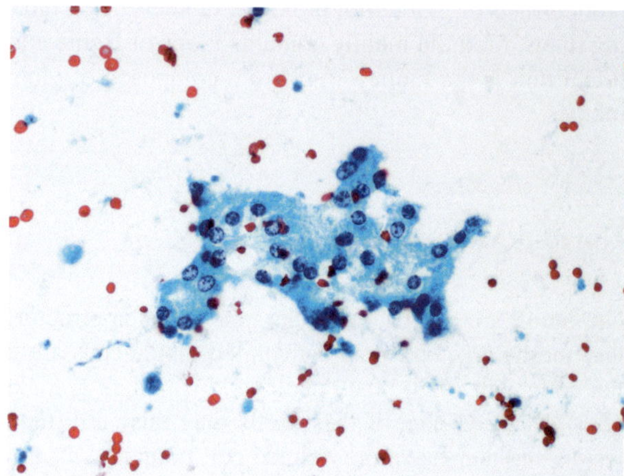

Renal Cystic Lesions

Background

Renal cysts lesions are common space-occupying lesions seen in the kidney. They
can be congenital or acquired and range from benign to neoplastic diagnoses. The
majority of renal cysts are usually benign, acquired, and unilateral [5–9]. Imaging
techniques are helpful to further characterize the cystic lesions by using the Bosniak
classification system to predict and classify renal cyst's likelihood of malignancy.
Bosniak I represents a benign simple renal cyst requiring no follow-up and no
FNA. Bosniak II represents a likely benign lesion requiring no follow-up. Bosniak
IIF represents mostly benign cystic masses with imaging follow-up. Bosniak III
cystic renal mass with an intermediate risk of malignancy. Bosniak IV cystic renal

masses are mostly (90%) malignant. FNA procedure helps to establish a diagnosis and can be used for Bosniak II or higher categories [6, 10].

Cytology and Cytologic Diagnosis

Renal cysts can be congenital or acquired. FNA of the renal cystic lesions is usually hypocellular specimens with macrophages and rarely cyst lining epithelial cells and renal tubular cells. No atypia should be seen in benign cysts, and the cell block material is usually helpful for further characterization by immunohistochemical staining. Simple benign renal cysts of various etiologies can have overlapping cytologic findings. However, the correlation of the cytomorphologic findings with the clinical history and imaging findings is essential [6, 11, 12] (see Table 15.1).

Simple Cysts

It represents the Bosniak Category I cysts; radiologically, they are solitary, thin walled, with no density. Those cysts usually yield clear fluid, and cytologically, the specimen is hypocellular with mostly cysts content and rare bland epithelial cells with any atypia.

Table 15.1 Normal variables and non-neoplastic lesions with differential diagnosis

Variables	Cytomorphologic features	Differential diagnosis
Normal kidney cells	Renal glomerulus cells with architecture distortion (procedure related)	Vascular lesion or papillary lesion
	Proximal tubular cells with granular cytoplasm	Oncocytic lesion/tumor
Renal cysts	Macrophages, cyst lining cells, renal parenchymal cells, and cells with atypical/degenerative changes	Multilocular cystic renal cell neoplasm Cystic clear cell renal cell carcinoma
		Cystic partially differentiated nephroblastoma
Xanthogranulomatous pyelonephritis	Foamy histiocyte and multinucleated giant cells	Clear cell renal cell carcinoma
Renal abscess	Acute inflammatory cells and reactive epithelial cells	Malignancy

Multicystic Processes

Autosomal Dominant Polycystic Kidney Disease

ADPKD is the most common inheritable form of cystic renal disease, with an approximate incidence between 1 in 1000 and 2500 [13]. It can cause gradual impairment in renal function and may result in renal failure later in life. Mutations in the genes *PKD1* or *PKD2 are usually seen in ADPKD*. Specimens show variable cellularity with macrophages and some scattered cyst lining epithelial cells. Papillary hyperplasia can often pose diagnostic challenges [6]. In such cases, correlation with imaging features would provide additional information [4, 6].

Multicystic Kidney Disease (Multicystic Dysplastic Kidney, MCDK)

This developmental anomaly results in multiple cysts of varying sizes replacing the renal parenchyma [14, 15]. This condition is usually unilateral but has a more aggressive course if bilateral [15]. Immature-appearing cartilage and glomeruli can be present. The differential diagnosis includes polycystic kidney disease, which has larger cysts as compared to this entity [16]. MCDK can rare associated with malignancies such as Wilms tumor and renal cell carcinoma [14].

Other Multilocular Cyst

Other multiloculated cystic processes include cystic nephroma, which shows bimodal age distribution younger than 4 or older than 30 years. Smears are hypocellular with epithelial lining cells and stromal cells [17, 18]. Epithelial cells can show some atypia [7]. Such cases require careful evaluation and correlation with clinical/imaging features to avoid overinterpretation as renal cell carcinoma. The diagnostically challenging cases can be characterized in an atypical category.

Inflammatory/Infectious Renal Diseases

Xanthogranulomatous Pyelonephritis

It is a chronic inflammatory process causing pyelonephritis due to infection or prolonged obstruction. It can affect any age group with a mean age range between the fourth and fifth decade of life. Like chronic pyelonephritis, it presents with the triad of flank pain, fever, and abdominal mass. *Proteus mirabilis* and *Escherichia coli* are identified in the majority of the cases [19]. Clinically, it can mimic infectious etiologies as well as malignancies. Smears are usually variably cellular, with a collection of foamy histiocytes, inflammatory cells, and multinucleated giant cells. The differential diagnosis includes clear cell renal cell carcinoma [20, 21]. In challenging cases, the role of the cell block is critical to differentiate between these two entities by doing immunohistochemical stains such as epithelial markers, and CD68. Vimentin is not helpful as it stains positive in both processes [19].

Renal Abscess

It can be either within the kidney or acquired from a perinephric site due to urinary tract infection from obstruction, renal stones, and diabetes. Fine needle aspirate shows a mixture of abundant acute and chronic inflammatory cells with occasional sloughed-off epithelial cells with atypical features, which may raise the possibility of malignancy [9]. In an inflammatory background, a cautious approach is suggested to avoid overinterpretation.

The Adrenal Glands

Normal Morphology

The adrenal gland contains the cortex and medulla. The adrenal cortex is subdivided into zona glomerulosa (present beneath the capsule with a short cord of cells with stainable/weak amphophilic cytoplasm), zona fasciculata (middle layer clusters of cells with distinct cell membranes and vacuolated/lipid-containing cytoplasm), and zona reticularis (deep layer with cells having acidophilic granular cytoplasm and lipofuscin pigment). The adrenal medulla consists of clusters of cells with variations in nuclear size and basophilic cytoplasm. FNA of the adrenal gland yields small groups or cords of uniform polygonal cells with a centrally located round nucleus and lipid-rich foamy cytoplasm if they are from zona glomerulosa or fasciculata (Figs. 15.3, 15.4, and 15.5).

Adrenal Rest

Adrenal tissue (mostly adrenal cortical) can be seen in other locations such as the kidney, liver, lung, mediastinum, spinal canal, testis, placenta, and other sites [22–25]. The differential diagnosis is discussed in Table 15.2.

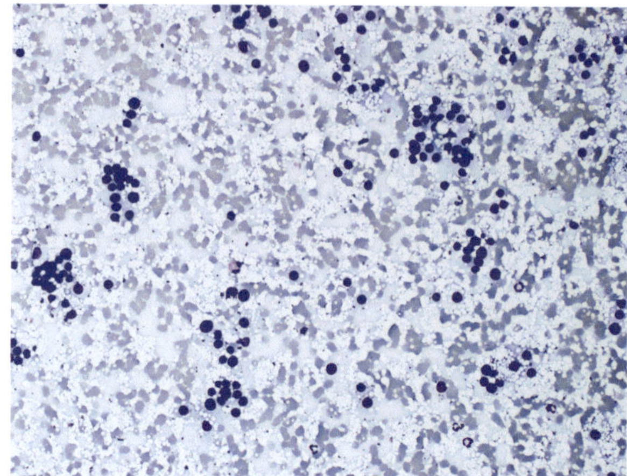

Fig. 15.3 Adrenal cortical cells with scattered round nuclei with background bubbly (lipid) material (Diff-Quik stain ×200)

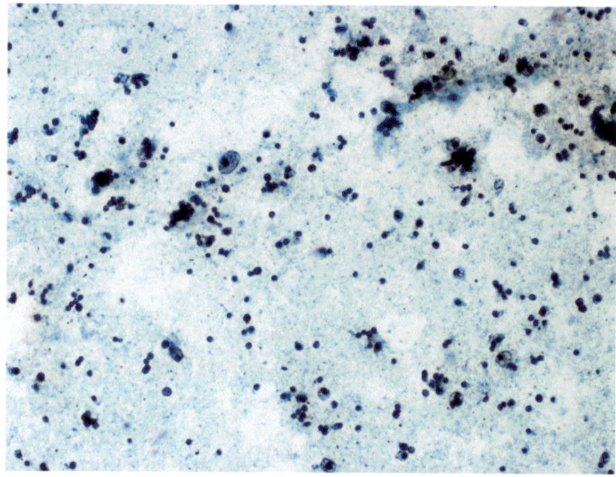

Fig. 15.4 Adrenal cortical cells with stripped nuclei and some are in clusters with indistinct borders (Papanicolaou stain ×200)

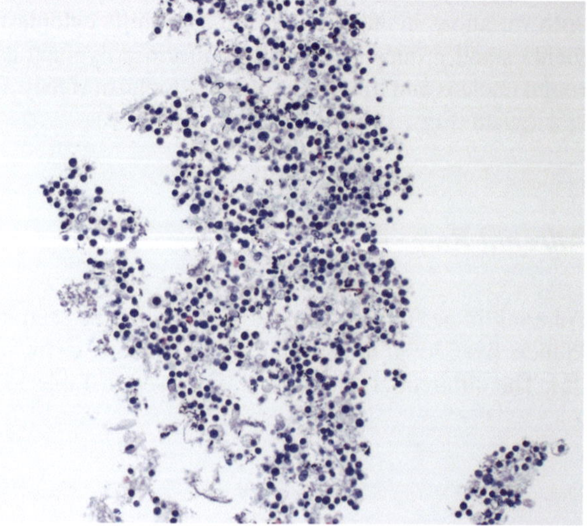

Fig. 15.5 Scattered discohesive adrenal cortical cells, may raises a concern for malignant process (Cell block, eosin and hematoxylin stain, ×200)

Table 15.2 Adrenal tissue cells and differential diagnosis

Normal adrenal tissue cells	Adrenal cortical nodular disease
	Adrenal cortical neoplasm (adenoma or carcinoma)
	Clear cell renal cell carcinoma
	Hepatocytes
Adrenal rest	Clear cell renal cell carcinoma, steroid cell tumor, Leydig cell tumor, hepatocellular carcinoma, metastatic adrenal tumor/carcinoma

Adrenal Gland Cysts

Adrenal cysts are benign and uncommon lesions and should be differentiated from neoplastic processes. The cyst includes pseudocysts, endothelial cysts, epithelial cysts, mesothelial cysts, and parasitic cysts [26–30].

Pseudocysts

Pseudocysts are benign and more common than other benign cysts. They lack cyst lining and have fibrous cyst walls. Specimens are hypocellular with fibrinoid material, macrophages, and cholesterol clefts formation.

Endothelial Lined Cysts

These cysts are usually simple, asymptomatic, incidentally discovered, and have an endothelial lining. They can be either lymphatic or vascular types. FNAs are generally performed to exclude malignancy and may show a paucicellular specimen with cyst contents and blood and rarely have lining cells. These cysts usually stain for at least one of the endothelial markers, such as CD31, D2-40, or CD34.

Epithelial Cysts

Epithelial cysts usually stain for an epithelial marker of mesothelial markers (such as calretinin) [31]. These cysts should be differentiated from adrenal cortical neoplasms and can show cystic degeneration.

Parasitic Cysts

The parasitic cyst is rare in the adrenal gland and is usually caused by Echinococcus infection, called Hydatid disease [32].

Acknowledgments None.

Conflict of Interest None.

References

1. Martignoni G, Pea M, Brunelli M, Chilosi M, Zamó A, Bertaso M, Cossu-Rocca P, Eble JN, Mikuz G, Puppa G, Badoual C, Ficarra V, Novella G, Bonetti F. CD10 is expressed in a subset of chromophobe renal cell carcinomas. Mod Pathol. 2004;17(12):1455–63.
2. Tong GX, Yu WM, Beaubier NT, Weeden EM, Hamele-Bena D, Mansukhani MM, O'Toole KM. Expression of PAX8 in normal and neoplastic renal tissues: an immunohistochemical study. Mod Pathol. 2009;22(9):1218–27.
3. Thedieck C, Kuczyk M, Klingel K, Steiert I, Müller CA, Klein G. Expression of Ksp-cadherin during kidney development and in renal cell carcinoma. Br J Cancer. 2005;92(11):2010–7.
4. Ozcan A, Zhai J, Hamilton C, Shen SS, Ro JY, Krishnan B, Truong LD. PAX-2 in the diagnosis of primary renal tumors: immunohistochemical comparison with renal cell carcinoma marker antigen and kidney-specific cadherin. Am J Clin Pathol. 2009;131(3):393–404.
5. Masoom S, Venkataraman G, Jensen J, Flanigan RC, Wojcik EM. Renal FNA-based typing of renal masses remains a useful adjunctive modality: evaluation of 31 renal masses with correlative histology. Cytopathology. 2009;20:50–5.
6. Renshaw AA, Granter SR, Cibas ES. Fine-needle aspiration of the adult kidney. Cancer. 1997;81(2):71–88.
7. Truong LD, Todd TD, Dhurandhar B, Ramzy I. Fine-needle aspiration of renal masses in adults: analysis of results and diagnostic problems in 108 cases. Diagn Cytopathol. 1999;20(6):339–49.
8. Scanga LR, Maygarden SJ. Utility of fine-needle aspiration and core biopsy with touch preparation in the diagnosis of renal lesions. Cancer Cytopathol. 2014;122(3):182–90.
9. Kelley CM, Cohen MB, Raab SS. Utility of fine-needle aspiration biopsy in solid renal masses. Diagn Cytopathol. 1996;14(1):14–9.
10. Silverman SG, Pedrosa I, Ellis JH, Hindman NM, Schieda N, Smith AD, Remer EM, Shinagare AB, Curci NE, Raman SS, Wells SA, Kaffenberger SD, Wang ZJ, Chandarana H, Davenport MS. Bosniak classification of cystic renal masses, version 2019: an update proposal and needs assessment. Radiology. 2019;292(2):475–88.
11. Volpe A, Kachura JR, Geddie WR, Evans AJ, Gharajeh A, Saravanan A, Jewett MA. Techniques, safety and accuracy of sampling of renal tumors by fine needle aspiration and core biopsy. J Urol. 2007;178(2):379–86.
12. Barwari K, Kummerlin IP, ten Kate FJ, Algaba F, Trias I, Wijkstra H, De la Rosette JJ, Laguna P. What is the added value of combined core biopsy and fine needle aspiration in the diagnostic process of renal tumours? World J Urol. 2013;31(4):823–7.
13. Cornec-Le Gall E, Alam A, Perrone RD. Autosomal dominant polycystic kidney disease. Lancet. 2019;393(10174):919–35.
14. Cardona-Grau D, Kogan BA. Update on multicystic dysplastic kidney. Curr Urol Rep. 2015;16(10):67.
15. Meyers ML, Treece AL, Brown BP, Vemulakonda VM. Imaging of fetal cystic kidney disease: multicystic dysplastic kidney versus renal cystic dysplasia. Pediatr Radiol. 2020;50(13):1921–33.
16. Chen RY, Chang H. Renal dysplasia. Arch Pathol Lab Med. 2015;139(4):547–51.
17. Cavıldak İK, Çakıcı MÇ, Karakoyunlu N, Ersoy H. Cystic nephroma: a case report in adult patients. Turk J Urol. 2018;44(4):373–6.

18. Ozturk H, Karaaslan S. Uretheral invagination of multilocular cystic nephroma; a case report of a new pathologic variant. Int J Clin Exp Pathol. 2014;7(8):5271–9.
19. Li L, Parwani AV. Xanthogranulomatous pyelonephritis. Arch Pathol Lab Med. 2011;135(5):671–4.
20. Kumar N, Jain S. Aspiration cytology of focal xanthogranulomatous pyelonephritis: a diagnostic challenge. Diagn Cytopathol. 2004;30(2):111–4.
21. Pegas KL, Edelweiss MI, Cambruzzi E, Zettler CG. Liesegang rings in xanthogranulomatous pyelonephritis: a case report. Pathol Res Int. 2010;2010:602523.
22. Enjoji M, Sanada K, Seki R, Ito T, Maeda M. Adrenal rest tumor of the liver preoperatively diagnosed as hepatocellular carcinoma. Case Rep Surg. 2017;2017:8231943.
23. Tarçın G, Ercan O. Emergence of ectopic adrenal tissues—what are the probable mechanisms? J Clin Res Pediatr Endocrinol. 2022;14(3):258–66.
24. Yousif MQ, Salih ZT, DeYoung BR, Qasem SA. Differentiating intrarenal ectopic adrenal tissue from renal cell carcinoma in the kidney. Int J Surg Pathol. 2018;26(7):588–92.
25. Corica D, Bottari A, Aversa T, Caudo D, Galletta K, Micalizzi MF, Pajno GB, Wasniewska M, Ascenti G. An unusual epididymal localization of Testicular Adrenal Rest Tumor in an adolescent with congenital adrenal hyperplasia. Endocrine. 2019;66(3):695–8.
26. Erickson LA, Lloyd RV, Hartman R, Thompson G. Cystic adrenal neoplasms. Cancer. 2004;101(7):1537–44.
27. Zheng W, Fung KM, Cheng L, Osunkoya AO. Benign vascular tumors, cysts, and pseudocysts of the adrenal gland: a contemporary multi-institutional clinicopathological analysis of 55 cases. Hum Pathol. 2018;82:95–102.
28. Sebastiano C, Zhao X, Deng FM, Das K. Cystic lesions of the adrenal gland: our experience over the last 20 years. Hum Pathol. 2013;44(9):1797–803.
29. Rozenblit A, Morehouse HT, Amis ES Jr. Cystic adrenal lesions: CT features. Radiology. 1996;201(2):541–8.
30. Chien HP, Chang YS, Hsu PS, Lin JD, Wu YC, Chang HL, Chuang CK, Tsuei KH, Hsueh C. Adrenal cystic lesions: a clinicopathological analysis of 25 cases with proposed histogenesis and review of the literature. Endocr Pathol. 2008;19(4):274–81.
31. Erickson LA, Whaley RD, Gupta S. Adrenal epithelial cysts. Mayo Clin Proc. 2023;98(2):353–4.
32. Bouchaala H, Mejdoub I, Mseddi MA, Kammoun O, Rebai N, Slimen MH. Giant primary hydatid cyst of the adrenal gland: a rare case report. Urol Case Rep. 2021;36:101580.

Chapter 16
Soft Tissue

Juan Xing

Introduction

Soft tissue lesions can be found throughout the human body and can range from palpable subcutaneous/superficial masses to deep seated masses. While sarcomas are a major concern for patients with soft tissue lesions, many soft tissue masses are benign, and not every soft tissue mass is neoplastic. Clinical history, presentation, and specific radiological characteristics are helpful in narrowing down the differential diagnoses, but tumor-like non-neoplastic soft tissue masses can closely resemble sarcomas. Therefore, pathology is often necessary to confirm the final diagnosis. Minimally invasive procedures such as fine needle aspiration (FNA) or core needle biopsy (CNB) are cost-effective modalities for tissue sampling. In contrast to CNB, which is the preferred method for initial workup, the utility of FNA in soft tissue masses has been controversial due to variable cellularity and lack of intact architecture. However, FNA of soft tissue masses has its own unique advantages. Compared to other sampling techniques, superficial soft tissue masses can be easily aspirated at FNA clinics, which are usually accessible as same-day procedures. FNA is an inexpensive method that patients can tolerate well. Rapid on-site evaluation (ROSE) ensures an adequate sample and triages the specimens for appropriate ancillary tests. For instance, obtaining fresh sterile material for microbiology is critical when infections are suspected. Despite FNA being a cost-effective method, soft tissue lesions encountered by cytology service are rare, and practicing cytopathologists might not be familiar with their cytomorphology, clinical features, and radiographic characteristics. We will address non-neoplastic lesions caused by metabolic disorders, trauma, procedures, infectious/inflammatory/autoimmune diseases, and others.

J. Xing (✉)
Cleveland Clinic Pathology & Laboratory Medicine Institute, Cleveland, OH, USA
e-mail: xingj@ccf.org

© The Author(s), under exclusive license to Springer Nature Switzerland AG 2023
S. M. Gilani, G. Cai (eds.), *Non-Neoplastic Cytology*,
https://doi.org/10.1007/978-3-031-44289-6_16

Metabolic Conditions

Amyloidoma

Deposition of amyloid may form a mass (amyloidoma, amyloid tumor, or tumoral amyloidosis), and these localized deposits have been reported in almost all anatomic sites. Amyloidoma may arise in patients with malignancy, including multiple myeloma, lymphoma, and rarely carcinoma [1]. Amyloidoma-associated benign conditions include long-term hemodialysis, chronic infectious, and inflammatory diseases [2, 3]. Rarely, amyloidoma occurs in patients with no preexisting diseases, and these lesions are mainly found in the soft tissues of the extremities [4]. Amyloidoma is a slow-growing non-neoplastic lesion that can clinically and radiographically mimic both benign and malignant neoplasms. Radiologically, amyloidomas show variable features. While some of them exhibit benign imaging features, others have aggressive features that resemble infection or malignant neoplasms [5].

Morphologically, amyloid presents as amorphous material that is homogeneous and waxy. On Diff-Quik (DQ) stain, amyloid appears deep blue to purple colored (Fig. 16.1a), and on Papanicolaou (PAP) stain, it appears green to light blue

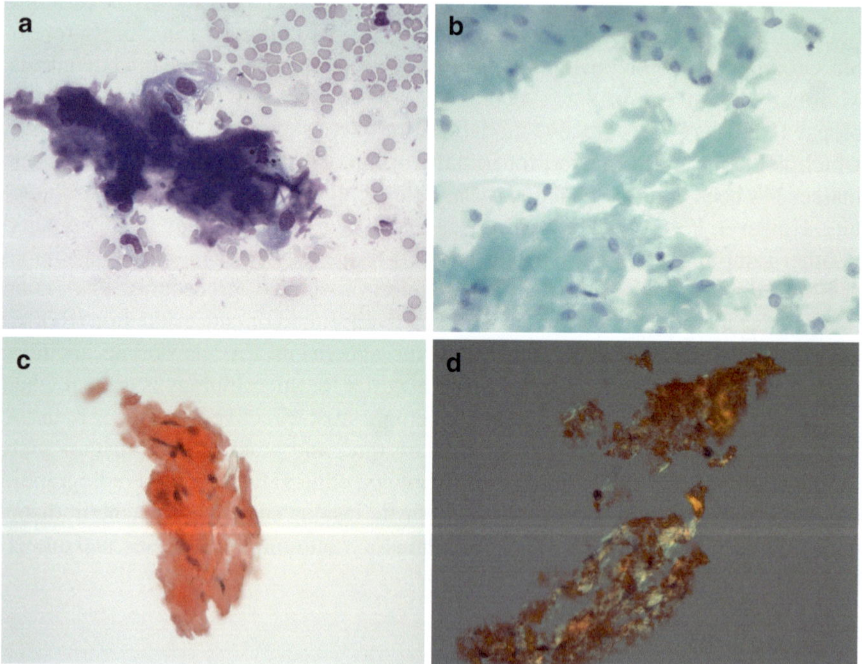

Fig. 16.1 An amyloidoma displays amorphous waxy material: (**a**) Diff-Quik stain (×400). (**b**) Papanicolaou stain (×400). (**c**) Cell block, Congo red stained (×400). (**d**) Cell block, Congo red stain under polarized light (×400)

(Fig. 16.1b). Under a light microscope, it displays a salmon pink color (Fig. 16.1c) and exhibits an apple-green color birefringence under polarized light with a Congo red stain (Fig. 16.1d). The cellularity is variable and consists of histiocytes, multinucleated giant cells, with or without a variable amount of lymphoplasmacytic cells. The presence of a foreign body-type granulomatous reaction may be misinterpreted as a giant cell tumor of soft tissue or a giant cell reparative granuloma. Mimics of extracellular material that may be mistaken for amyloid include calcifications, chondromyxoid matrix, hyalinizing collagen, thick mucin, and thick colloid (Table 16.1).

Table 16.1 Differential diagnosis of extracellular material

	Cytomorphology	Associated diseases	Ancillary studies
Amyloid	Variable sizes of amorphous, homogeneous, and waxy material	Multiple myeloma, lymphoma, rarely carcinoma, chronic hemodialysis, infectious/ inflammatory diseases, localized amyloidoma without preexisting conditions, systemic amyloidosis	Congo red stain: salmon pink color under a light microscope and apple-green color birefringence under polarized light
Calcifications	Finely granular debris, irregular-shaped large chunk, psammoma body-like structures	Tumoral calcinosis, microcalcifications in breast lesions/neoplasms, psammoma bodies in thyroid and ovarian lesions/neoplasms	von Kossa stain: black or brown-black color
Chondromyxoid matrix	Metachromatic fibrillary material, gumball-like spheres, amorphous granular or film-like myxoid material, chunky chondroid material with sharp borders	Salivary gland neoplasms, myxoid lesions/neoplasms, chondroid lesions/ neoplasms	Chondrocytes positive for S100 immunohistochemistry, ancillary studies in the cellular component for specific diagnosis
Collagen fibers	Strands of thick material with vague linear lines, often with crush artifact	Hyalinizing fibrous lesions/neoplasms	Trichrome stain: blue color
Thick mucin	Thick amorphous material in the center with fibrillary edge	Mucocele, mucinous neoplasms	Mucicarmine stain: red color PAS stain: magenta color
Thick colloid	Homogeneous, well-defined round, oval, or irregular border	Thyroid lesions/ neoplasms	Positive for thyroglobulin immunohistochemistry

Abdominal Fat Pad Fine Needle Aspiration for Systemic Amyloidosis

Systemic amyloidosis is much more common than amyloidoma and has a worse prognosis [6]. It is a life-threatening condition that leads to organ dysfunction and ultimately death. Prompt diagnosis and treatment are critical in managing these patients. Thus, it is worthwhile to discuss the utility of abdominal fat pad fine needle aspiration (AFP-FNA) for diagnosing systemic amyloidosis, even in the absence of mass lesion formation. AFP-FNA was introduced in the 1970s as a diagnostic procedure for systemic amyloidosis and has since become a preferred outpatient method for evaluating clinically suspicious patients [7]. The reported sensitivity of AFP-FNA ranges from 19% to 93%, and specificity is close to 100% [8–11]. Possible causes of false-negative results include insufficient adipose tissue, difficulty in interpreting Congo red stain, and lack of experience of cytopathologists [12].

To procure adequate tissue, larger gauge needles (e.g., 22 G to 18 G) are used. The area about 2 in. away from the umbilicus is aspirated. On-site evaluation of smears to look for at least 5–6 lobules of adipose tissue with associated blood vessels is adequate. In general, 4–5 FNA passes are needed to obtain an adequate sample if a 22 G needle is used. Aspirate smears are prepared from the first 1 or 2 passes to assess the adequacy, and the same smears can be used for Congo red stain. Needle rinse and 2–3 dedicated passes are collected in preservatives for cell block. An adequate cell block is prudent because amyloid subtyping is required for clinical management. Congo red-stained smear slides show a salmon pink color under a light microscope (Fig. 16.2a) and an apple-green color birefringence under polarized light (Fig. 16.2b). Congo red-stained cell block sections have similar findings (Fig. 16.2c, d). In contrast to amyloidoma, amyloid precipitate within the blood vessel walls and fibrous tissue surrounding the adipocytes instead of forming large amorphous material. A potential pitfall is mistaking elastic fibers of blood vessel walls as amyloid deposition. Elastic fibers demonstrate bright yellow to orange color and fibrillary, while amyloid shows an apple-green color and appears homogeneous under polarized light. Sometimes, amyloid deposits are focal, making a definitive diagnosis difficult. AFP-FNA is a simple, safe, and highly specific diagnostic method for suspected systemic amyloidosis although negative results do not exclude the possibility, and additional diagnostic modalities should be considered if clinical suspicion is high.

Tumoral Calcinosis

Tumoral calcinosis is a non-neoplastic disorder and characterized by tumor-like periarticular soft tissue deposition of calcium hydroxyapatite. It mainly presents in large joints and involves soft tissue in the regions of the hip, shoulder, and elbow [13]. There are three forms of tumoral calcinosis [14]. The most common form is

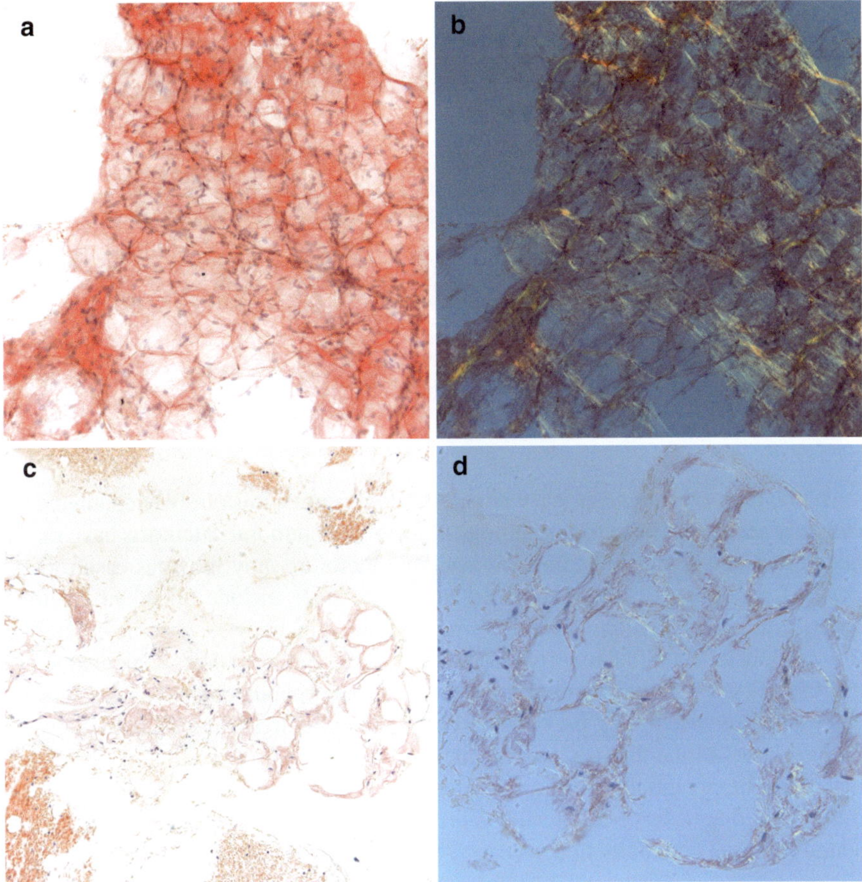

Fig. 16.2 Systemic amyloidosis detected through abdominal fat pad fine needle aspiration: (**a**) Congo red stain (×200). (**b**) Congo red under polarized light (×200). (**c**) Cell block, Congo red stained (×200). (**d**) Cell block, Congo red stain under polarized light (×400)

sporadic and idiopathic. The second form is familial, inherited in an autosomal recessive manner, and consists of hyperphosphatemic and normophosphatemic tumoral calcinosis. There is also a secondary form of tumoral calcinosis due to the overproduction of ectopic calcifications, which includes a wide variety of conditions such as chronic renal failure and primary hyperparathyroidism, among many others. Radiologically, the differential diagnosis is broad and includes benign conditions and sarcomas. Plain film radiographs, computed tomography (CT), and magnetic resonance imaging (MRI) reveal a large conglomerate of amorphous cloud-like densities separated by radiolucent lines within the soft tissue, imparting a chicken-wire pattern of lucencies with a distinct fluid level in some of the nodules [15, 16].

Fig. 16.3 Tumoral calcinosis shows calcifications of various shapes (Cell block, Hematoxylin Eosin stain, ×400)

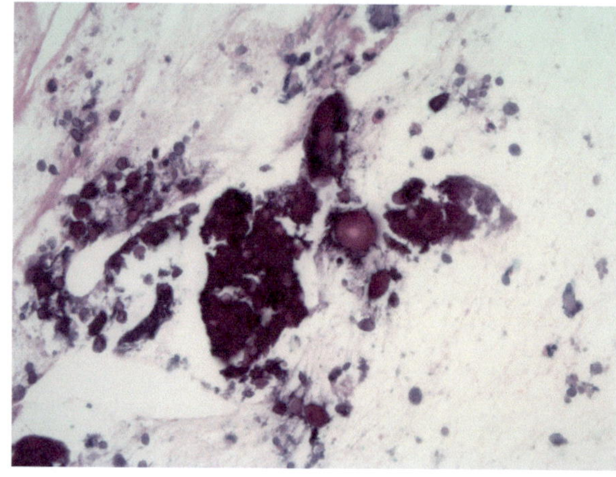

While tumoral calcinosis is a distinct histologic entity, it is rarely encountered by cytology services. The cytomorphological features of tumoral calcinosis have rarely been described in cytology, and the available literature only includes case reports [17–21]. Common features described in the literature include abundant calcified amorphous material, mononuclear or multinucleated histiocytes, chronic inflammatory cells, osteoclast-like multinucleated giant cells, and fibroblasts. Calcified material can present as finely granular debris, large amorphous chunks and laminated calcospherites resembling psammoma body-like structures (Fig. 16.3). Depending on the phases of the disease, lesions could have a florid proliferation of fibroblasts that could be potentially misdiagnosed as a calcifying spindle cell neoplasm. The differential diagnosis of calcifications includes amyloid, ova of parasites, and ultrasound (US) gel contamination.

Tophaceous Gout

Tophaceous gout is the most severe form of gout and occurs when monosodium urate (MSU) crystals form masses. MSU crystal-induced soft tissue masses are known as tophi, which usually develop around the joints and soft tissue in patients with longstanding chronic hyperuricemia but may manifest as an initial presentation when they occur subcutaneously [22]. Tophi are commonly found in fingers, elbows, toes, and other locations such as the Achilles tendon and the knees [15]. Clinically, soft tissue tophi may be mistaken as a soft tissue neoplasm, and pathology may be required, especially in patients without a previous history of gout. Radiologically, a tophus often shows classic features of gout on plain radiographs, which demonstrate a well-defined dense mass with the presence of well-defined/punched-out erosions with overhanging edges and sclerotic margins with a marginal distribution [15].

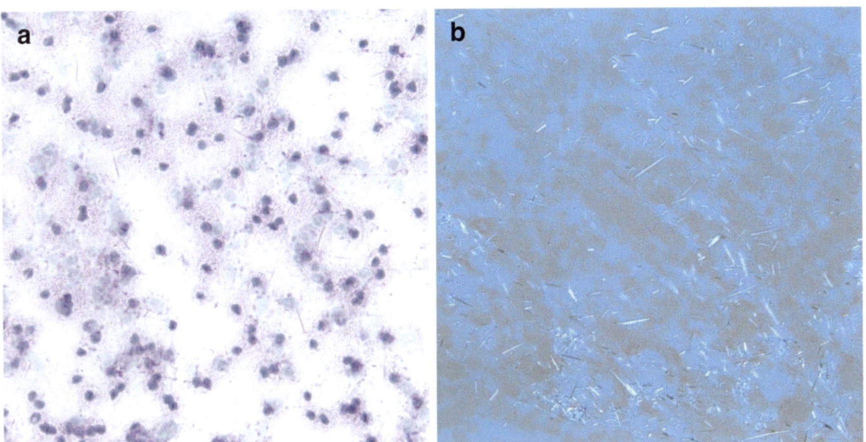

Fig. 16.4 Tophi with needle-shaped crystals: (**a**) Diff-Quik stain (×600). (**b**) Unstained smear slide under polarized light (×600)

FNA is a valuable tool as it is easier and less painful than biopsy. When tophi are aspirated, the material expelled on the glass slides demonstrates a white chalky consistency. A crunchy or squeaking-sand sound can be appreciated when preparing the smear slides. Awareness of these features is helpful during the procedure, as a portion of fresh specimen can be sent to the clinical laboratory for crystal analysis for confirmation. Microscopically, MSU crystals are readily detectable as characteristic needle-shaped, negatively birefringent microcrystals under polarization. They can be seen on a variety of cytology preparations, including unstained slides (Fig. 16.4a), DQ-stained air-dried smears (Fig. 16.4b) and PAP-stained alcohol-fixed smears or ThinPrep slides. MSU crystals are usually lost in formalin-fixed cell blocks. In addition to numerous MSU crystals, histiocytes, multinucleated giant cells, and inflammatory cells can be variably present. The differential diagnosis includes other crystal-induced arthritis such as pseudogout and infectious or inflammatory arthritis, which will be discussed in detail below in non-neoplastic bone lesions.

Traumatic and Procedure-Related Conditions

Hematoma

Hematomas are caused by localized collections of blood and are often associated with traumatic muscle injury, muscle strain, contusions, anticoagulant therapy, clotting disorders, and occasionally iatrogenic conditions. They are slowly growing expanding masses and account for 5% of soft tissue masses [23].

Fig. 16.5 A hematoma exhibits degenerated red blood cells, fibrin, and occasional hemosiderin-laden macrophages (ThinPrep slide, Papanicolaou stain, ×400)

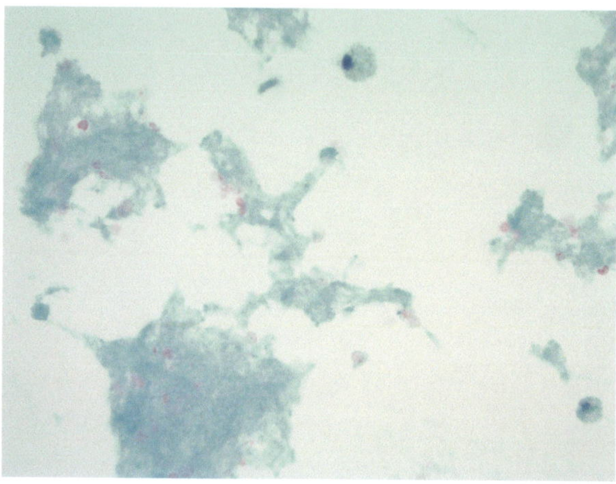

Radiologically, the appearance of hematomas changes over time depending on their stages. In the later stage, an organizing hematoma could form, demonstrating a heterogeneous pseudo-solid mass. Its complex appearance may be indistinguishable from an aggressive tumor [15]. Therefore, for deeply seated hematomas, tissue sampling is often performed to exclude the possibility of neoplastic process.

The amount of material sampled from hematomas by FNA depends on the stages and ranges from scanty to abundant blood. Cytology specimens are usually hypocellular with lysed/degenerated blood, fibrin, and occasional hemosiderin-laden macrophages (Fig. 16.5). When an organizing hematoma is aspirated, reactive fibroblasts may be seen. Clinical history and radiological findings are helpful for further classification. In patients who are diagnosed with a hematoma by FNA or CNB, clinical and radiological correlation, as well as close follow-up, are required to ensure the gradual resolution of the masses. It is important to exclude intratumoral hemorrhage associated with malignancy. The differential diagnosis includes benign vascular tumors and arteriovenous malformation.

Postoperative Seroma

Seromas are fluid collections caused by the leakage of serous exudate. They are commonly associated with surgery and formed in the surgical tracts. Seromas typically manifest as enlarging and sometimes painful swelling near the surgical sites. Acute or non-infected seromas can be diagnosed using US, and tissue sampling may not be necessary. On the other hand, complicated or chronic seromas may exhibit non-enhancing/peripheral enhancing fluid collection of variable complexity on radiology studies, which may raise the possibility of neoplasm or tumor recurrence [15].

FNA can be both diagnostic and therapeutic by draining the fluid. It can yield a variable amount of clear or straw-colored fluid from non-infected seromas and cloudy yellow-colored or rarely pus-like fluid in infected seromas. FNA cytology findings are nonspecific. Aspirate smears and cell blocks are usually acellular or hypocellular with a few macrophages and lymphocytes. Aspirates may show a variable amount of acute inflammation or mixed acute and chronic inflammation when seromas are infected. When infection is suspected during ROSE, it is important to submit a portion of the specimen for microbiology and obtain adequate material for special stains. Seromas usually take 2–6 months for seromas to resolve. It is also important to closely follow-up with patients who undergo surgery for malignancy to avoid mistaking tumor recurrence as a seroma.

Fat Necrosis

Fat necrosis is a non-neoplastic inflammatory lesion that is presumably related to trauma. It can occur in various areas such as the breasts, thighs and over sites of bony prominences, forming a mass lesion [24]. In patients who have undergone prior surgical procedures, it may occur in the surrounding fibroadipose tissue near the surgical sites. Clinically, patients present with a painful or asymptomatic mass lesion that can mimic a neoplasm. Some patients do not recall a preceding history of trauma. Radiologically, a focal area containing fat lobules with varying degrees of surrounding inflammatory changes can be identified on US and MRI [15]. Foci of fat necrosis can also be detected in a large lipomatous mass of concern on radiology [15]. Often, the diagnosis of fat necrosis is based on clinical presentation with support from radiology. However, in patients with a prior history of surgery for malignancy or in female patients presenting with an asymptomatic breast mass without previous history of surgery or trauma, it may be sampled for pathology to exclude the possibility of malignancy.

FNA can be used as an initial modality to sample these lesions. Aspirate smear slides show necrotic adipocytes with associated foamy macrophages, multinucleated giant cells, and variable amount of chronic inflammation (Fig. 16.6). In the late stages, varying degrees of fibrosis with fibroblast proliferation and calcifications may occur and persist for years. While the diagnosis is typically easy and straightforward, obtaining an adequate sample is important to prevent sampling errors, particularly in large lesions. FNA can be helpful as it allows for obtaining tissue from multiple portions of the mass by altering the direction of the needle. The differential diagnosis includes benign and malignant lipomatous tumors, xanthomas histiocytic disease such as Erdheim-Chester disease, fibroblastic tumors in cases of long-standing fat necrosis, and foreign body granulomas.

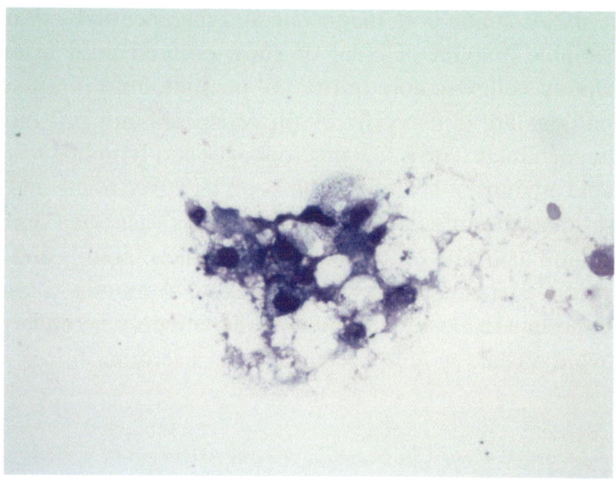

Fig. 16.6 Fat necrosis is characterized by necrotic adipocytes with surrounding foamy macrophages (Diff-Quik stain, ×400)

Foreign Body Granuloma

Foreign body reaction is an inflammatory response to an exogenous substance that is recognized as foreign material by the immune system. The most common manifestation of foreign body reaction is foreign body granuloma (FBG), which is characterized by granulomatous inflammation surrounding the foreign body. It can occur at any site, but sites of the cutaneous injuries are most commonly affected. Many substances can induce a foreign body reaction, including silica from traumatic inoculation, silicone from cosmetic procedures, cotton gauge or suture from surgeries, and tattoos, among others. In some cases, FBG may present as a soft tissue mass and accounts for less than 1% of soft tissue tumor mimics [23]. Clinically, patients typically present with a nonspecific painful or painless mass, and many of them have a recent history of surgical procedure or penetrating soft tissue injury. US is the preferred diagnostic test as it can detect radiolucent foreign bodies and often reveal a hyperechoic linear structure within a hypoechoic mass [15].

Microscopically, aspirate smears and cell block sections show epithelioid histiocytes singly or in aggregates, foreign body type multinucleated giant cells, and varying amount of lymphoplasmacytic cells. Well-formed granulomas may or may not be present. The definitive diagnosis is established by identifying the specific foreign body material (Fig. 16.7a, b), and examination under polarized light is necessary (Table 16.2). The differential diagnosis includes fat necrosis, infectious/inflammatory granulomatous reactions, and lipomatous tumors.

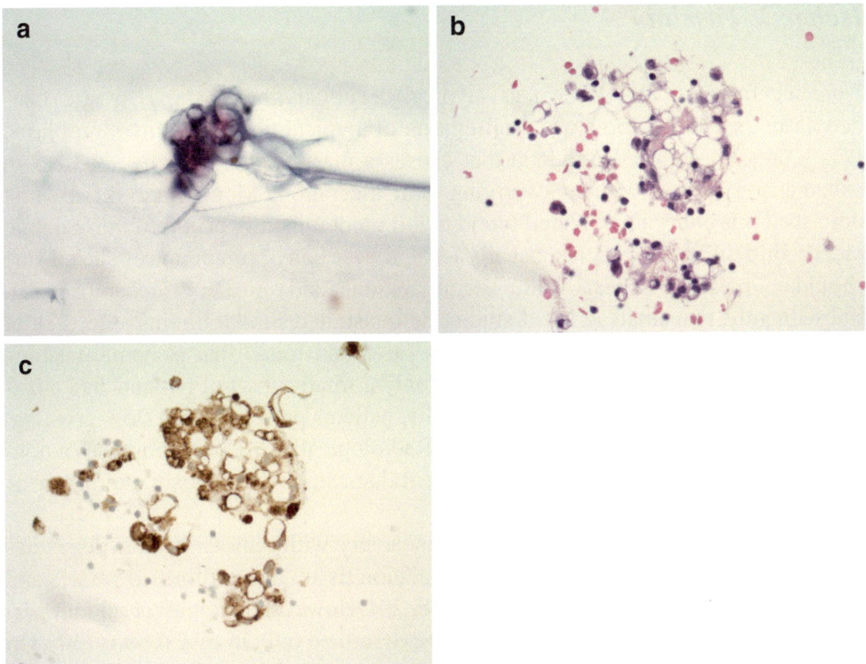

Fig. 16.7 Silicon-induced foreign body reaction displays round, clear intracytoplasmic droplets, resulting in a Swiss cheese-like pattern on the cell block: (**a**) Papanicolaou stain (×400). (**b**) Cell block, Hematoxylin Eosin stain (×400). (**c**) CD68 immunostain (×400)

Table 16.2 Patterns of foreign bodies that may be encountered by cytology

Foreign body	Morphology	Polarizable	Ancillary studies
Tattoo	Extracellular pigment and pigment laden macrophages	No	No
Silicone	Cystic spaces of varying size (Swiss cheese) due to intracytoplasmic clear round-shaped droplets	No	Stain with oil red O on fresh tissue
Paraffin	Cystic spaces of varying size (Swiss cheese) due to intracytoplasmic clear round-shaped droplets	No	Do not stain with oil red O on fresh tissue
Silica	Crystalline particles or amorphous	Yes	No
Talc	Thin, flat plates or flake-like particles	Yes	No
Starch	Maltese cross-shaped pattern	Yes	Positive for PAS
Suture	Vary depending on the type of suture, can be glassy and sharply circumscribed	Yes	No

Ischemic Fasciitis

Ischemic fasciitis, also known as atypical decubital fibroplasia, is a rare non-neoplastic, pseudosarcomatous proliferation of atypical fibroblasts/myofibroblasts. It is a pressure-induced ischemia that causes a mass-forming reactive process in subcutaneous tissue without overlying skin ulceration. Montgomery et al. first described this entity in 1992 and found that it predominantly occurred in immobile elderly or deliberated patients, usually located over bony protuberances such as the shoulder, posterior chest wall, sacral region, and greater trochantor [25]. Subsequently, two small series of studies demonstrated similar findings [26, 27]. In 2008, Liegl et al. reported a series of 44 cases and found that ischemic fasciitis could also be seen in young patients, and only a small subset of patients had a history of physical deliberation [28]. Clinically, patients present with a slow-growing, painless mass located at a pressure point. Radiologically, MRI demonstrates a non-specific mass with a central fluid component that can be erroneously interpreted as a necrotic sarcoma [15].

Histology shows characteristic zonal appearance with central fibrinoid degeneration/necrosis surrounded by a ring of granulation tissue-like neoformed vessels and proliferating fibroblasts/myofibroblasts [28, 29]. However, cytology is seldom performed, and cytomorphological features are described only in case reports [30]. On cytology, fibroblasts/myofibroblasts present as spindled or oval cells with ample cytoplasm. It is advised to be conservative and request CNB if atypical fibroblasts/myofibroblasts are seen during ROSE. FNA and CNB complement each other and help to reduce false-positive diagnosis of sarcoma. Fibroblasts/myofibroblasts show focal positivity for smooth muscle action (SMA) and desmin, but these stains are not helpful for further classification. The differential diagnosis includes proliferative fasciitis, proliferative myositis, nodular fasciitis, and sarcomas with fibroblastic proliferation. Table 16.3 summarizes the clinical, radiological, and cytomorphological features of pseudosarcomatous fibroblastic/myofibroblastic proliferation. Overall, ischemic fasciitis is a rare non-neoplastic lesion that can be confused with a sarcoma radiologically and microscopically. A clinical history of a subcutaneous mass at a pressure point in an immobile elderly or physically deliberated patient is a tip-off to a diagnosis although it can also be seen in young patients without physical deliberation.

Proliferative Fasciitis and Proliferative Myositis

Proliferative fasciitis (PF) and proliferative myositis (PM) are the same disease process involving the subcutaneous tissue (PF) and skeletal muscle (PM), respectively. They are considered as mass-forming inflammatory pseudosarcomatous lesions. However, recent studies have shown that PF/PM harbors *FOS* gene rearrangement, similar to nodular fasciitis, which has a characteristic *USP6* gene rearrangement

Table 16.3 Clinical, radiological, and cytomorphological features of benign pseudosarcomatous lesions

	Ischemic fasciitis	Proliferative fasciitis	Proliferative myositis	Nodular fasciitis
Reactive vs. neoplastic	Reactive	May be neoplastic	May be neoplastic	Neoplastic
Anatomic sites	Pressure points at subcutaneous tissue of shoulder, posterior chest wall, sacral region, greater trochanter	Subcutaneous tissue of upper extremities, particularly forearm, lower extremities, trunk	Skeletal muscle of trunk, shoulder girdles, upper extremities, less likely in the thighs	Most common in subcutaneous tissue throughout body, common in extremities, head and neck, trunk
Patient age	Mostly in elder patients, may occur in young patients	Predominantly in middle aged adults, rarely in children	Predominantly in middle aged adults, rarely in children	Predominantly in young adults, can occur at any age
Presentation	Slow growing painless mass in immobile elder or deliberated patients, also occurs in young patients without deliberation	Rapid-growing firm mass, about 2/3 of patients with pain or tenderness	Rapid-growing firm mass, about 2/3 of patients with pain or tenderness	Rapid-growing firm mass, may be tender, mildly painful, or asymptomatic
Radiology	A nonspecific mass with a central fluid component on MRI that can be mistaken as a necrotic sarcoma	Enhancing mass lesion with features suggestive of a benign inflammatory process, but nonspecific	Enhancing mass lesion with features suggestive of a benign inflammatory process, but nonspecific	Nonspecific, difficult to differentiate from sarcoma
Cytology	Spindled cells or oval-shaped cells with ample cytoplasm	Spindled or plump oval cells with round to oval nuclei, hallmark ganglion-like cells, myxoid background with lymphocytes	Spindled or plump oval cells with round to oval nuclei, hallmark ganglion-like cells, myxoid background with lymphocytes	Spindled or plump oval cells, mitosis may be seen but not atypical, myxoid background with scattered lymphocytes and macrophages
Gene rearrangement	None	Recent studies reveal *FOS* gene rearrangement in epithelioid cells	Recent studies reveal *FOS* gene rearrangement in epithelioid cells	USP6 gene rearrangement in more than 90% cases

[31–34]. This suggests that PF/PM may be a neoplastic clonal process. The most common anatomical sites involved by PF include the upper extremities, particularly forearm, lower extremities, and trunk. PM often occurs in the trunk, shoulder

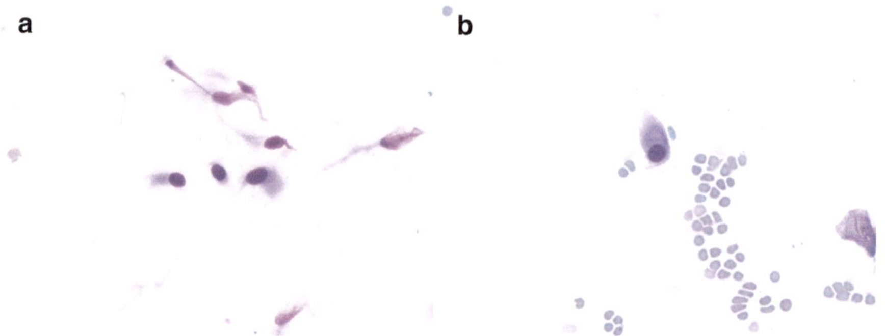

Fig. 16.8 Touch preparation of a core biopsy of proliferative myositis shows rare plump fibroblasts (**a**) and a ganglion-like cell (**b**) (Diff-Quik stain ×600). (Courtesy from Dr. Lajara)

girdles, upper extremities, and less likely in the thighs [35, 36]. Clinically, patients present with a rapid growing firm mass that mimics a sarcoma. PF masses are always less than 5 cm, while PM may be slightly larger. Pain or tenderness is noted in about two-thirds of the patients [35]. MRI demonstrates an enhancing mass lesion with features suggestive of a benign inflammatory process, but a definitive diagnosis cannot be made by radiology [37]. Thus, tissue sampling is required to confirm the diagnosis.

Cytological features of PF/PM lesions have been reported in case reports [38–40]. Cytology shows variable cellularity and usually hypocellular due to fibrosis. Fibroblasts/myofibroblasts demonstrate spindled cells with long cytoplasmic processes and ample cytoplasm or plump oval cells with round to oval nuclei (Fig. 16.8a). The hallmark cells are round cells with eccentrically located large nuclei, prominent nucleoli, and abundant cytoplasm, known as ganglion-like cells (Fig. 16.8b). The large nuclei are cytologically benign with smooth nuclear membranes and fine, even chromatin. The background is myxoid with lymphocytes and erythrocytes. The differential diagnosis includes ischemic fasciitis, nodular fasciitis, and sarcomas with fibroblastic proliferation. Overall, PF/PM can be mistaken clinically as a sarcoma due to its rapidly growing firm mass. Recent studies suggest that it is probably a neoplastic clonal process with *FOS* gene rearrangement.

Infections, Inflammation, and Autoimmune Diseases

Abscess

Abscess is a localized collection of pus that can develop at any anatomic sites and in patients of all age groups. It accounts for approximately 7% of soft tissue pseudotumors [23]. Soft tissue abscesses usually result from the direct extension of cutaneous infections or complications of trauma or surgery. Risk factors for abscess

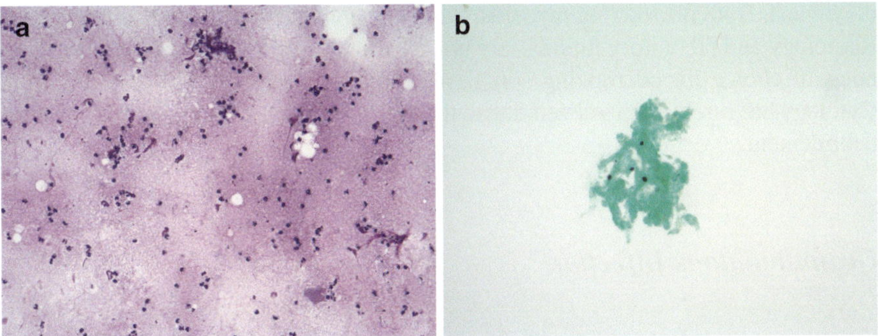

Fig. 16.9 An abscess displays nonspecific acute inflammation, and teardrop-shaped histoplasmas are revealed by the GMS stain (**a**) Diff-Quik stain (×200). (**b**) GMS stain (×400)

formation include post-surgery, immunocompromise/immunodeficiency, diabetes, and coexisting systemic infections. The most common causative agent is *Staphylococcus aureus* although various microorganisms can lead to abscess formation. Clinically, patients with abscesses typically present with fever and a painful fluctuant mass. The overlying skin usually appears pink/red and warm. Radiologically, US is a useful tool for identifying abscesses, demonstrating a cystic mass with peripheral and surrounding soft tissue vascularity [15].

FNA of an abscess can be particularly helpful as it is less painful. Cytology diagnosis is usually straightforward, with specimens showing abundant acute inflammation and inflammatory exudates (Fig. 16.9a). Sometimes, bacteria can be readily identifiable on the smear slides. When an abscess is suspected during ROSE, it is critical to submit fresh sterile material for microbiology cultures. Unstained smear slides can also be used for special stains, including Gram stain, acid-fast bacillus (AFB) stain, and Grocott's methenamine silver (GMS) stain. Occasionally, PAP stained ThinPrep slides can be reused for special stains when microbiology findings are non-contributory, particularly for fungal infection (Fig. 16.9b). In patients with a history of surgery for malignancy, specimens should be carefully examined to exclude tumor recurrence with superimposed abscess formation.

Necrotizing Soft Tissue Infections

Necrotizing soft tissue infections include necrotizing forms of fasciitis, myositis, and cellulitis. They are rare but rapidly progressive, causing fulminant tissue destruction. These infections are life-threatening infection and can be fatal if left untreated. Early recognition and intervention are crucial, as even with treatment, there is 15% mortality [41]. They are usually caused by group A *streptococcus*, but other bacteria or fungi can also be the causative agents, including zygomycosis [42]. Necrotizing fasciitis is characterized by extensive fascial necrosis and difficult to distinguish from necrotizing myositis, which is an infection of the skeletal muscle. Radiology and laboratory findings are nonspecific. Surgical exploration is the diagnosis of choice for necrotizing soft tissue infections and should not be delayed. Cytology has rarely been utilized due to the rapid clinical course and urgent need for debridement.

Granulomatous Infection

Granulomatous infection is a pathologic description characterized by aggregates of histiocytes with variable inflammatory cells, with or without multinucleated giant cells. It exhibits the same morphology at any sites. It is further divided into necrotizing and non-necrotizing granulomatous inflammation. While necrotizing granulomatous inflammation is mainly due to infections, it can also be seen in non-infectious diseases such as granulomatosis with polyangiitis. Granulomatous infections of soft tissue can form a mass lesion, which can potentially pose diagnostic challenges clinically and radiologically [15]. Various bacterial and fungal microorganisms are capable of forming a soft tissue mass, including *Mycobacterium tuberculosis*, atypical *Mycobacterium* species, *Actinomyces* species, mucormycosis, histoplasmosis, among others [43–46]. FNA can be of great value in obtaining tissue for diagnosis, and smear slides can be used for special stains. Since granulomas are morphologically similar and the differential diagnosis is broad, ancillary studies including microbiology cultures, special stains, and clinical information are required to identify the underlying etiology.

Epidermal Inclusion Cyst

Epidermal inclusion cyst is the most common cutaneous cystic lesion. It is caused by obstructed hair follicles or deep implantation of epidermal elements into dermis. It can occur anywhere in the body but are most commonly seen in the head and neck region, trunk, and extremities. Patients present with a slow growing, firm to fluctuant, dome-shaped mass, and the diagnosis is often made on clinical assessment. US is helpful and shows a well-circumscribed, heterogeneous filiform lesion that often exhibits posterior acoustic enhancement and no vascular signal [15]. Manipulation or trauma can induce inflammation and/or rupture of the cyst. Inflamed or ruptured cyst can involve the surrounding soft tissue and may lead to fat necrosis with foreign body granulomatous reaction and variable amount of inflammation. Radiologically, an inflamed or ruptured epidermal inclusion cyst may have an appearance similar to that of an aggressive lesion such as sarcoma.

FNA is the preferred sampling method. The aspirated material has a soft, whitish, cheesy consistency with an odor. The smear slides show anucleate squamous cells, as well as cholesterol crystals and keratin flakes (Fig. 16.10). Acute and/or

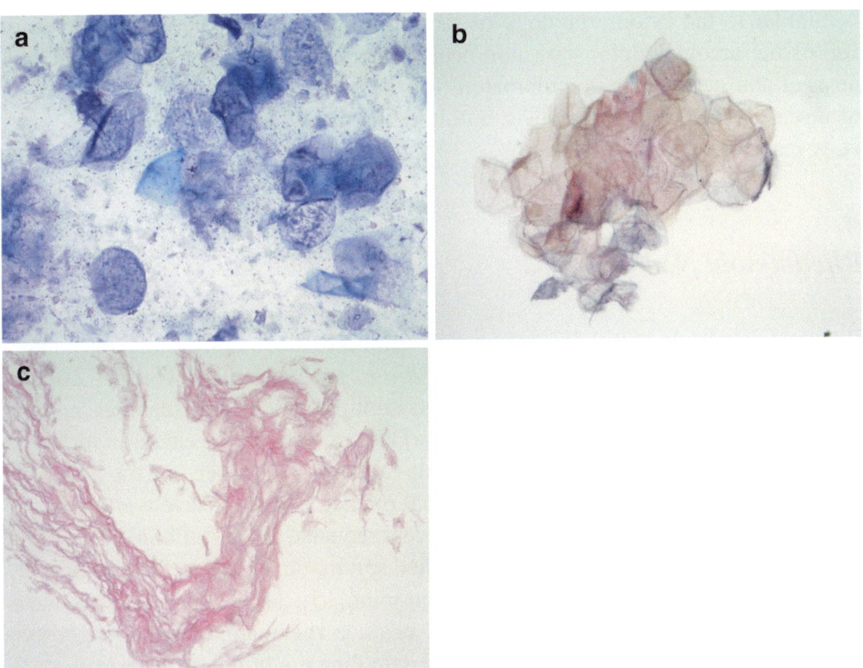

Fig. 16.10 Epidermal inclusion cyst shows anucleated squamous cells with cholesterol crystals and keratin flakes (**a**) Diff-Quik stain (×400). (**b**) ThinPrep slide, Papanicolaou stain (×400). (**c**) Cell block, Hematoxylin Eosin stain (400×)

granulomatous inflammation may be observed if the cyst is inflamed or ruptured. The differential diagnosis includes necrotic keratin debris associated with squamous cell carcinoma, other squamous lined cystic lesions, and foreign body granulomas.

Sarcoid Nodule

Sarcoidosis is a multisystem granulomatous inflammatory disease of unclear etiology. Soft tissue involvement by sarcoidosis is common [47]. In patients with sarcoidosis, non-necrotizing granulomas have been frequently detected in muscle biopsies, but tumor-like sarcoid nodules are relatively rare [47–49]. In addition to skeletal muscle, sarcoid nodules can also be seen in subcutaneous tissue and tendon sheets [50, 51]. Clinically, patients present with painless subcutaneous/soft tissue masses, mimicking soft tissue tumors. A clinical history of preexisting sarcoidosis or characteristic pulmonary sarcoid is helpful in making the diagnosis. US reveals a hypoechoic nodule without internal vascularity, but the features are not specific.

Similar to the cytomorphology of sarcoidosis in other organ systems, FNA of soft tissue sarcoid nodules show non-necrotizing granulomas. The differential diagnosis of non-necrotizing granulomatous inflammation can be seen in a wide variety of diseases, including sarcoidosis, autoimmune disorders, drug reactions, foreign body reactions, and malignancies.

Rheumatoid Nodule

Rheumatoid nodules are the most common extra-articular manifestation of rheumatoid arthritis and commonly arise in the skin as subcutaneous/soft tissue nodules [52, 53]. Clinically, they present as single or multiple solitary subcutaneous nodules near-pressure point and prominent bone surfaces, mostly on the extensor surface at sites of frequent trauma [54, 55]. The nodules are firm, nontender, and movable. The presence of rheumatoid nodules is a clinical predictor of more severe arthritis, and more aggressive treatment is needed to prevent sequalae [56, 57]. Plain radiographs, US and MRI show a nonspecific, noncalcified soft tissue mass, and features of rheumatoid arthritis may be seen in the adjacent joint [15]. The presence of subcutaneous/soft tissue nodules in a patient with positive rheumatoid factors suggests a diagnosis of rheumatoid nodule, and tissue sampling might not be necessary.

Cytologic features of subcutaneous/soft tissue rheumatoid nodules have been described in the literature [58]. Cytology specimens show many macrophages, epithelioid histocytes, occasional multinucleated giant cells, and variable inflammatory cells in a background of necrosis. Well-formed granulomas are less common [59]. Occasionally, florid fibroblast/myofibroblast proliferation with cytological atypia may be seen and may be misdiagnosed as a spindle cell malignancy [60]. The differential diagnosis includes infectious and other inflammatory granulomatous diseases.

Miscellaneous

Brown Adipose Tissue

Brown adipose tissue (normal brown fat) is a specialized type of adipose tissue that regulates body temperature in newborns. It has been believed that brown adipose tissue is replaced by white adipose tissue over time, and minimal residual brown fat is present in adults. However, recent studies have shown that substantial amounts of metabolically active brown adipose tissue can be present in healthy adult humans [61, 62]. Medical conditions can also lead to increased brown adipose tissue in adults, such as alcohol abuse, malnourishment and cachexia, and cardiovascular diseases [63]. Common locations of brown adipose tissue in the human body include the interscapular region, neck, mediastinum, axilla, and retroperitoneum. They are mostly incidental findings in patients who undergo positron-emission tomography (PET) and CT for the diagnosis of neoplasms and metastases. Due to high glucose uptake on PET-CT and the common location for metastasis, brown adipose tissue can be mistaken as a neoplasm or metastatic deposit [61].

Cytology specimens show flat sheets or lobules of adipocytes separated by fibrous septa. Brown adipocytes are smaller than white adipocytes, polygonal shaped, and contain abundant multivacuolated and/or granular cytoplasm with peripherally located bland appearing nuclei (Fig. 16.11a, b). The cells are positive for S100 (Fig. 16.11c) but negative for keratin and other soft tissue markers. The differential diagnosis includes benign and malignant neoplasms exhibiting clear cell features, such as clear cell renal cell carcinoma. Hibernoma, a benign neoplasm of brown adipose tissue, poses challenges in distinguishing it from normal brown adipose tissue through cytology.

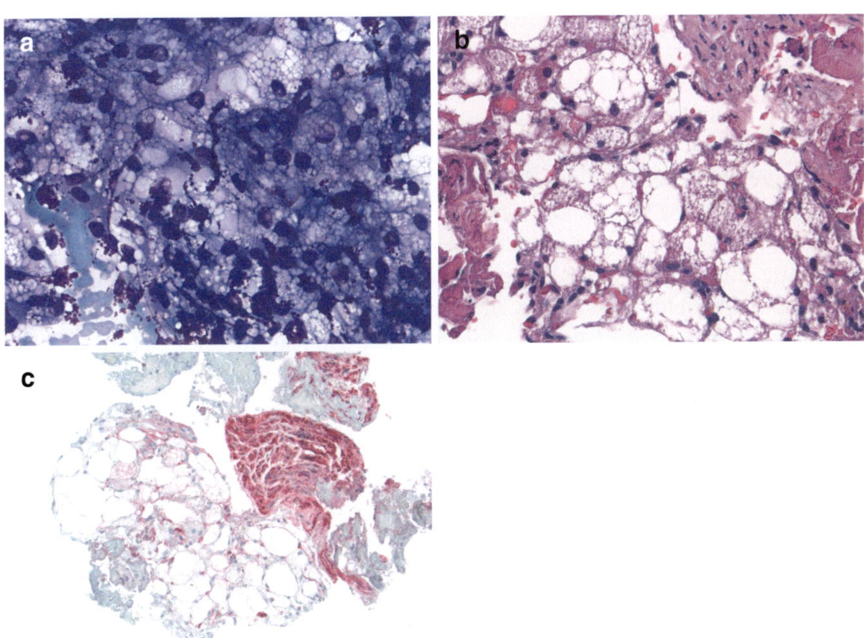

Fig. 16.11 Brown adipose tissue exhibits lobules of adipose tissue with polygonal-shaped cells containing multivacuolated cytoplasm. S100 stain confirms the adipocytes. (**a**) Diff-Quik stain (×400). (**b**) Cell block, Hematoxylin Eosin stain (400×). (**c**) S100 immunostain (×200). (Courtesy from Dr. Lajara)

Ancillary Studies

In contrast to neoplastic lesions, special stains are often used to aid in the diagnosis of non-neoplastic lesions. For instance, GRAM, AFB, and GMS stains are utilized to identify microorganisms. Congo red stain is employed for amyloid, and Oil red O is used for silicone material and adipose tissue. Examination of specimens under polarized light is warranted for crystals and foreign bodies. Immunohistochemistry is less frequently used and is often employed to exclude the possibility of a neoplastic process. Caution should be exercised when interpreting immunohistochemical stains. Fibroblasts/myofibroblasts can be focally positive for SMA and desmin, but this is not indicative of a neoplasm. Occasionally, they can exhibit focal positivity for keratin stains, but this should not be interpreted as malignancy. Non-neoplastic pseudosarcomatous lesions can morphologically mimic benign soft tissue tumors and sarcomas. Fluorescent in situ hybridization (FISH) and next-generation sequencing (NGS) might be performed to exclude an aggressive process.

Conclusions

FNA is a valuable and cost-effective method for sampling soft tissue lesions, especially certain non-neoplastic entities. Cytopathologist's familiarity with these entities can greatly benefit patients. However, non-neoplastic soft tissue lesions are not commonly sampled by cytology, and the cytomorphological descriptions of some entities in this section are primarily based on case reports. Additionally, non-neoplastic inflammatory pseudosarcomatous lesions can closely resemble sarcomas, and FNA yields may be low in such cases. Therefore, it is important to note that accurate diagnosis of these lesions requires clinical, radiological, and pathological correlation.

Acknowledgments Dr. Sigfred Lajara for providing images.

Conflict of Interest None.

References

1. Azzopardi JG, Lehner T. Systemic amyloidosis and malignant disease. J Clin Pathol. 1966;19(6):539–48.
2. Glenn GG. Amyloid deposits and amyloisosis. The Beta-fibrilloses (first of two parts). N Engl J Med. 1980;302(23):1283–92.
3. Glenn GG. Amyloid deposits and amyloisosis. The Beta-fibrilloses (second of two parts). N Engl J Med. 1980;302(23):1333–43.

4. Pasternak S, Wright BA, Walsh N. Soft tissue amyloidoma of the extremities: report of a case and review of the literature. Am J Dermatopathol. 2007;29(2):152–5.
5. Parmar H, Rath T, Castillo M, Gandhi D. Imaging of focal amyloid depositions in the head, neck, and spine: amyloidoma. AJNR Am J Neuroradiol. 2010;31(7):1165–70.
6. Picken MM. New insights into systemic amyloidosis: the importance of diagnosis of specific type. Curr Opin Nephrol Hypertens. 2007;16(3):196–203.
7. Westermark P, Stenkvist B. A new method for the diagnosis of systemic amyloidosis. Arch Intern Med. 1973;132(4):522–3.
8. Halloush RA, Lavrovskaya E, Mody DR, Lager D, Truong L. Diagnosis and typing of systemic amyloidosis: the role of abdominal fat pad fine needle aspiration biopsy. Cytojournal. 2009;6:24.
9. Gertz MA, Li CY, Shirahama T, Kyle RA. Utility of subcutaneous fat aspiration for the diagnosis of systemic amyloidosis (immunoglobulin light chain). Arch Intern Med. 1988;148(4):929–33.
10. van Gameren II, Hazenberg BP, Bijzet J, van Rijswijk MH. Diagnostic accuracy of subcutaneous abdominal fat tissue aspiration for detecting systemic amyloidosis and its utility in clinical practice. Arthritis Rheum. 2006;54(6):2015–21.
11. Guy CD, Jones CK. Abdominal fat pad aspiration biopsy for tissue confirmation of systemic amyloidosis: specificity, positive predictive value, and diagnostic pitfalls. Diagn Cytopathol. 2001;24(3):181–5.
12. van Gameren II. The role of abdominal fat tissue FNA for early detection and typing of systemic amyloidosis. Cancer Cytopathol. 2015;123(3):139–40.
13. Pakasa NM, Kalengayi RM. Tumoral calcinosis: a clinicopathological study of 111 cases with emphasis on the earliest changes. Histopathology. 1997;31(1):18–24.
14. Goldblum JR, Folpe AL, Weiss SW. Miscellaneous benign soft tissue tumors and pseudotumor. In: Enzinger and Weiss's soft tissue tumors. Philadelphia: Saunders/Elsevier; 2014.
15. Shah A, Paramesparan K, Robinson P, Rennie WJ. Non-neoplastic soft tissue tumors and tumor-like lesions. Semin Musculoskelet Radiol. 2020;24(6):645–66.
16. Fletcher CD, Unni KK, Mertens F. Pathology and genetics of tumors of soft tissue and bone. Lyon, France: IARC Press; 2002.
17. Zaharopoulos P, Di Patre PL. Aspiration cytology of a case of tumoral calcinosis. Diagn Cytopathol. 1995;13(4):339–44.
18. Saleh HA, Baker H. Aspiration biopsy cytology of tumoral calcinosis: a case report. Acta Cytol. 2009;53(3):323–6.
19. Snitchler AN, Silverman JF. Cytologic diagnosis of tumoral calcinosis: a case report. Acta Cytol. 2011;55(5):478–80.
20. Gupta RK, Naran S, Cheung YK. Fine-needle aspiration cytology of soft-tissue calcinosis presenting as an enlarging mass in the chest wall. Diagn Cytopathol. 1998;19(6):465–7.
21. Gupta RK, Naran S, Lallu S, Fauck R, Johnston P. Fine needle aspiration cytology of soft tissue calcinosis presenting as an enlarging mass in the neck. Acta Cytol. 2001;45(3):476–8.
22. Iglesias A, Londono JC, Saaibi DL, Peña M, Lizarazo H, Gonzalez EB. Gout nodulosis: widespread subcutaneous deposits without gout. Arthritis Care Res. 1996;9(1):74–7.
23. Crundwell N, O'Donnell P, Saifuddin A. Non-neoplastic conditions presenting as soft-tissue tumours. Clin Radiol. 2007;62(1):18–27.
24. Robinson P, Farrant JM, Bourke G, Merchant W, McKie S, Horgan KJ. Ultrasound and MRI findings in appendicular and truncal fat necrosis. Skelet Radiol. 2008;37(3):217–24.
25. Montgomery EA, Meis JM, Mitchell MS, Enzinger FM. Atypical decubital fibroplasia. A distinctive fibroblastic pseudotumor occurring in debilitated patients. Am J Surg Pathol. 1992;16(7):708–15.
26. Perosio PM, Weiss SW. Ischemic fasciitis: a juxta-skeletal fibroblastic proliferation with a predilection for elderly patients. Mod Pathol. 1993;6(1):69–72.
27. Baldassano MF, Rosenberg AE, Flotte TJ. Atypical decubital fibroplasia: a series of three cases. J Cutan Pathol. 1998;25(3):149–52.

28. Liegl B, Fletcher CD. Ischemic fasciitis: analysis of 44 cases indicating an inconsistent association with immobility or debilitation. Am J Surg Pathol. 2008;32(10):1546–52.
29. Ilaslan H, Joyce M, Bauer T, Sundaram M. Decubital ischemic fasciitis: clinical, pathologic, and MRI features of pseudosarcoma. AJR Am J Roentgenol. 2006;187(5):1338–41.
30. Kendall BS, Liang CY, Lancaster KJ, McCabe KM, Solanki PH. Ischemic fasciitis. Report of a case with fine needle aspiration findings. Acta Cytol. 1997;41(2):598–602.
31. Makise N, Mori T, Motoi T, Shibahara J, Ushiku T, Yoshida A. Recurrent FOS rearrangement in proliferative fasciitis/proliferative myositis. Mod Pathol. 2021;34(5):942–50.
32. Vargas AC, Ma L, Talbot J, Gill AJ, Maclean FM. Preliminary exploration of the role of FOS immunohistochemistry in proliferative fasciitis and myositis. Histopathology. 2022;81(3):414–7.
33. Erickson-Johnson M, Chou M, Evers B, et al. Nodular fasciitis: a novel model of transient neoplasia induced by *MYH9-USP6* gene fusion. Lab Investig. 2011;91:1427–33.
34. Oliveira AM, Chou MM. USP6-induced neoplasms: the biologic spectrum of aneurysmal bone cyst and nodular fasciitis. Hum Pathol. 2014;45(1):1–11.
35. Chung EB, Enzinger FM. Proliferative fasciitis. Cancer. 1975;36(4):1450–8.
36. Enzinger FM, Dulcey F. Proliferative myositis. Report of thirty-three cases. Cancer. 1967;20(12):2213–23.
37. Gan S, Xie D, Dai H, Zhang Z, Di X, Li R, Guo L, Sun Y. Proliferative myositis and nodular fasciitis: a retrospective study with clinicopathologic and radiologic correlation. Int J Clin Exp Pathol. 2019;12(12):4319–28.
38. Wong NL. Fine needle aspiration cytology of pseudosarcomatous reactive proliferative lesions of soft tissue. Acta Cytol. 2002;46(6):1049–55.
39. Chow LT, Chow WH, Lee JC. Fine needle aspiration (FNA) cytology of proliferative fasciitis: report of a case with immunohistochemical study. Cytopathology. 1995;6(5):349–57.
40. Anglo-Henry MR, Seaquist MB, Marsh WL Jr. Fine needle aspiration of proliferative fasciitis. A case report. Acta Cytol. 1985;29(5):882–6.
41. Dworkin MS, Westercamp MD, Park L, McIntyre A. The epidemiology of necrotizing fasciitis including factors associated with death and amputation. Epidemiol Infect. 2009;137(11):1609–14.
42. Jain D, Kumar Y, Vasishta RK, Rajesh L, Pattari SK, Chakrabarti A. Zygomycotic necrotizing fasciitis in immunocompetent patients: a series of 18 cases. Mod Pathol. 2006;19(9):1221–6.
43. Androulaki A, Papathomas TG, Liapis G, Papaconstantinou I, Gazouli M, Goutas N, Bramis K, Papalambros A, Lazaris AC, Papalambros E. Inflammatory pseudotumor associated with Mycobacterium tuberculosis infection. Int J Infect Dis. 2008;12(6):607–10.
44. Kumar C, Shrivastava K, Singh A, Chauhan V, Varma-Basil M. Skin and soft-tissue infections due to rapidly growing mycobacteria: an overview. Int J Mycobacteriol. 2021;10(3):293–300.
45. Zeeshan M, Fatima S, Farooqi J, Jabeen K, Ahmed A, Haq A, Arif MO, Zafar A. Reporting of mycetoma cases from skin and soft tissue biopsies over a period of ten years: a single center report and literature review from Pakistan. PLoS Negl Trop Dis. 2022;16(7):e0010607.
46. Peghin M, Ruiz-Camps I. Recent concepts in fungal involvement in skin and soft tissue infections. Curr Opin Infect Dis. 2022;35(2):103–11.
47. Takami K, Suzuki M, Horiuchi T. Muscular sarcoidosis. Nihon Rinsho. 1994;52(6):1599–602.
48. Stjernberg N, Cajander S, Truedsson H, Uddenfeldt P. Muscle involvement in sarcoidosis. Acta Med Scand. 1981;209(3):213–6.
49. Zisman DA, Biermann JS, Martinez FJ, Devaney KO, Lynch JP III. Sarcoidosis presenting as a tumorlike muscular lesion. Case report and review of the literature. Medicine (Baltimore). 1999;78(2):112–22.
50. Morganroth PA, Chaffins ML, Lim HW. Subcutaneous nodules on the fingers. JAMA Dermatol. 2013;149(2):223.
51. Al-Ani Z, Oh TC, Macphie E, Woodruff MJ. Sarcoid tenosynovitis, rare presentation of a common disease. Case report and literature review. J Radiol Case Rep. 2015;9(8):16–23.
52. García-Patos V. Rheumatoid nodule. Semin Cutan Med Surg. 2007;26(2):100–7.

53. Bang S, Kim Y, Jang K, Paik SS, Shin SJ. Clinicopathologic features of rheumatoid nodules: a retrospective analysis. Clin Rheumatol. 2019;38(11):3041–8.
54. Chua-Aguilera CJ, Möller B, Yawalkar N. Skin manifestations of rheumatoid arthritis, juvenile idiopathic arthritis, and spondyloarthritides. Clin Rev Allergy Immunol. 2017;53(3):371–93.
55. Veys EM, De Keyser F. Rheumatoid nodules: differential diagnosis and immunohistological findings. Ann Rheum Dis. 1993;52(9):625–6.
56. Jorizzo JL, Daniels JC. Dermatologic conditions reported in patients with rheumatoid arthritis. J Am Acad Dermatol. 1983;8(4):439–57.
57. Ting PT, Barankin B. Dermacase. Rheumatoid nodules. Can Fam Physician. 2005;51(1):35, 41, 43.
58. Kalugina Y, Petruzzelli GJ, Wojcik EM. Fine-needle aspiration of rheumatoid nodule: a case report with review of diagnostic features and difficulties. Diagn Cytopathol. 2003;28(6):322–4.
59. Vass L, Limjoco JM, Gupta PK. Fine needle aspiration of a rheumatoid nodule. Acta Cytol. 1992;36(1):107–8.
60. Youngberg GA, Farnum JB. Cellular atypia in a rheumatoid nodule: a diagnostic pitfall of aspiration biopsy. J Dermatol Surg Oncol. 1984;10(2):128–32.
61. Virtanen KA, Lidell ME, Orava J, Heglind M, Westergren R, Niemi T, Taittonen M, Laine J, Savisto NJ, Enerbäck S, Nuutila P. Functional brown adipose tissue in healthy adults. N Engl J Med. 2009;360(15):1518–25.
62. Søberg S, Löfgren J, Philipsen FE, Jensen M, Hansen AE, Ahrens E, Nystrup KB, Nielsen RD, Sølling C, Wedell-Neergaard AS, Berntsen M, Loft A, Kjær A, Gerhart-Hines Z, Johannesen HH, Pedersen BK, Karstoft K, Scheele C. Altered brown fat thermoregulation and enhanced cold-induced thermogenesis in young, healthy, winter-swimming men. Cell Rep Med. 2021;2(10):100408.
63. Santos GC, Araujo MR, Silveira TC, Soares FA. Accumulation of brown adipose tissue and nutritional status. A prospective study of 366 consecutive autopsies. Arch Pathol Lab Med. 1992;116(11):1152–4.

Chapter 17
Bone

Sigfred Lajara

Bone is a type of specialized tissue of the body that provides structural support and performs metabolic functions. The bone has a combination of organic and inorganic components, which distinguishes it from the rest of the body. The bone matrix is composed of proteins and minerals, and the cellular components include osteoblasts, osteocytes, and osteoclasts. These cells interact and regulate bone remodeling, mineral homeostasis and they perform endocrine functions [1–3]. The bone also houses bone marrow, which is composed of varying quantities of adipose tissue and hematopoietic elements. The amount and distribution of hematopoietic elements is age-dependent; there is decreasing proportion and more limited distribution with increasing age.

The evaluation of bone lesions, similar to other organ systems, involves the synthesis of clinical, radiologic, and pathologic information. Radiologists also integrate clinical findings and information from different imaging studies to narrow down the differential diagnosis and provide a prediction for risk of pathologic fracture [4]. Unless unequivocally benign by clinical and radiologic evaluation, most bone lesions would need image-guided sampling [5]. Several clinically significant questions with drastically different management implications can arise in the clinical and radiologic evaluation of patients presenting with bone lesions. These include differentiating a benign stress fracture from a pathologic fracture, infection versus tumor, and benign hematoma versus tumor with hemorrhage [5]. These issues could also carry over in the examination of biopsies. Reparative changes related to fracture can mimic the appearance of some bone malignancies [5, 6]. Although there are radiologic features that have been described to be associated with infections and neoplasms, the distinction between an infectious and a neoplastic process based on imaging can be difficult [7].

S. Lajara (✉)
Department of Pathology, University of Pittsburgh Medical Center, Pittsburgh, PA, USA
e-mail: lajaras@upmc.edu

S. M. Gilani, G. Cai (eds.), *Non-Neoplastic Cytology*,
https://doi.org/10.1007/978-3-031-44289-6_17

More recently, the Society of Skeletal Radiology released guidelines for the diagnostic management of incidentally identified solitary bone lesions identified on CT or MRI in adults. They use an algorithmic approach to classify bone lesions based on their CT or MRI features, which ultimately provide a bone reporting and data system (Bone-RADS) score with appropriate management recommendations [8].

Adequacy and Reporting

There are no set adequacy criteria and universally accepted reporting scheme in bone FNA. Adequacy follows the general rule in non-gynecologic cytology assessing whether or not the samples are representative of the targeted lesion, which raises the importance of correlating with clinical and imaging findings. We cannot exclude the possibility of sampling bias when faced with a negative or non-diagnostic sample in patients with suspicious imaging findings. However, several studies have shown that even non-diagnostic biopsies could guide clinical decision-making when interpreted together with clinical and radiologic features, and when discussed during multidisciplinary team meetings [9, 10]. One series has shown that up to 98% of negative biopsies of suspicious bone lesions had truly benign follow-up after 2 years, suggesting that a negative bone biopsy is a valid indicator for the absence of bone metastasis [11].

Technical Considerations

Open biopsy is still the gold standard, but core needle biopsy (CNB) is the preferred method for sampling musculoskeletal lesions because of its good accuracy and better safety profile [5]. The preferred imaging modality for the biopsy of deeper soft tissues and bone is CT scan [5, 12]. A recently published paper by Ariizumi et al. evaluated FNA and CNB, both with and without image guidance [13]. They did not provide a separate analysis for bone lesions, and in their cohort, there generally was no difference between the accuracy rate between image guided and blindly performed procedures. However, as expected, cases with no palpable lesions had higher sampling error rate when performed blindly (40%) versus with image guidance (8.2%). The reported accuracy rate for bone and soft tissue FNA varies, but multiple papers have reported more than 90% accuracy, sensitivity, and specificity [14–18]. Köster et al. reported somewhat lower accuracy for FNA at 88%, and CNB at 90%, but their analysis was limited to primary lesions with histologic follow-up [17]. In addition, when it comes to their bone only cohort, the sensitivity and specificity for FNA was at 85% and 83%. Yang and Damron reported a better accuracy rate for CNB compared to FNA when determining the nature of the lesion (benign vs. malignant), specific diagnosis, histologic grading and typing [19]. They also noted that there was better performance of both modalities in high-grade tumors compared to low-grade and benign tumors. Cardona and Dodd in their review of bone cytology, recognize the limitation of FNA, especially in situations where there is thickening of the cortex, extensively sclerotic lesions, and largely cystic lesions, since the yield in these cases is likely low [20]. A recent meta-analysis showed that for both bone and soft tissue lesions, FNA was better in determining the nature of the lesion, compared to providing a specific diagnosis [21]. However, when analyzed separately, bone FNA was better than soft tissue FNA at determining the nature of lesions, while the reverse is true for providing a specific diagnosis.

Normal Components of Bone and Marrow and Pitfalls

The ground substance of the bone is mineralized and brittle. When aspirated, it can cause difficulty in smearing due to poor contact between slides. It appears amorphous, almost like broken bits of glass (Fig. 17.1a, b). Osteoblasts are round to polygonal cells with abundant granular cytoplasm and eccentrically placed nuclei with conspicuous nucleoli (Fig. 17.2a, b). They contain a characteristic perinuclear clearing or hof, which represents the Golgi body. On quick examination, osteoblasts can be mistaken for plasma cells, or even poorly differentiated carcinomas, which is especially important during rapid on-site evaluation. Osteoblasts are generally larger than plasma cells and their clearing or hof is farther from the nucleus, in contrast to the hof of plasma cells (Fig. 17.3a). Also, plasma cells have the characteristic clumped chromatin that imparts a clock-face appearance. Osteoblasts can sometimes cluster [22], and poorly differentiated carcinomas can appear as single cells with eccentric nuclei (Fig. 17.3b). However, the nuclei of carcinomas are large and atypical, and if they have cytoplasmic vacuoles, these usually have well-delineated borders, in contrast to the hof seen in osteoblasts.

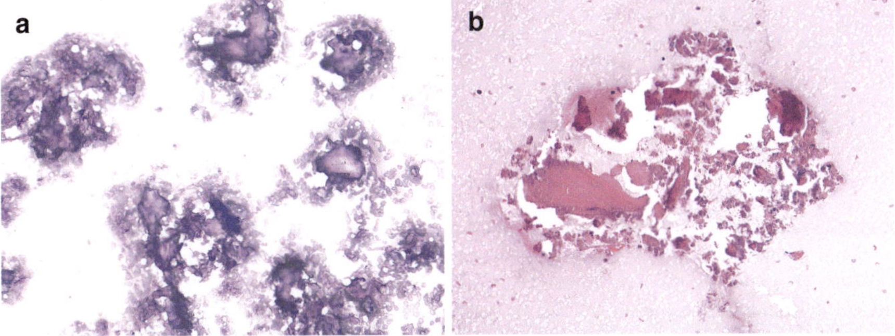

Fig. 17.1 Acellular irregular fragments of calcified amorphous bone matrix. (**a**) Air-dried smear, Diff-Quik, 20× magnification. (**b**) Cell block, hematoxylin and eosin, 20× magnification

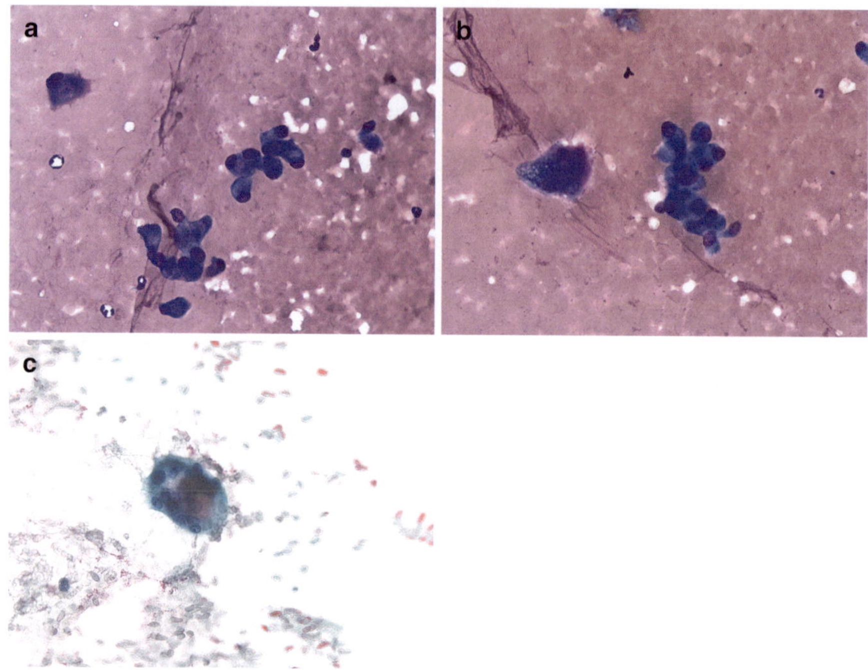

Fig. 17.2 Loose clusters of osteoblasts and an osteoclast. The osteoblasts have round uniform nuclei that usually forms the edge of the cell and a cytoplasmic hof that is away from the nucleus. The osteoclasts contain uniform nuclei with conspicuous nucleoli that are haphazardly arranged within the cytoplasm. (**a**, **b**) Air-dried touch preparation smear, Diff-Quik, 40× magnification. (**c**) Alcohol-fixed smear, Papanicolaou stain, 40× magnification

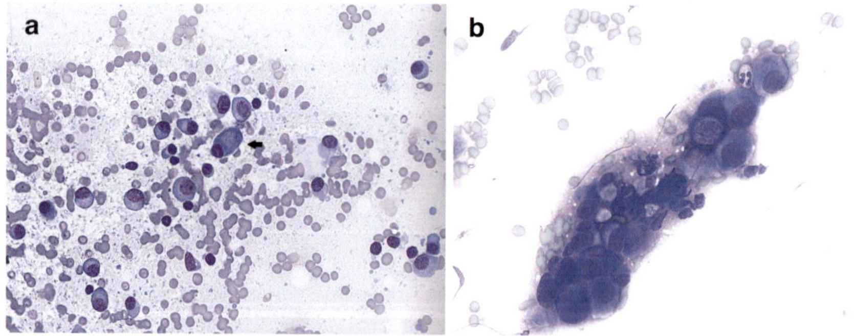

Fig. 17.3 Morphologic mimics of osteoblasts. (**a**) A single non-neoplastic osteoblast surrounded by neoplastic plasma cells. The osteoblast has a very low n/c ratio, and the hof does not touch the nucleus. The plasma cells have higher n/c ratio, a characteristic clock-face chromatin, and perinuclear hof adjacent to the nuclei. (**b**) A cluster of poorly differentiated adenocarcinoma cells. There is a moderate amount of cytoplasm with mucin vacuoles. The nuclei are enlarged, with prominent nucleoli. Air-dried touch preparation smear, Diff-Quik, 40× magnification

Osteocytes, which differentiate from osteoblasts, comprise 90–95% of all bone cells [23]. However, despite their number, they are not usually seen in cytology specimens. They reside in lacunar spaces, which are surrounded by mineralized matrix, which makes them inaccessible by FNA [24].

Osteoclasts appear as large multinucleated cells with abundant cytoplasm with uniform, round to ovoid nuclei with conspicuous nucleoli (Fig. 17.2b, c). Osteoclasts are derived from the progenitor cells of the granulocytic-macrophage colony-forming units and macrophage colony-forming units [1]. These cells are morphologically similar to giant cells associated with certain infections or neoplastic conditions. Multinucleated giant cells in infections would have an inflammatory background with acute and chronic inflammation. When numerous, these cells can signify sampling of giant cell-rich tumors. The overall cellularity, and the presence of other cell types, as well as correlation with the imaging findings would indicate a more specific etiology [22, 25].

Bone marrow cells can be seen in bone aspirates, appearing as different hematopoietic lineages of various degrees of maturation (Fig. 17.4). The presence of occasional blasts should not be overinterpreted as part of a neoplastic process in the background of maturing trilineage hematopoiesis. Megakaryocytes give rise to platelets. They appear as large cells with multilobated and hyperchromatic nuclei, which can be mistaken for atypical or bizarre epithelial or stromal cells (Fig. 17.4). However, these cells are often scattered singly in a background of other hematopoietic cells and mature fat. Table 17.1 summarizes the different normal elements of bone and periarticular tissue, and the associated pitfalls.

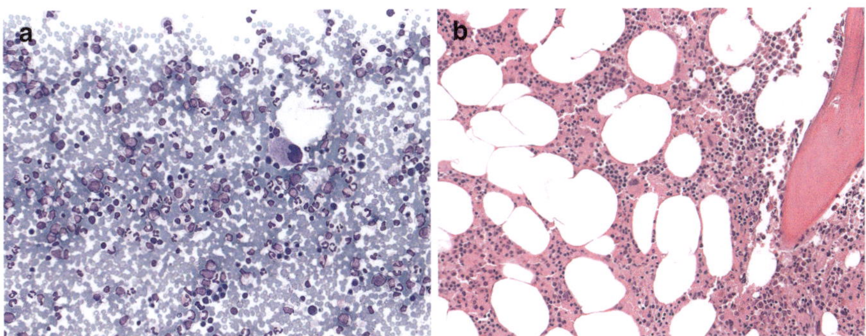

Fig. 17.4 Bone marrow elements. (**a**) The bone marrow elements show trilineage hematopoiesis with lymphoid, erythroid, and myeloid cells of varying maturity. A large megakaryocyte with a lobated nucleus is present. Air-dried smear, Diff-Quik, 20× magnification. (**b**) Bone marrow elements including fat and adjacent bone. Hematoxylin and eosin, 20× magnification

Table 17.1 Normal elements of bone and periarticular tissue and pitfalls

Normal elements	Morphology	Pitfalls
Osteoblasts	Polygonal to round cells with moderate to abundant cytoplasm. Characteristic clearing or "hof," and round nucleus with conspicuous nucleolus	Can mimic plasma cells or carcinoma
Osteoclasts	Large multinucleated cells with multiple monomorphic round to ovoid nuclei with conspicuous nucleoli. Fine granules can be seen in Romanowsky-based preparations	If numerous, can raise the possibility of giant cell-rich tumors Multinucleated giant cells associated with infection have acute and chronic inflammation and debris
Bone marrow elements	Maturing trilineage hematopoiesis, fat, and occasional blasts and megakaryocytes	Megakaryocytes can appear bizarre and mimic atypical epithelial or stromal cells
Cartilage	Hypocellular abundant extracellular hyaline/glassy material with chondrocytes in lacunae	Inadvertent sampling of articular cartilage during bone FNA may be confused for a low-grade chondroid lesion

Cystic Lesions of Bone

Unicameral or simple bone cyst (UBC) is a lytic, fluid-filled lesion that is usually seen in the metaphysis of long bones of children and adolescents and occurs more in males [26–28]. UBC is classically thought to be a reactive, rather than a neoplastic process; the pathogenesis is unclear, and theories include venous obstruction, intraosseous synovial cyst, and local growth aberration [26–28]. However, there are reports of UBC with associated translocation [27]. Most UBCs are asymptomatic until a fracture occurs. Imaging findings show a centrally expansile lesion along the longitudinal axis. The development of a fracture can be seen as "fallen fragment" sign, which is floating bone fragments on X-ray or CT scans [27]. UBCs are rarely resected, and they show a unilocular cyst filled with fluid, and lined by a thin fibrous tissue that can contain material that can have a cementum-like appearance [28]. However, oftentimes, these lesions are curetted instead, and specimens are composed of fragmented bones with associated thin fragmented fibrous tissue. The cytologic features of UBCs are not extensively described, as they are expected to show non-specific findings. In a series by Jorda et al., UBC was the most frequently encountered tumor-like lesion in FNA cytology of bone [16]. They found these cases to show hemosiderin, granulation tissue, macrophages, and rare lymphocytes, which were correlated with clinical and radiologic findings to make the diagnosis.

Juxta-articular bone cyst or intraosseous ganglion is a non-neoplastic subchondral cyst that is not related to other joint pathology, especially degenerative changes [29]. These lesions are uncommon and could be confused with other entities [30]. The most common location is the medial malleolus, hip, tibia, fibula, shoulder, wrist and carpal bones, and they appear as sharply demarcated rounded lucencies within bone, often with sclerotic borders on imaging [28]. The histologic and cytologic features of these lesions are similar to their soft tissue counterparts [30, 31].

Epidermoid bone cysts are squamous-lined intramedullary and unilocular cysts with keratin debris [32]. Those that arise in the terminal phalanges are thought to be due to traumatic implantation of epidermal tissue that causes them to proliferate within the bone [33, 34]. The histologic features of these lesions are similar to those arising in other parts of the body [32, 33]. There are no reports of the cytologic findings, but they are likely similar to those found elsewhere in the body.

Metabolic Bone Diseases

Metabolic bone disease is a general term referring to a group of disorders that are due to alterations in bone remodeling and/or mineralization [35]. The etiology of these diseases vary from genetic disorders, nutritional causes, or acquired conditions [36]. The presentation varies; biochemical testing and bone imaging are often diagnostic, but the gold standard is tetracycline-labeled undecalcified bone biopsy of the anterior iliac crest [35]. Cytology has limited value in the evaluation of these lesions, unless they exhibit mass lesions such as brown tumors in hyperparathyroidism.

Hyperparathyroidism

Primary hyperparathyroidism is a disorder of calcium metabolism due to hypersecretion of parathyroid hormone by one or more parathyroid glands. The patients are mostly asymptomatic with less patients having clinical manifestations such as bone pain, fractures, kidney stones, and muscle weakness [37]. Secondary and tertiary hyperparathyroidism is often due to end-stage renal disease. Bone disease in primary hyperparathyroidism, described as osteitis fibrosa cystica, is due to overactivity of osteoclasts that leads to breakdown of bone and thinning of cortex [38]. Brown tumors, seen in up to 3% of primary hyperparathyroid, and 1.5–1.7% of secondary hyperparathyroid patients, are focal lytic lesions due to a localized area of bone loss [39]. Brown tumors can be single or multiple, and the most common locations are the pelvis, mandible, ribs, long bones, hands, and vertebrae [39]. Although classically regarded as non-neoplastic or reactive bone lesion, a couple of recent papers have shown that up to 54% and 62% of brown tumors demonstrated pathogenic *KRAS* mutations, suggesting that they could be true neoplasms [40]. Histologically, they appear as a giant cell-rich lesion with a lobulated pattern, richly vascular connective tissue with fibroblastic stroma and hemosiderin deposition [41]. The cytopathologic findings of brown tumor includes bland spindled stromal cells, histiocytes, multinucleated, osteoclast-like giant cells and hemosiderin pigment [42–45]. These findings are not at all specific for the diagnosis of brown tumor, and the differential diagnosis would include other giant cell-rich tumors such as aneurysmal bone cyst, giant cell tumor, and giant cell reparative granuloma. The specific diagnosis would rely heavily on correlation with clinical and radiologic parameters.

Inflammatory, Reactive, and Infectious Conditions

Fracture

Fracture healing is a complex process with different phases, beginning with hematoma formation to eventually fracture callus formation and remodeling [46]. Fractures can be associated with benign and malignant conditions. It is important to be aware of fracture healing since these can potentially lead to a misdiagnosis if one is not familiar with its associated morphologic changes. A fracture callus in cases of stress fractures can potentially mimic malignancy on imaging and histology, especially in the absence of relevant or distinct history of trauma or a known history of an underlying lesion [6]. Histologically, fracture callus and stress fractures show periosteal and endosteal active new bone formation, necrotic lamellar bone, osteoid and calcified woven bone (Fig. 17.5) [47]. These features of stress fractures and fracture callus can sometimes raise the differential diagnosis of osteosarcoma [6]. The FNA of a fracture callus due to the presence of bone may yield very little material including osteoblasts, osteoclasts, or stromal cells. Koh et al. describe the cytomorphologic features of late-stage fracture callus in stress fracture in an 18-year-old patient, who presented with right lower leg pain [48]. The authors noted the presence of dispersed oval to round cells with eccentrically located nuclei with fine chromatin and indistinct nucleolus and no pleomorphism. Few osteoclast-like giant cells were present, as well as few fibroblastic clusters.

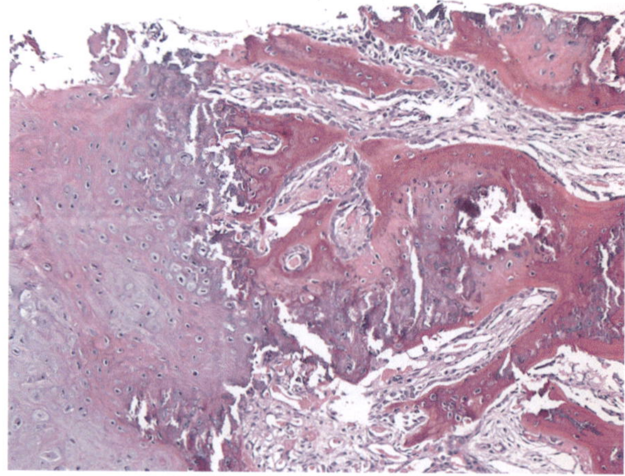

Fig. 17.5 Fracture callus showing cartilage undergoing endochondral ossification, reactive stromal cells, and bone. Hematoxylin and eosin, 10× magnification

Osteomyelitis

Osteomyelitis is an infection involving the bone, which can be acute or chronic, and may be due to hematogenous spread of organisms, or direct inoculation. Hematogenous spread is more commonly seen in the pediatric population [20]. There could be overlap with the imaging findings between an infectious and a neoplastic process, with Ewing sarcoma being known to be difficult to distinguish from osteomyelitis [5]. In acute osteomyelitis, FNA usually demonstrates high cellularity, with neutrophilic predominance, debris, necrosis, and foci of histiocytic inflammation (Fig. 17.6) [20]. Chronic osteomyelitis is characterized by chronic inflammation, with fibrosis of the marrow, erosion of bone, necrotic bone, and reactive bone formation. The cytologic diagnosis of chronic osteomyelitis may be more difficult given the presence of marrow fibrosis and necrotic bone. The smears from chronic osteomyelitis showed varying amounts of acute and chronic inflammation in one series, while lymphocytes, neutrophils, macrophages, and fragments of dead bone were present in another [16, 49]. Chronic granulomatous osteomyelitis can

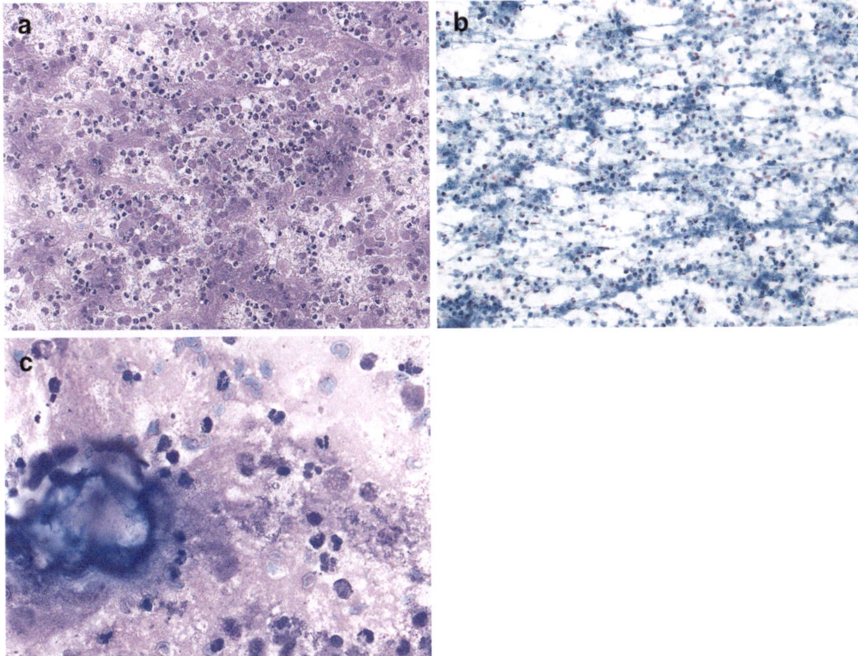

Fig. 17.6 Acute bacterial osteomyelitis. (**a, b**) There are abundant neutrophils and necroinflammatory debris. Air-dried smear, Diff-Quik (**a**) and alcohol-fixed smear, Papanicolaou stain (**b**), 20× magnification. (**c**) A small fragment of bone is seen adjacent to clusters of coccal bacteria. Air dried smear, Diff-Quik, 60× magnification

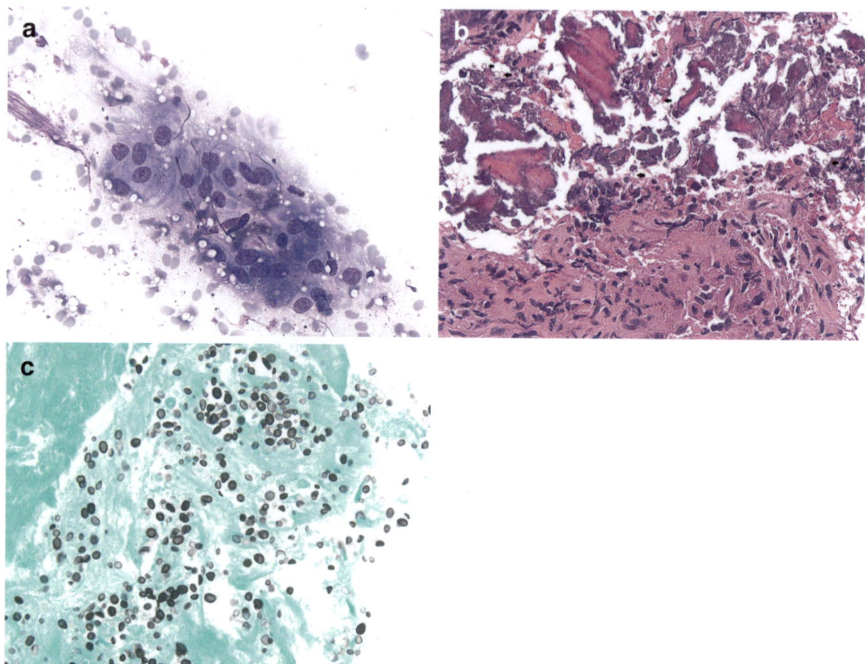

Fig. 17.7 Cryptococcal granulomatous osteomyelitis. (**a**) An aggregate of epithelioid histiocytes and many yeast forms of *Cryptococcus neoformans*. The yeast forms appear as empty round spaces with faint light violet staining in the middle. Air-dried touch preparation smear, Diff-Quick, 40× magnification. (**b**) Granulomatous inflammation, dead bone, and scattered yeasts, appearing as small ovoid empty structures. Hematoxylin and eosin, 20× magnification. (**c**) Numerous fungal yeast forms are highlighted. Grocott Methenamine Silver stain, 60× magnification

yield necrosis, lymphocytes, epithelioid histiocytes, and granulomas (Fig. 17.7). Given the importance of clinicopathologic correlation in these cases, it is important to also acquire material for microbiological studies.

Joint and Synovial Fluid

Cellular Elements of Joint and Fluid

The joint comprises the ends of contiguous bones, cartilage, ligaments, and synovium. Hyaline cartilage covers the ends of bones in diarthrodial joins except for the sternoclavicular and temporomandibular joints, which are covered by fibrocartilage [50]. Hyaline cartilage is hypocellular and composed of chondrocytes in

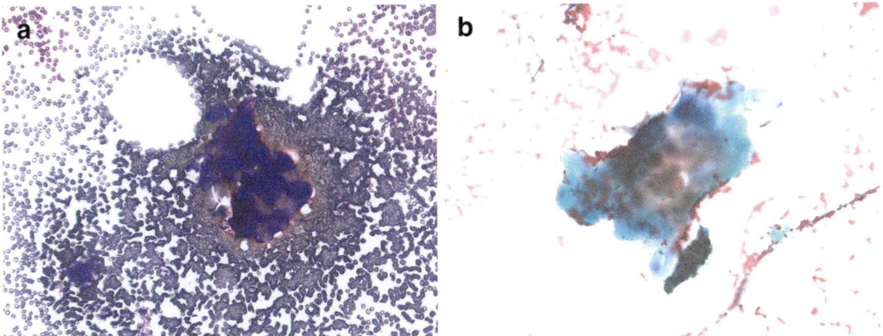

Fig. 17.8 Normal cartilage. (**a**) Hypocellular dense dark purple matrix material. Air-dried smear, Diff-Quik, 20×. (**b**) Light blue green to light pink matrix material. Alcohol-fixed smear, Papanicolaou stain, 20×

lacunae within abundant hyaline extracellular matrix. Cartilage in air-dried Romanowsky-stained smear preparations appear as glassy, dense, blue to purple, while it appears blue green to blue gray to light pink and dense in Pap-stained preparations (Fig. 17.8). The synovium is composed of a single layer of synoviocytes lining the joint space (Type A, macrophage-like), while the second component provides a supportive backing layer (Type B, connective tissue derived, secretes hyaluronate) [50]. Ligaments and tendons are composed of dense collagenous connective tissue.

Normally, the joint space only contains a small amount of synovial fluid to provide lubrication, and supply oxygen and nutrients to the articular cartilage. Synovial fluid is an ultrafiltrate of plasma, which is normally viscous, hypocellular and does not clot. Joint aspiration or arthrocentesis is performed when there is joint effusion or inflammation. In addition to confirming the presence of infection or crystal arthropathy, removal of fluid can provide symptomatic relief. Synoviocytes are one of the least common cells found in synovial fluid [51]. They can be sampled during joint fluid aspiration or during FNAs for lesions near the joint space. Type A synoviocytes (Fig. 17.9a, b) are large cells with foamy cytoplasm, eccentric nuclei, and lower nucleus to cytoplasmic ratio compared to macrophages [52]. Type B synoviocytes are usually not seen in synovial fluid specimens, unless there is disruption of the synovium. They are bland, with higher nucleus to cytoplasmic ratio, fibroblastic appearing with ovoid nuclei (Fig. 17.9c) [24]. In addition to the other cytopreparatory methods, synovial fluid can be examined to look for crystals and other debris using a "Wet Prep" method. This is done by placing a small amount of fluid on a slide. It is then coverslipped and examined under light and polarizing microscopy.

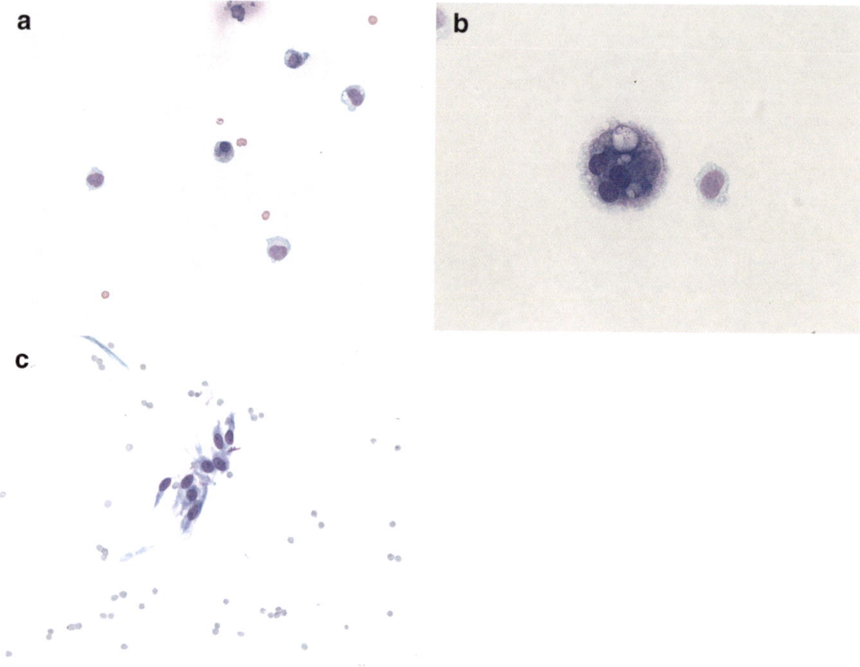

Fig. 17.9 Synoviocytes. (**a**) The synovial fluid shows a type A synoviocyte (center of the image) has a low n/c ratio, with eccentrically placed nucleus. The surrounding macrophages have larger nuclei. (**b**) Multinucleated synoviocyte. Air-dried cytospin preparation, Diff-Quik, 40× (**a**) and 60× (**b**) magnification. (**c**) FNA of a joint shows type B synoviocytes with a bland fibroblastic appearance. Air-dried smear, Diff-Quik, 40× magnification

Arthritides

Septic Arthritis

Septic arthritis, an inflammatory arthritis, is a rheumatologic emergency that can lead to septicemia. It refers to the infection of a joint (most commonly the knee) and is commonly due to Gram-positive bacteria, with *Staphylococcus aureus* being the most common etiologic agent, followed by *Streptococci* [53]. Gonococcal arthritis used to be a leading cause of septic arthritis in young adults in the United States, but it now accounts for 1% of cases [53]. The synovium lacks a protective membrane, which makes it vulnerable to bacteremic seeding, although some cases are due to direct, penetrating trauma [53]. An important risk factor for developing septic arthritis is a pre-existing joint disease. Aspirates from bacterial infections demonstrate abundant neutrophils (Fig. 17.10), while mycobacterial infections can have increased lymphocytes. Bacteria can be identified in majority of cases, but a significant number of cases would have negative cultures due to antibiotic treatment prior to aspiration [51].

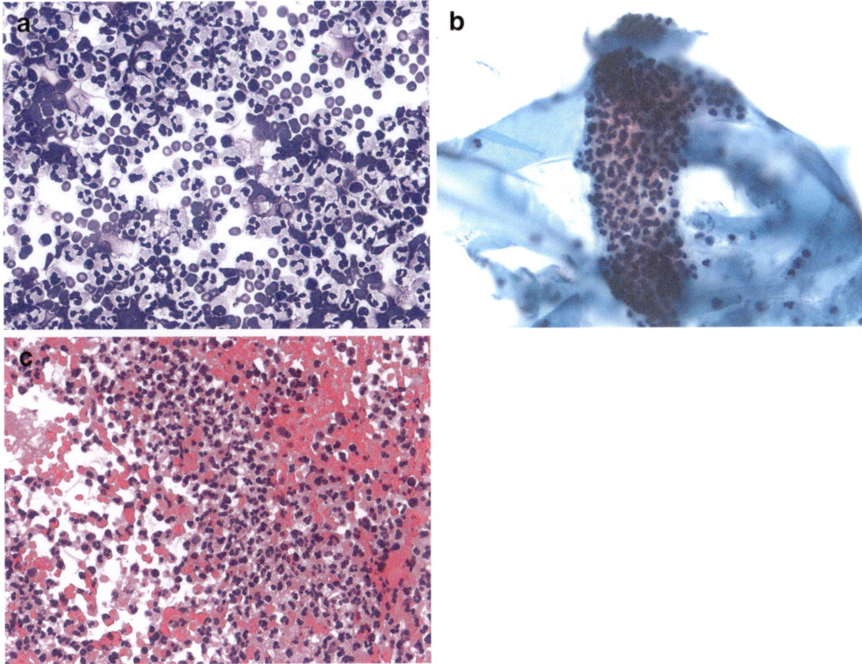

Fig. 17.10 Septic arthritis, synovial fluid. Abundant neutrophils. Air-dried cytospin preparation, Diff-Quik (**a**); ThinPrep preparation, Papanicolaou stain (**b**); cell block, hematoxylin and eosin (**c**), 40× magnification

Rheumatoid Arthritis

Rheumatoid arthritis (RA) is an autoimmune chronic inflammatory disease that primarily involves the joints, but also presents with extraarticular disease. Genome-wide studies have identified loci implicating immune mechanisms that are associated with RA risk, while epigenetics contribute to pathogenesis, and some environmental factors have been associated with development of RA [54]. Clinically, the diagnosis of RA is not straightforward, as it shares signs and symptoms with other autoimmune/connective tissue diseases. The criteria in the diagnosis of RA include joint involvement, serological testing, acute phase reactants, and chronicity of symptoms [55]. Histologically, early-stage RA presents with synovial hyperplasia with infiltration by plasma cells and lymphocytes, with formation of lymphoid follicles, while end-stage RA resembles OA [56]. The pathology of RA shares the general features with psoriatic arthritis and other arthritides [57] (Fig. 17.11). Mononuclear cells, such as lymphocytes and plasma cells are usually present in joints affected by autoimmune arthritides. Neutrophils can be present in rheumatoid arthritis, and one should be cautious before making a diagnosis of infection. Fragments of cartilage, bone and hydroxyapatite crystals can be found in joint fluids due to the ongoing

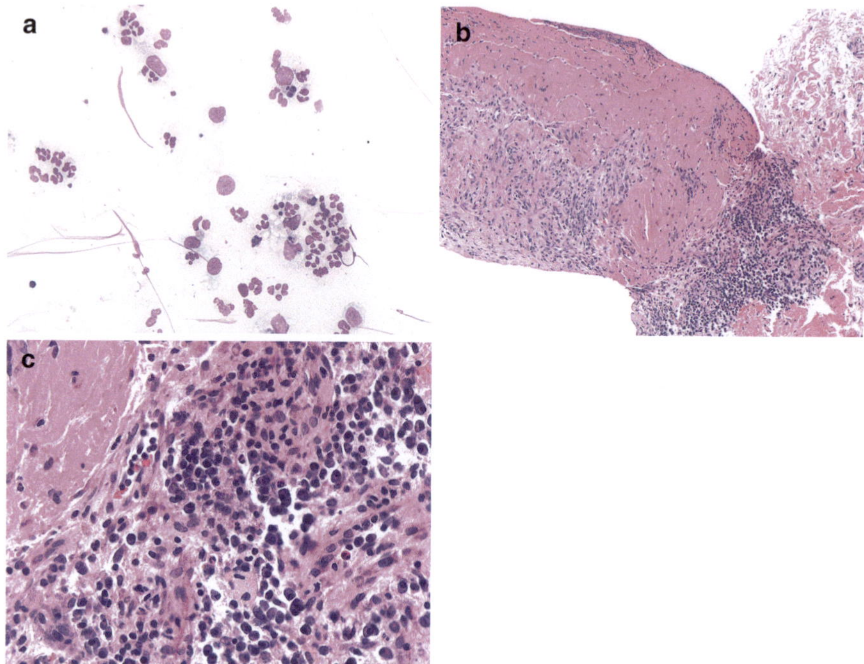

Fig. 17.11 Inflammatory arthritis, patient with psoriasis. (**a**) Mixed inflammatory cells with neutrophils, lymphoid cells, and macrophages. Air-dried touch preparation smear, Diff-Quik, 40× magnification. (**b**) Synovium with fibrinous degeneration, fibrosis, and increased lymphoplasmacytic infiltrates. (**c**) Higher magnification highlights the increased plasma cells. Hematoxylin and eosin, 10× magnification (**b**) and 40× magnification (**c**)

erosive process [58]. Examination of a wet mount preparation can reveal ragocytes, which are cells that can be any type of phagocytes that contain one or more distinctive granules [58].

Osteoarthritis/Degenerative Joint Disease

Osteoarthritis (OA) is the most common type of arthritis and is due to the wear and tear of the articular cartilage. Risk factors include age, obesity, prior joint injury, and a family history of OA. Patients present with joint pain that is worse in the morning and feels better with activity. The classic imaging findings include joint space narrowing, development of osteophytes, and subchondral sclerosis and cysts [59]. Synovial fluids typically have a low number of inflammatory cells, but type A synoviocytes can be seen (Fig. 17.12). The synovium can undergo hyperplastic change (Fig. 17.13). Due to the loss of cartilage, and eventual articulation of bone on bone, various debris can be seen in the synovial fluid, including cartilage with

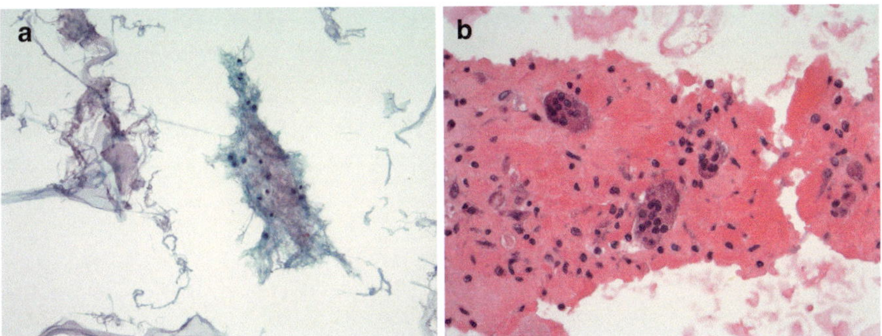

Fig. 17.12 Osteoarthritis, synovial fluid. (**a**) Fibrinous material with some entrapped synovio-cytes, lymphocytes, and macrophages. ThinPrep preparation, Papanicolaou stain, 20× magnification. (**b**) A small fragment of fibrotic synovium with multinucleated giant cells. Cell block, hematoxylin and eosin, 40× magnification. (Photos provided by Dr. Juan Xing)

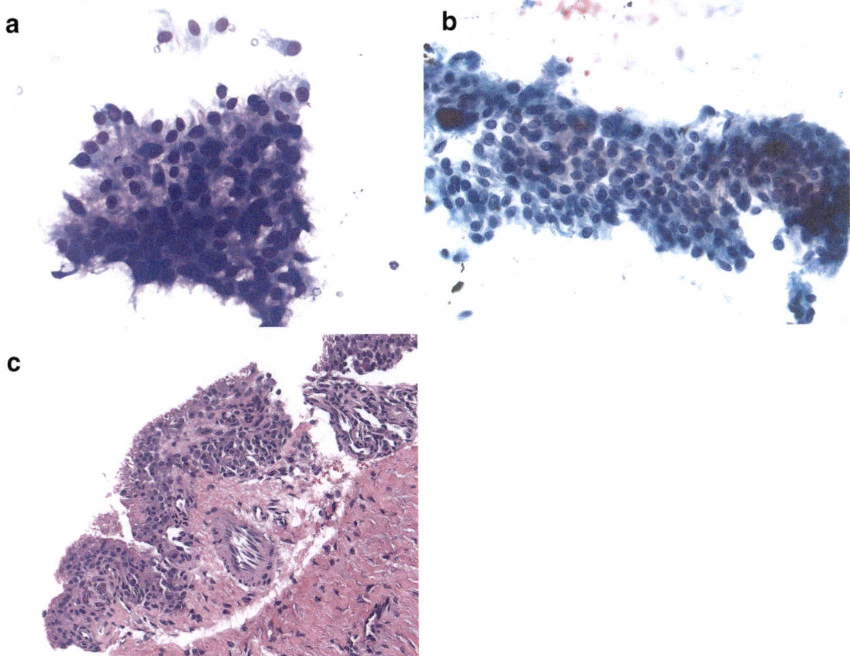

Fig. 17.13 Osteoarthritis, sternoclavicular joint FNA. Fragments of hyperplastic synovium, with proliferation of bland type B synoviocytes. (**a**) Air-dried smear, Diff-Quik, 40× magnification, (**b**) alcohol-fixed smear, Papanicolaou stain, 40× magnification, (**c**) hematoxylin and eosin, 20× magnification

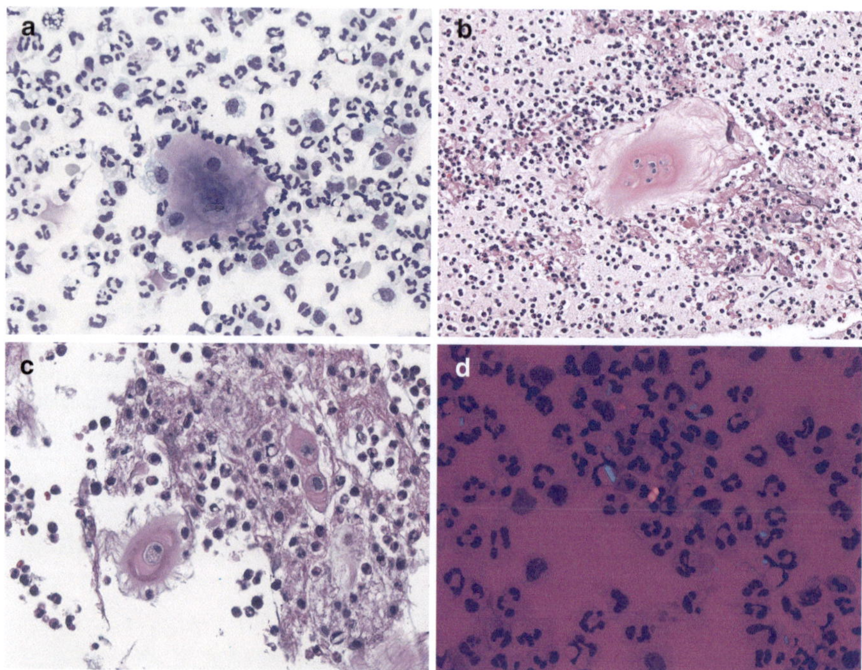

Fig. 17.14 Septic arthritis in a patient with osteoarthritis, synovial fluid. (**a**) Abundant neutrophils and a fragment of cartilage with two chondrocytes and fibrillated matrix. Air-dried cytospin preparation, Diff-Quik, 40× magnification. (**b**) Cartilage with chondrocyte cluster, and (**c**) cartilage with fibrillated matrix. Cell block, hematoxylin and eosin, 20× (**b**) and 40× (**c**) magnification. (**d**) Calcium pyrophosphate crystals. Air-dried cytospin preparation, Diff-Quik, 60× magnification, with compensated polarization

clusters of chondrocytes, fibrillary cartilage, apatite/bone debris, and calcium pyrophosphate crystals (Fig. 17.14) [58]. The presence of cartilage with chondrocyte clusters and fibrillated cartilage in synovial fluid are diagnostic of OA [51].

Pathology Related to Joint Replacement

Joint replacement surgery is indicated in patients who fail conservative management. However, the indications are expanding, and surgical joint replacement earlier in the course of disease may be offered even to younger patients [60]. Some of the patients will eventually require revision arthroplasties, and the most common indications are "dislocation, mechanical loosening, other mechanical problems, infection, osteolysis, periprosthetic fracture, wear and implant failure or breakage" [61]. Periprosthetic joint infections are relatively rare complications, and the diagnosis involves several criteria that includes culture studies, synovial fluid analysis (leukocyte count >3000/mL with >80% neutrophils) and histopathological assessment [62]. Prosthetic debris can be present in joint fluid aspirates [51]. Formation of pseudotumors, which are reactive soft tissue lesions composed of inflammatory cells and necrotic tissue, is another complication of arthroplasties, and is well-recognized in patients with metal-on-metal hip arthroplasty (Fig. 17.15 and Table 17.2) [63].

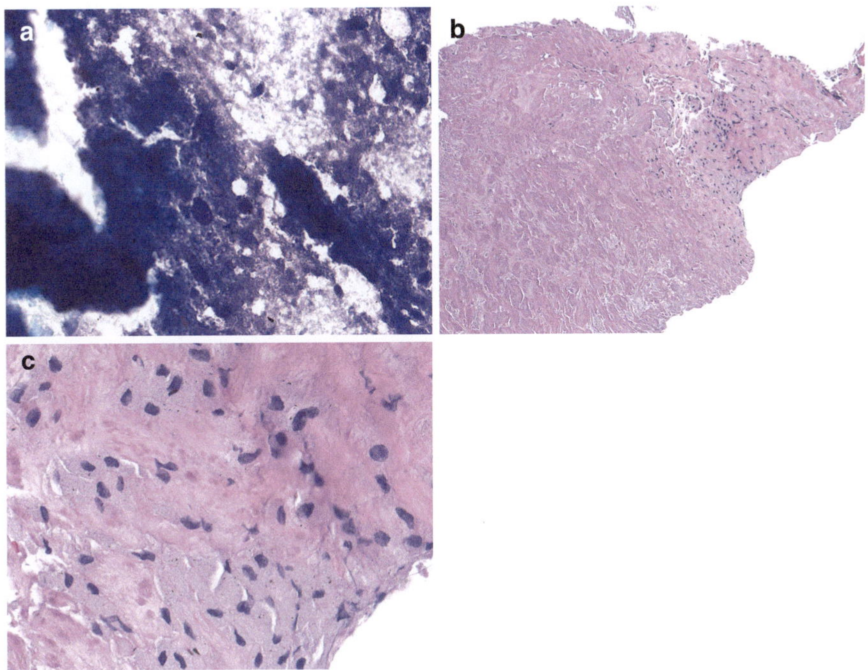

Fig. 17.15 Pseudotumor secondary to joint prosthesis. (**a**) Abundant granular necrotic debris with few inflammatory cells and black specks, compatible with prosthetic wear debris. Air-dried touch preparation smear, Diff-Quik, 60× magnification. (**b**) Extensively necrotic tissue with hyalinized fibrosis and (**c**) histiocyte aggregates with prosthetic wear debris. Hematoxylin and eosin, 10× (**b**) and 60× (**c**) magnification

Table 17.2 Crystal arthropathies

Crystal arthropathy	Clinical features	Site of involvement	Crystal	Crystal characteristics
Gout	Presents with gout flares; chronic tophaceous disease fairly common	First metatarsophalyngeal joint (most common), foot, ankle	Monosodium urate	Negatively birefringent needle-shaped crystals
Calcium pyrophosphate deposition disease (pseudogout)	Can be asymptomatic, or present with acute and chronic forms. Very rare tophaceous disease	Knee and wrist (most common); rare in first metatarsophalyngeal joint	Calcium pyrophosphate	Positively birefringent rhomboid crystals

Crystal Arthropathy

Gout

Gout is an inflammatory arthritis resulting from the inflammatory response to the chronic deposition of monosodium urate (MSU) crystals, which form due to increased urate concentrations. Patients present with symptoms of swelling, pain, warmth, and tenderness of the affected joints (gout flares). The most common site of involvement is the first metatarsophalangeal joint, but other sites in the foot or ankle are commonly affected. When the hyperuricemia is untreated, it can lead to formation of tophi or chronic gouty arthritis or both [64]. The gold standard in the diagnosis is demonstration of monosodium urate crystals in the synovial fluid (Fig. 17.16) or tophaceous material (Fig. 17.17) by polarizing microscopy. MSU crystals are needle-shaped, and negatively birefringent; when parallel to the axis of the polarizer under compensated polarizing microscopy, they appear yellow, and blue when they are perpendicular. FNA of gouty tophi yields more diagnostic crystals, as well as occasional foreign body-type giant cells (Fig. 17.18a, b).

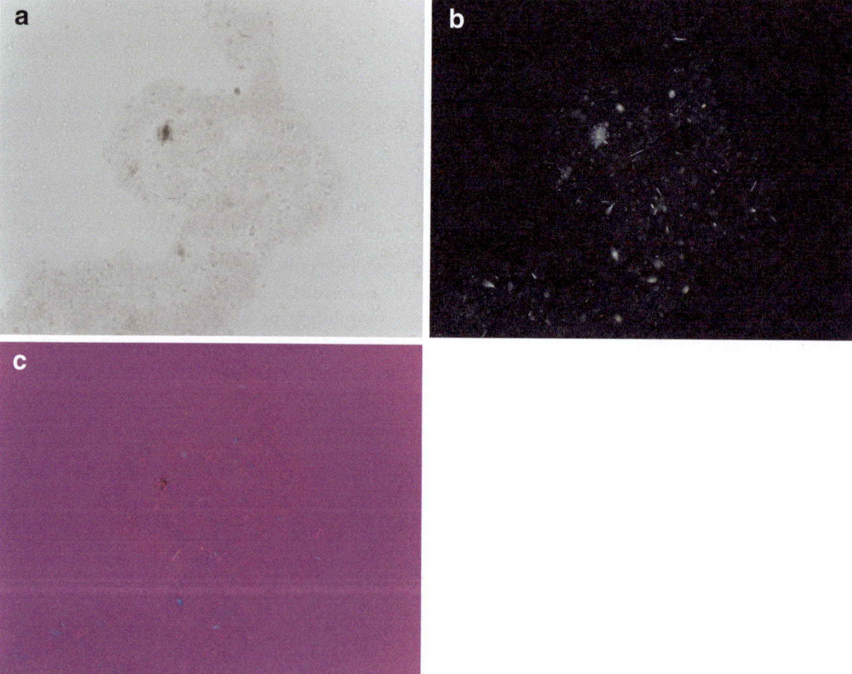

Fig. 17.16 Gout, synovial fluid. Monosodium urate crystals are seen as refractile, needle-shaped crystals within fibrin aggregates (**a**) that polarize (**b**). They appear yellow when parallel to axis of the polarizer under compensated polarizing microscopy (**c**). Wet prep preparation, 20× magnification, light microscopy without polarization (**a**), with polarization (**b**), with compensated polarization (**c**). (Photos provided by Dr. Matthew Then)

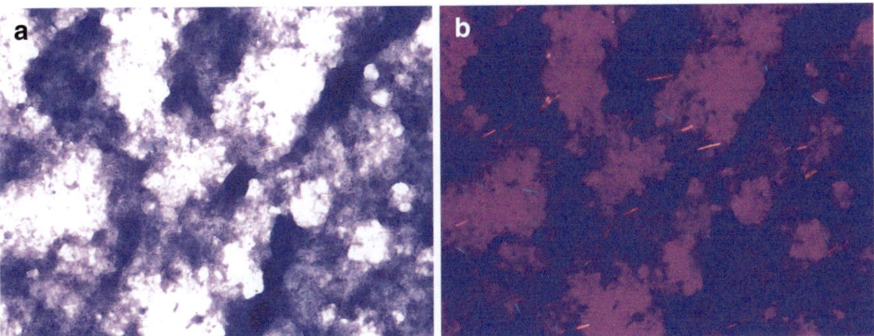

Fig. 17.17 Tophaceous gout, FNA. Abundant granular debris with refractile needle-shaped crystals that appear as empty spaces without polarization (**a**). The crystals appear yellow when parallel to the polarizer on compensated polarizing microscopy. Air-dried smear, Diff-Quik, 60× magnification, light microscopy without polarization (**a**), and with compensated polarization (**b**)

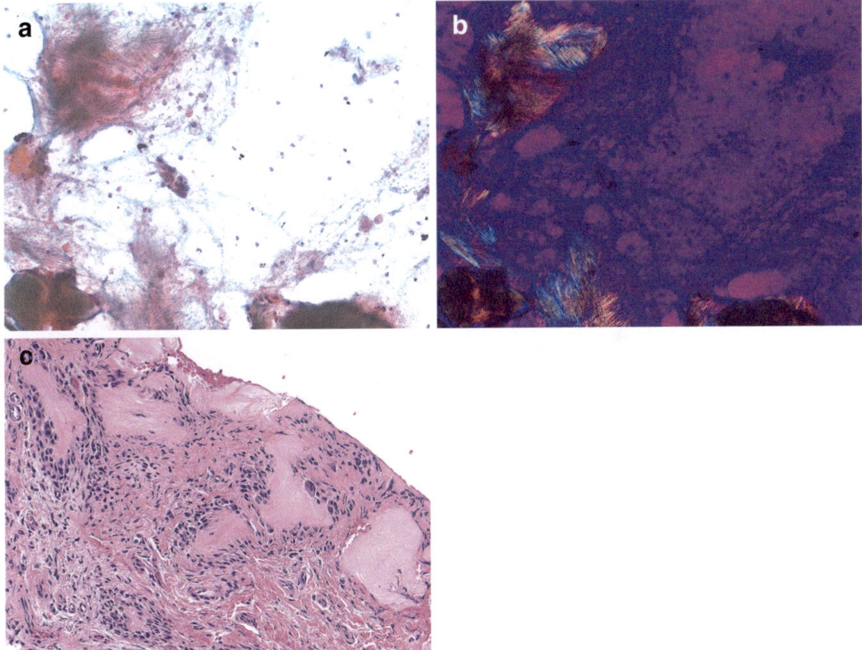

Fig. 17.18 Tophaceous gout. FNA shows abundant refractile, needle-shaped crystals with mixed inflammatory cells, debris, and multinucleated foreign-body type giant cells. Alcohol-fixed smear, Papanicolaou stain, 20× magnification, light microscopy without polarization (**a**), and with compensated polarization (**b**). (**c**) Gout appears feathery to fluffy with lightly eosinophilic to amphophilic material left after dissolution of MSU crystals post tissue processing. Gout elicits an inflammatory reaction, with the crystals surrounded by histiocytes and foreign body-type giant cells. Hematoxylin and eosin, 20× magnification

Histologically, MSU crystals are dissolved with conventional processing, leaving a fluffy and feathery area with surrounding histiocytes and foreign body-type giant cell reaction (Fig. 17.18c).

Calcium Pyrophosphate Deposition Disease (Pseudogout)

Calcium pyrophosphate deposition disease (CPPD) is arthritis caused by the accumulation of CPP crystals, usually in the pericellular matrix of the cartilage; they rarely form in non-cartilaginous tissues [65]. CPPD can be asymptomatic in some patients. Acute CPPD presents with monoarticular or oligoarticular disease that is clinically indistinguishable from gout, with the knee and wrist being the most commonly affected joints. Some chronic forms clinically resemble osteoarthritis, while rare examples resemble rheumatoid arthritis [65]. A very rare disease manifestation is a tumoral or tophaceous pseudogout [66]. CPPD is diagnosed by the confirmation of the presence of CPP crystals by polarizing microscopy. CPP crystals (Fig. 17.19a, b) are rhomboid and positively birefringent, in contrast to MSU crystals. Relative to

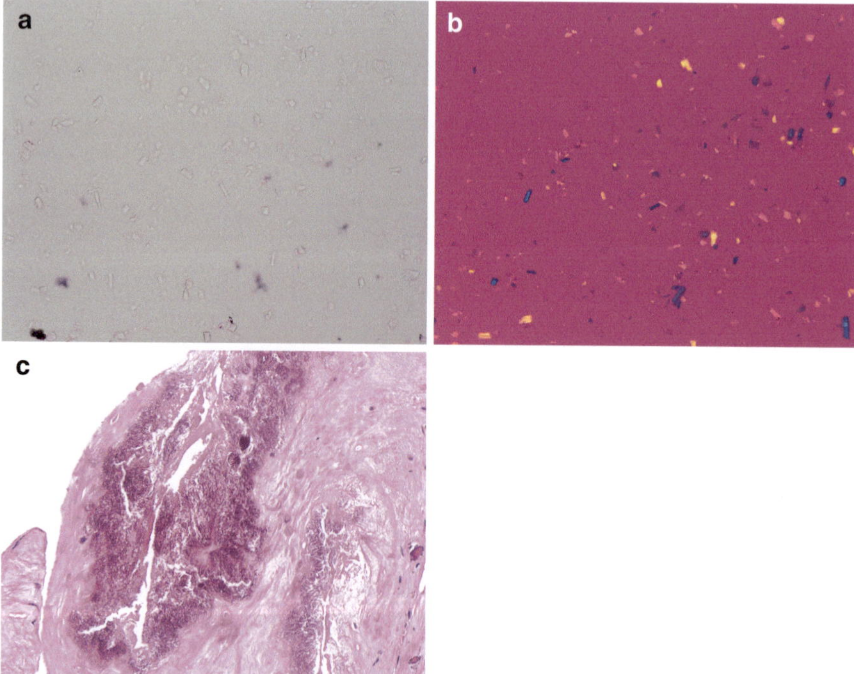

Fig. 17.19 Calcium pyrophosphate disease (pseudogout), synovial fluid. Abundant rhomboid refractile crystals on light microscopy without polarization (**a**). The crystals appear blue when parallel to the axis of the polarizer on compensated polarizing microscopy. Wet prep preparation, 40× magnification, with compensated polarization (**b**). (**c**) Pseudogout crystals appear basophilic on tissue sections, and they do not elicit an inflammatory reaction in contrast to gout. Hematoxylin and eosin, 20× magnification. (Figures **a** and **b** provided by Dr. Stacia Semple)

the axis of the polarizer under compensated polarizing microscopy, they appear blue when parallel, and they appear yellow when perpendicular. Histologically, in contrast to MSU crystals, CPP crystals typically appear basophilic, and do not elicit the same inflammatory response (Fig. 17.19c). Table 17.2 summarizes the difference between gout and pseudogout.

Cystic Lesions Around the Joint

Bursitis

A bursa is a fluid-filled, synovial-lined structure located around joints, which helps cushion moving structures and prevent wear and tear. The accumulation of synovial fluid and eventual bursal distention leads to bursitis [67]. Common causes include injury to adjacent structures, or acute or repetitive trauma, infection or inflammatory arthropathy [67]. FNA of bursitis can yield non-specific cystic findings with histiocytes, fibrinous material, and in infected bursitis, acute inflammatory cells (Fig. 17.20). Bursal cysts are thin-walled cysts filled with gelatinous material and the aspirates are usually hypocellular, with histiocytoid synovial cells, in a mucoid background, while some cases show pseudopapillary structures and inflammatory cells [68].

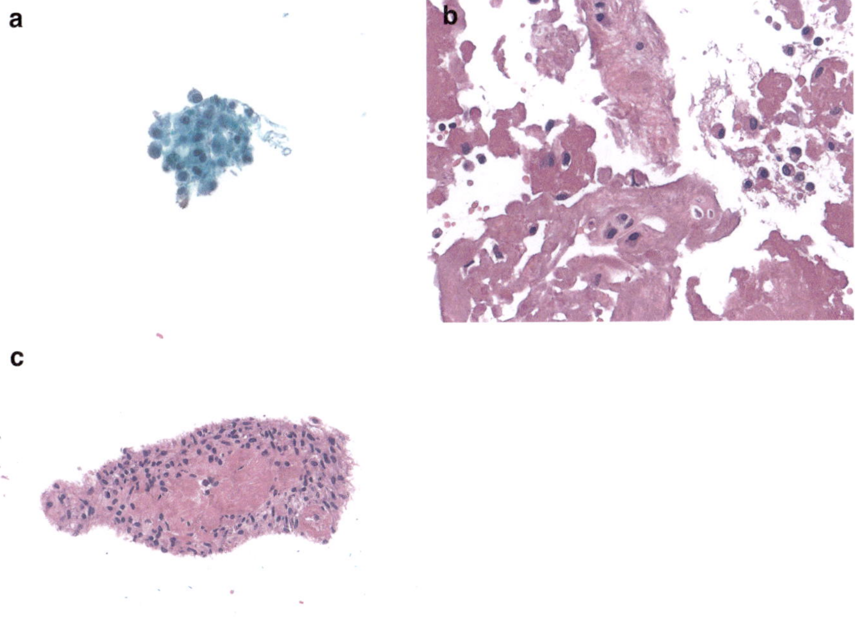

Fig. 17.20 Fibrinous bursitis, FNA. (**a**) A group of synoviocytes, lymphocytes, and macrophages. ThinPrep, Papanicolaou stain, 40× magnification. (**b**) Fibrinous debris and fragments of cartilage, with synoviocytes, macrophages, and lymphocytes. (**c**) A fragment of synovial lining with some hyperplastic change. Hematoxylin and eosin, 40× (**b**) and 20× (**c**) magnification

Synovial Cysts and Ganglion Cysts

Synovial cysts and ganglion cysts are both juxta-articular structures that have identical findings on MRI [69]. A synovial cyst is a juxta-articular synovium-lined fluid collection that is thought to form due to the herniation of the synovial membrane through a degenerative or traumatic defect [70]. The prime example of a synovial cyst is a Baker cyst (popliteal cyst), which is due to the posterior herniation of the synovial membrane. There is true synovial lining and cartilage may be seen within the wall [56]. An FNA of a synovial cyst is usually hypocellular and would show a proteinaceous granular background, synoviocytes and macrophages (Fig. 17.21). A report of an FNA of a Baker-type cyst of the arm resulting from a ruptured long head of the biceps tendon describes synovial fluid collection, with numerous macrophages and small lymphocytes with a proteinaceous background [71]. The same report also noted rare granulomas and cholesterol clefts.

Ganglion cysts are the most common soft tissue tumor of the hand, and they are thought to arise due to myxoid degeneration of collagen, and trauma or irritation leading to production of hyaluronic acid [72]. They can occur in the lower

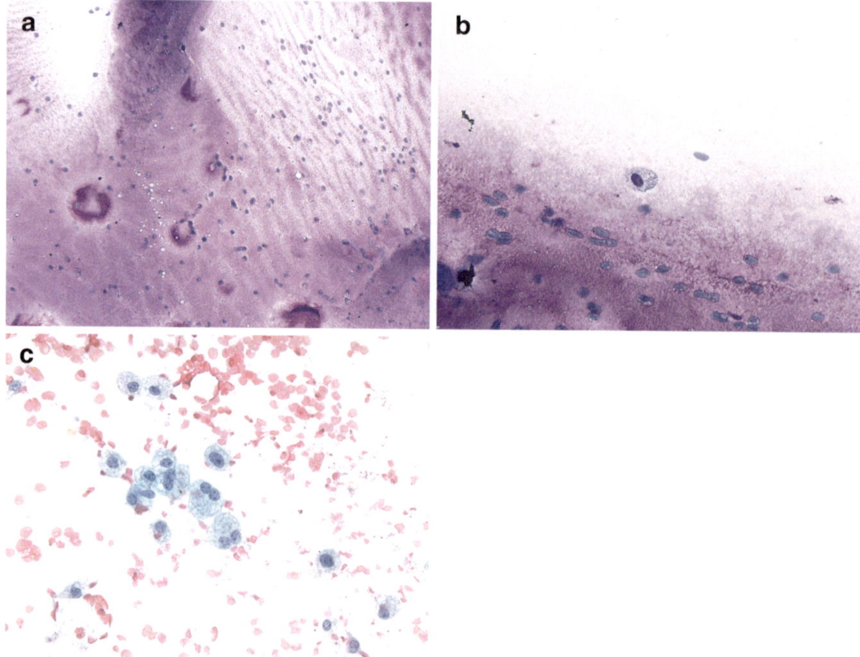

Fig. 17.21 Popliteal (Baker) cyst, FNA. (**a**) Abundant hypocellular granular proteinaceous material. (**b**, **c**) Few scattered synoviocytes with a couple of binucleated forms, and macrophages are present. The synoviocytes appear similar to macrophages, but with lower n/c ratio. Air-dried smear, Diff-Quik, 20× (**a**) and 40× (**b**) magnification. Alcohol-fixed smear, Papanicolaou stain, 40× magnification (**c**)

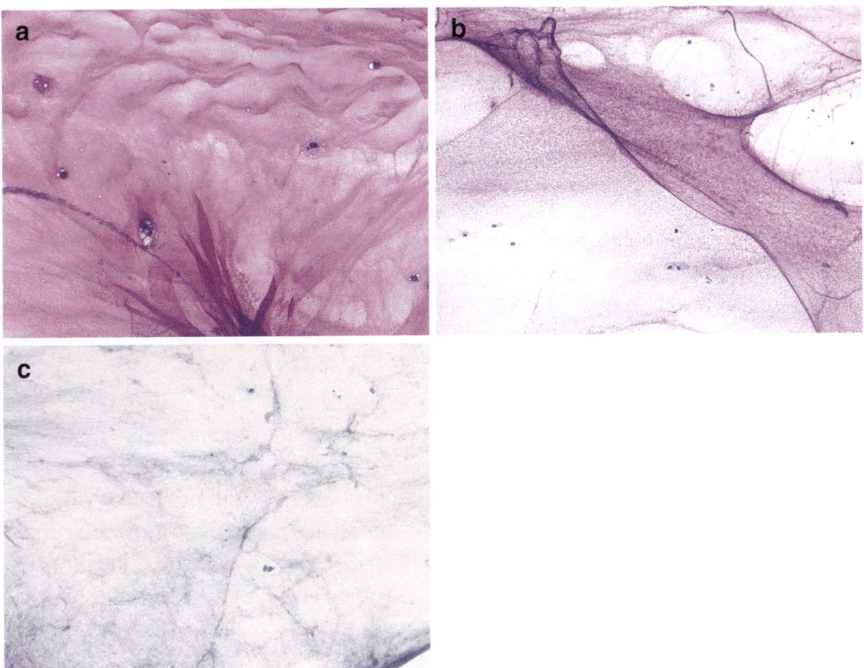

Fig. 17.22 Ganglion cyst, FNA. Abundant granular, myxoid material with few macrophages. The myxoid material appears purple to violet on Diff-Quik stain, while blue gray on Papanicolaou stain. Air-dried smear, Diff-Quik (**a**, **b**), alcohol-fixed smear, Papanicolaou stain (**c**), 20× magnification

extremities, including the foot, ankle, and knees [73]. Histologically, ganglion cysts are well-circumscribed lesions composed of a densely collagenous wall with no lining and often filled with hypocellular mucoid material. FNA of these lesions yield clear or whitish thick viscous material that smears easily [74]. This appears as hypocellular, granular myxoid material that folds, imparting a pleated plastic wrap or glaze-like crackle pattern with occasional histiocytes (Fig. 17.22) [74–76].

Approach to Diagnosis of Non-neoplastic Bone and Soft Tissue Lesions

Bone and soft tissue cytology specimens should be interpreted in the context of clinical and imaging studies. The clinical and radiologic information provide valuable clues to the diagnosis, and specimen adequacy, emphasizing the need for proper communication among clinicians, radiologists, and pathologists [77]. Employing Rapid On-Site Evaluation (ROSE) should be considered, which helps in ensuring specimen adequacy, while providing an opportunity to triage cases for additional

CNB or ancillary studies (flow cytometry, microbiology, etc.). Jorda et al. postulate that their high insufficient aspirate rate could be partially due to the absence of a cytopathologist on site [16]. On the other hand, Yu et al. credit their very low CNB inadequacy rate to the concurrent FNA to the use of ROSE [78]. On-site evaluation with imprint cytology is a viable tool for rapid assessment, but its value may be limited to patients with a suspicion of malignancy [79]. The same paper noted that benign lesions had a low success rate with imprint cytology, with most benign cases showing non-specific/non-diagnostic imprint cytology. This does not take into consideration the advantage of having the opportunity to triage specimen for culture studies and flow cytometry, which are only possible on fresh specimens.

The modern practice of cytology relies on the cell block as much as, if not more than conventional cytology preparations. The use of cell blocks unlocks the potential for specialized testing that used to only be available for surgical pathology specimens, including special histochemical stains, immunohistochemistry, molecular techniques, and proteomics [80]. These include special stains for identification of microorganisms and certain proteins. Immunohistochemical identification of infectious disease is also possible on cell block material. In addition, molecular techniques on paraffin-embedded material can be used for identification of microbiological organisms, including *Mycobacteria* and fungi [81, 82]. Proteomics assays with mass spectrometry allows for the confirmation and subclassification of amyloid in fat pad aspirates [83].

References

1. Kerr DA, Rosenberg AE. Bone. In: Mills SE, editor. Histology for pathologists. 5th ed. Lippincott Williams & Wilkins; 2020. p. 87–112.
2. Dirckx N, Moorer MC, Clemens TL, Riddle RC. The role of osteoblasts in energy homeostasis. Nat Rev Endocrinol. 2019;15(11):651–65.
3. Zhou R, Guo Q, Xiao Y, et al. Endocrine role of bone in the regulation of energy metabolism. Bone Res. 2021;9(1):1–19.
4. Bernard S, Walker E, Raghavan M. An approach to the evaluation of incidentally identified bone lesions encountered on imaging studies. Am J Roentgenol. 2017;208(5):960–70.
5. Meek RD, Mills MK, Hanrahan CJ, et al. Pearls and pitfalls for soft-tissue and bone biopsies: a cross-institutional review. Radiographics. 2020;40(1):266–90.
6. Hoch B, Montag A. Reactive bone lesions mimicking neoplasms. Semin Diagn Pathol. 2011;28(1):102–12.
7. Lex JR, Gregory J, Allen C, Reid JP, Stevenson JD. Distinguishing bone and soft tissue infections mimicking sarcomas requires multimodal multidisciplinary team assessment. Ann R Coll Surg Engl. 2019;101(6):405–10.
8. Chang CY, Garner HW, Ahlawat S, et al. Society of Skeletal Radiology—white paper. Guidelines for the diagnostic management of incidental solitary bone lesions on CT and MRI in adults: bone reporting and data system (Bone-RADS). Skelet Radiol. 2022;51(9):1743–64.
9. Didolkar MM, Anderson ME, Hochman MG, et al. Image guided core needle biopsy of musculoskeletal lesions: are nondiagnostic results clinically useful? Clin Orthop. 2013;471(11):3601–9.

10. Osman K, Hussain S, Downes F, Sumathi V, Botchu R, Evans S. A multidisciplinary team approach is highly effective in the management of nondiagnostic bone tumour biopsies: a 10-year retrospective review at a specialist sarcoma unit. Sarcoma. 2022;2022:1–8.
11. Lange MB, Petersen LJ, Nielsen MB, Zacho HD. Validity of negative bone biopsy in suspicious bone lesions. Acta Radiol Open. 2021;10(7):20584601211030662.
12. Espinosa LA, Jamadar DA, Jacobson JA, et al. CT-guided biopsy of bone: a radiologist's perspective. Am J Roentgenol. 2008;190(5):W283–9.
13. Ariizumi T, Kawashima H, Yamagishi T, et al. Diagnostic accuracy of fine needle aspiration cytology and core needle biopsy in bone and soft tissue tumor: a comparative study of the image-guided and blindly performed procedure. Ann Diagn Pathol. 2022;59:151936.
14. Vangala N, Uppin SG, Pamu PK, Hui M, Nageshwara Rao K, Chandrashekar P. Fine-needle aspiration cytology in preoperative diagnosis of bone lesions: a three-year study in a tertiary care hospital. Acta Cytol. 2020;65(1):75–87.
15. Bommer KK, Ramzy I, Mody D. Fine-needle aspiration biopsy in the diagnosis and management of bone lesions. Cancer Cytopathol. 1997;81(3):148–56.
16. Jorda M, Rey L, Hanly A, Ganjei-Azar P. Fine-needle aspiration cytology of bone. Cancer Cytopathol. 2000;90(1):47–54.
17. Köster J, Ghanei I, Domanski HA. Comparative cytological and histological assessment of 828 primary soft tissue and bone lesions, and proposal for a system for reporting soft tissue cytopathology. Cytopathology. 2021;32(1):7–19.
18. Khalbuss WE, Teot LA, Monaco SE. Diagnostic accuracy and limitations of fine-needle aspiration cytology of bone and soft tissue lesions. Cancer Cytopathol. 2010;118(1):24–32.
19. Yang YJ, Damron TA. Comparison of needle core biopsy and fine-needle aspiration for diagnostic accuracy in musculoskeletal lesions. Arch Pathol Lab Med. 2004;128(7):759–64.
20. Cardona DM, Dodd LG. Bone cytology: a realistic approach for clinical use. Surg Pathol Clin. 2012;5(1):79–100.
21. Chambers M, O'Hern K, Kerr DA. Fine-needle aspiration biopsy for the diagnosis of bone and soft tissue lesions: a systematic review and meta-analysis. J Am Soc Cytopathol. 2020;9(5):429–41.
22. Samedi VG, Bocklage T. Bone and soft tissue cytology. In: Pitfalls in diagnostic cytopathology with key differentiating cytologic features, Essentials in cytopathology. 1st ed. Springer International Publishing; 2016. p. 201–39.
23. Bonewald LF. The amazing osteocyte. J Bone Miner Res. 2011;26(2):229–38.
24. Cantley RL, Pantanowitz L. Musculoskeletal system (bone, cartilage, muscle, soft tissue) and skin. In: Lew M, Pang J, Pantanowitz L, eds. Normal cytology—an illustrated, practical guide. Springer International Publishing; 2022:131–142.
25. Jager L, Johnson DN, Sukhanova M, Streich L, Chapa AR, Alexiev BA. Diagnosis of giant cell-rich bone tumors on core needle biopsy: a practical approach. Pathol Res Pract. 2022;231:153777.
26. Mascard E, Gomez-Brouchet A, Lambot K. Bone cysts: unicameral and aneurysmal bone cyst. Orthop Traumatol Surg Res. 2015;101(1):S119–27.
27. Noordin S, Allana S, Umer M, Jamil M, Hilal K, Uddin N. Unicameral bone cysts: current concepts. Ann Med Surg. 2018;34:43–9.
28. Remotti F, Feldman F. Nonneoplastic lesions that simulate primary tumors of bone. Arch Pathol Lab Med. 2012;136(7):772–88.
29. Olvi LG, Lembo GM, Velan O, Santini-Araujo E. Juxta-articular bone cyst. In: Santini-Araujo E, Kalil RK, Bertoni F, Park YK, editors. Tumors and tumor-like lesions of bone: for surgical pathologists, orthopedic surgeons and radiologists. 1st ed. Springer; 2015. p. 683–99.
30. Selvaraj S, Keloth T, Stephen NS, Gochhait D, Siddaraju N. Intraosseous ganglion diagnosed on cytology: a familiar entity in an exotic location. Cytopathology. 2020;31(1):81–2.
31. Chen KTK. Fine needle aspiration cytology of intraosseous ganglion: a case report. Acta Cytol. 2011;52(4):451–3.

32. Olvi LG, Gonzalez ML, Velan O, Santini-Araujo E. Epidermoid bone cyst. In: Santini-Araujo E, Kalil RK, Bertoni F, Park YK, editors. Tumors and tumor-like lesions of bone: for surgical pathologists, orthopedic surgeons and radiologists. 1st ed. Springer; 2015. p. 701–3.
33. Wang BY, Eisler J, Springfield D, Klein MJ. Intraosseous epidermoid inclusion cyst in a great toe. Arch Pathol Lab Med. 2003;127(7):e298–300.
34. Richardson MP, Foster JR, Logan DB. Intraosseous epidermal inclusion cyst of the proximal phalanx of the fifth toe and review of the literature: a case study. Foot Ankle Spec. 2017;10(5):470–2.
35. Walker MD, Weber TJ. Metabolic bone diseases. In: Wing EJ, Schiffman FJ, editors. Cecil essentials of medicine. 10th ed. Elsevier Inc; 2022. p. 748–65.
36. Chang CY, Rosenthal DI, Mitchell DM, Handa A, Kattapuram SV, Huang AJ. Imaging findings of metabolic bone disease. Radiographics. 2016;36(6):1871–87.
37. Oberger Marques JV, Moreira CA. Primary hyperparathyroidism. Best Pract Res Clin Rheumatol. 2020;34(3):101514.
38. Yang Q, Li J, Yang Z, et al. Skeletal lesions in primary hyperparathyroidism. Am J Med Sci. 2015;349(4):321–7.
39. Bennett J, Suliburk JW, Morón FE. Osseous manifestations of primary hyperparathyroidism: imaging findings. Int J Endocrinol. 2020;2020:e3146535.
40. Turek D, Haefliger S, Ameline B, et al. Brown tumors belong to the spectrum of KRAS-driven neoplasms. Am J Surg Pathol. 2022;46(11):1577.
41. Olvi LG, Santini-Araujo E. "Brown tumor" of hyperparathyroidism. In: Santini-Araujo E, Kalil RK, Bertoni F, Park YK, editors. Tumors and tumor-like lesions of bone: for surgical pathologists, orthopedic surgeons and radiologists. 1st ed. Springer; 2015. p. 815–25.
42. Pavlovic S, Valyi-Nagy T, Profirovic J, David O. Fine-needle aspiration of brown tumor of bone: cytologic features with radiologic and histologic correlation. Diagn Cytopathol. 2009;37(2):136–9.
43. Ojha SS, Valecha J, Sharma A, Nilkanthe R. Role of fine needle aspiration cytology in diagnosis of brown tumor secondary to parathyroid adenoma. J Lab Physicians. 2018;10(01):118–20.
44. Kemp AMC, Bukvic M, Sturgis CD. Fine needle aspiration diagnosis of osteitis fibrosa cystica (brown tumor of bone). Acta Cytol. 2008;52(4):471–4.
45. Agnihotri M, Kothari K, Naik L. Ω Brown tumor of hyperparathyroidism. Diagn Cytopathol. 2017;45(1):43–4.
46. Whittle AP. General principles of fracture treatment. In: Azar FM, Canale ST, Beaty JH, editors. Campbell's operative orthopaedics. 14th ed. Elsevier Inc; 2021. p. 2758–811.
47. Olvi LG, Gonzalez ML, Santini-Araujo E. Stress fracture. In: Santini-Araujo E, Kalil RK, Bertoni F, Park YK, editors. Tumors and tumor-like lesions of bone: for surgical pathologists, orthopedic surgeons and radiologists. 1st ed. Springer; 2015.
48. Koh JS, Chung JH, Kweon MS, Lee SS, Lee SY, Lee JH. Fine needle aspiration cytology of late-stage callus in stress fracture. Acta Cytol. 2001;45(3):445–8.
49. Handa U, Bal A, Mohan H, Bhardwaj S. Fine needle aspiration cytology in the diagnosis of bone lesions. Cytopathology. 2005;16(2):59–64.
50. Maclean F. Joints. In: Mills SE, editor. Histology for pathologists. 5th ed. Lippincott Williams & Wilkins; 2020. p. 113–32.
51. Hermansen P, Freemont T. Synovial fluid analysis in the diagnosis of joint disease. Diagn Histopathol. 2017;23(5):211–20.
52. Oliviero F, Galozzi P, Ramonda R, et al. Unusual findings in synovial fluid analysis: a review. Ann Clin Lab Sci. 2017;47(3):253–9.
53. Ross JJ. Septic arthritis of native Joints. Infect Dis Clin N Am. 2017;31(2):203–18.
54. Smolen JS, Aletaha D, McInnes IB. Rheumatoid arthritis. Lancet. 2016;388(10055):2023–38.
55. Aletaha D, Neogi T, Silman AJ, et al. 2010 Rheumatoid arthritis classification criteria: an American College of Rheumatology/European League Against Rheumatism collaborative initiative. Arthritis Rheum. 2010;62(9):2569–81.

56. Reith JD. Bone and Joints. In: Goldblum J, Lamps LW, McKenney JK, Myers JL, editors. Rosai and Ackerman's surgical pathology, vol. 2. 11th ed. Elsevier Inc; 2017. p. 1740–809.

57. Tenazinha C, Barros R, Fonseca JE, Vieira-Sousa E. Histopathology of psoriatic arthritis synovium—a narrative review. Front Med. 2022;9:860813.

58. Freemont AJ, Denton J. Atlas of synovial fluid cytopathology, vol. 18. Springer Book Archive; 1991.

59. Glyn-Jones S, Palmer AJR, Agricola R, et al. Osteoarthritis. Lancet. 2015;386(9991):376–87.

60. Katz JN, Earp BE, Gomoll AH. Surgical management of osteoarthritis. Arthritis Care Res. 2010;62(9):1220–8.

61. Harkess JW, Crockarell JR. Arthroplasty of the hip. In: Azar FM, Beaty JH, editors. Campbell's operative orthopaedics, vol. 1. 14th ed. Elsevier Inc; 2021. p. 178–333.

62. Patel R. Periprosthetic joint infection. N Engl J Med. 2023;388(3):251–62.

63. Kleeman LT, Goltz D, Seyler TM, et al. Association between pseudotumor formation and patient factors in metal-on-metal total hip arthroplasty population. J Arthroplast. 2018;33(7 Suppl):S259–64.

64. Dalbeth N, Merriman TR, Stamp LK. Gout. Lancet. 2016;388(10055):2039–52.

65. Rosenthal AK, Ryan LM. Calcium pyrophosphate deposition disease. N Engl J Med. 2016;374(26):2575–84.

66. Park HJ, Chung HW, Oh TS, Lee JS, Song JS, Park YK. Tumoral pseudogout of the proximal interphalangeal joint of a finger: a case report and literature review. Skelet Radiol. 2016;45(7):1007–12.

67. Vicentini JRT, Chang CY. MR imaging of the knee bursae and bursal pathology. Magn Reson Imaging Clin N Am. 2022;30(2):241–60.

68. Punia RS, Gupta S, Handa U, Mohan H, Garg S. Fine needle aspiration cytology of bursal cyst. Acta Cytol. 2002;46(4):690–2.

69. Ilaslan H, Sundaram M. Radiologic evaluation of soft tissue tumors. In: Goldblum J, Folpe AL, Weiss SW, editors. Enzinger and Weiss's soft tissue tumors. 7th ed. Elsevier Inc; 2020. p. 32–83.

70. Diehn FE, Benson JC, Maus TP. Radiologic assessment of patient with spine pain. In: Benzon H, editor. Practical management of pain. 6th ed. Elsevier Inc; 2023. p. 232–89.

71. Fels Elliott DR, Ljung BM, Patel R, Iezza G. Primary diagnosis of ruptured biceps tendon "Baker's-type cyst" using fine needle aspiration biopsy: a case report. Diagn Cytopathol. 2018;46(10):870–2.

72. Lowden CM, Attiah M, Garvin G, Macdermid JC, Osman S, Faber KJ. The prevalence of wrist ganglia in an asymptomatic population: magnetic resonance evaluation. J Hand Surg. 2005;30(3):302–6.

73. Rozbruch SR, Chang V, Bohne WH, Deland J. Ganglion cysts of the lower extremity: an analysis of 54 cases and review of the literature. Orthopedics. 1998;21(2):141–8.

74. Layfield LJ, Dodd L, Klijanienko J. Myxoid neoplasms of bone and soft tissue: a pattern-based approach. J Am Soc Cytopathol. 2021;10(3):278–92.

75. Dodd LG, Layfield LJ. Fine-needle aspiration cytology of ganglion cysts. Diagn Cytopathol. 1996;15(5):377–81.

76. Wakely PE, Bos GD, Mayerson J. The cytopathology of soft tissue mxyomas: ganglia, juxta-articular myxoid lesions, and intramuscular myxoma. Am J Clin Pathol. 2005;123(6):858–65.

77. Bush CH. Bone tumor radiology 101 for pathologists. Surg Pathol Clin. 2012;5(1):1–13.

78. Yu GH, Maisel J, Frank R, Pukenas BA, Sebro R, Weber K. Diagnostic utility of fine-needle aspiration cytology of lesions involving bone. Diagn Cytopathol. 2017;45(7):608–13.

79. Kubik MJ, Mohammadi A, Rosa M. Diagnostic benefits and cost-effectiveness of on-site imprint cytology adequacy evaluation of core needle biopsies of bone lesions. Diagn Cytopathol. 2014;42(6):506–13.

80. Shidham VB. Cell-blocks and other ancillary studies (including molecular genetic tests and proteomics). CytoJournal. 2021;18:4.

81. Jillwin J, Rudramurthy SM, Singh S, et al. Molecular identification of pathogenic fungi in formalin-fixed and paraffin-embedded tissues. J Med Microbiol. 2021;70(2):001282.
82. Schulz S, Cabras AD, Kremer M, et al. Species identification of mycobacteria in paraffin-embedded tissues: frequent detection of nontuberculous mycobacteria. Mod Pathol. 2005;18(2):274–82.
83. Vrana JA, Theis JD, Dasari S, et al. Clinical diagnosis and typing of systemic amyloidosis in subcutaneous fat aspirates by mass spectrometry-based proteomics. Haematologica. 2014;99(7):1239–47.

Chapter 18
Brain and Cerebrospinal Fluid

Armine Darbinyan, Anita Huttner, and Minhua Wang

Introduction

The brain and the spinal cord form the Central Nervous System (CNS). Anatomical structures of the brain include supratentorial (above tentorium cerebelli) components: cerebral hemispheres connected by corpus callosum, and infratentorial components: cerebellum and brainstem (the midbrain, the pons, and the medulla oblongata). Within the brain is the ventricular system, consisting of four interconnected ventricles, lined by ependymal cells (two lateral, third and fourth ventricles) and cerebral aqueduct in which cerebrospinal fluid (CSF) is circulated (Fig. 18.1). Several important structures of the brain, including the thalamus, the hypothalamus, the hippocampus, the amygdala, the basal ganglia, the pineal and pituitary glands control proper complex function of the brain via processing and integrating the

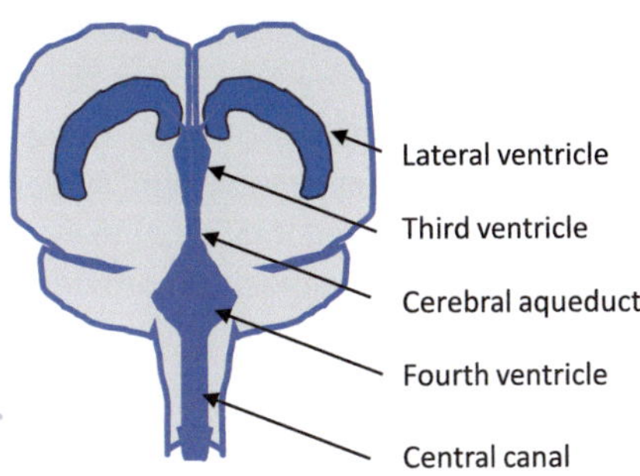

Fig. 18.1 A schematic presentation of the cerebral ventricular system

A. Darbinyan (✉) · A. Huttner · M. Wang
Department of Pathology, Yale School of Medicine, New Haven, CT, USA
e-mail: armine.darbinyan@yale.edu; anita.huttner@yale.edu; minhua.wang@yale.edu

S. M. Gilani, G. Cai (eds.), *Non-Neoplastic Cytology*,
https://doi.org/10.1007/978-3-031-44289-6_18

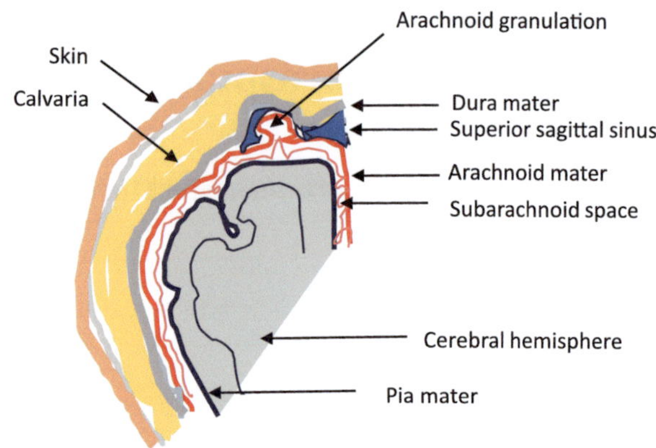

Fig. 18.2 A schematic presentation of dural structures

information it receives from sensory structures and coordinating and executing the response. Cellular components of the human brain include neurons, glial cells (astrocytes, ependymal cells, and oligodendrocytes), microglia, neural stem cells, and cells forming blood vessels. The brain and spinal cord are covered by the meninges which are formed by the dura mater, the outermost thick membrane (closest to the bone of skull and vertebrae), the arachnoid mater (the middle layer), and the pia mater, a delicate membrane adhered to the surfaces of the brain and spinal cord (Fig. 18.2). The subarachnoid space lies between the arachnoid and the pia mater. It communicates with the ventricular system and contains CSF.

Brain

Cytologic Examination, Advantages, and Disadvantages

Cytologic examination of brain tissue and frozen sections are used primarily for intraoperative consultation with major purpose to answer questions required for directing surgery and treatment: to establish the presence of representative tissue, to render a specific diagnosis, to provide diagnostic material for cultures, flow cytometry, electron microscopy, molecular and genetic studies. Adequate, representative, well-prepared specimen is essential for proper evaluation of the specimen. It is critical to have knowledge about clinical setting, including clinical presentation, imaging appearance, and treatment history (chemotherapy or radiation therapy) prior to intraoperative consultation. Intraoperative diagnosis should be formulated along algorithm: (1) is the tissue abnormal? (2) is the lesion neoplastic? (3) if neoplastic, what is the type and grade of the neoplasm? (4) is the pathological diagnosis consistent with clinical and radiological findings? [1] Diagnoses should be brief and include only the information necessary (e.g., "no tumor present" or "metastatic cancer present"). Abbreviations should not be used. To note, histologic type or grade of the tumor should be rendered when it is possible, however in some cases diagnostic precision is not possible and is expected from evaluation of "permanent sections."

Advantages of cytologic examination Cytologic preparations are widely recognized by many neuropathologists as extremely valuable in the morphologic assessment of CNS lesions [2–4]. Often neuropathologists perform smear only when specimen's size is limited, and intraoperative diagnosis is essential [1]. Cytologic examination provides additional information over that provided by frozen section because of optimal preservation of nuclear and cellular detail, demonstration of cytoplasmic processes, and absence of ice crystal artifact. Evaluation of cellular cohesion and sampling of multiple areas of specimen are additional important advantages of cytologic examination of brain tissue. Fine needle aspiration biopsies (FNAB) of the CNS are also used to identify infectious agents, particularly in immunosuppressed patients [5, 6]. Studies suggest that CT-guided FNAB procedures are associated with lower morbidity (intraparenchymal hemorrhage) and mortality, with a small decrease in the diagnostic accuracy. FNAB was shown to be most effective in diagnosing high-grade glial tumors, metastatic carcinomas, lymphomas, and abscesses [7].

Disadvantages of cytologic examination include requirement of knowledge of cytopathology and insufficient architectural information. Diagnostic ability is especially limited in pauci-cellular lesions and lesions with dense stroma. Evaluation of lesion/tumor-brain interface is difficult or not possible.

Types of Cytologic Preparations

Cytologic preparations can be prepared as touch Imprints and smears/squash preparations.

Touch Imprints

Touch imprints are suggested to be used for specimens which are very small or very fragmented to be scraped to create smear preparations. Most appropriate specimens for touch imprints are highly cellular lesions that freely release individual cells (pituitary adenoma, lymphomas, cellular metastatic lesions, and meningiomas). Touch imprints are not satisfactory for gliomas or schwannomas. In touch imprints, it is more likely to produce monolayers and cytoplasm of cells tends to be better preserved than in scrape/smear technique. In addition, touch imprints may replicate architectural features (e.g., lymphoid follicles).

Technique

1. Touch clean and dry glass slide to freshly cut tissue surface. Do not apply pressure or movement.
2. Immediately immerse in fixative (95% alcohol) prior to H&E or Papanicolaou staining.

Smears/Squash Preparation

This is the preferred technique for stereotactic biopsies because of demonstration of single cell morphology, particularly of cells with long cytoplasmic processes. Often produce tissue fragments that may allow evaluation of both cytological and histological features.

Technique

1. Place small piece of abnormal tissue (<1 × 1 mm) near labeled end of slide.
2. Using another slide, firmly squash tissue and spread it along slide longitudinally.
3. Separate two slides and immediately place in fixative.
4. Both slides are stained and covered with cover slip slide.

To note: If lesion is heterogeneous, multiple small fragments can be placed side-by-side. Excessive manipulation should be avoided to prevent damage of cells. Strong pressure may result in rupture of cells with small amount of cytoplasm (e.g., lymphomas or medulloblastomas).

Normal Cytology and Potential Misinterpretation as Abnormalities

In normal white matter glial cells (oligodendrocytes and astrocytes) are monomorphous and cytologically bland (Fig. 18.3a). The neuropil has a "fluffy" appearance. Oligodendrocytes tend to have small round nuclei with dense chromatin. Astrocytes have long fine processes, relatively large round, or elongated nuclei with less dense chromatin. Neurons are identified by their prominent nucleoli (Fig. 18.3b). The size and shape of neurons varies depending on the location (the cortex vs. deep grey nuclei). The cytoplasm of neurons is fragile and can be lost during the smearing process. Abundance of normal neurons (thick smears) can be misinterpreted as evidence of glioneuronal neoplasm. Similarly, high number of glial cells in thick smear can be suggestive of glioma. Evaluation of monolayer smear is optimal.

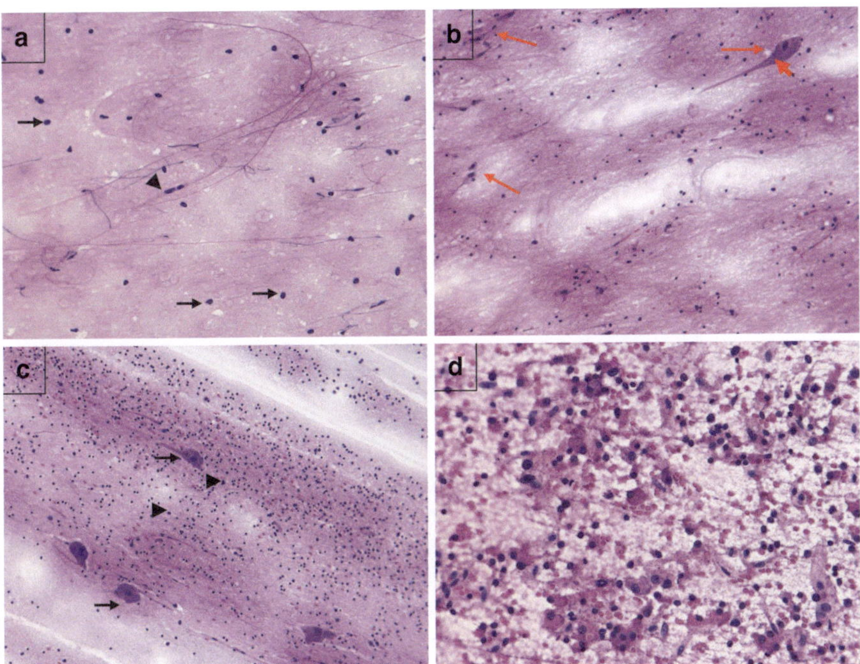

Fig. 18.3 (**a**) Smear of normal white matter with glial cells (black arrow) and capillaries (black arrowhead). Glial cells, predominantly oligodendrocytes, of normal white matter are well spread. Cellularity is low. Oligodendrocytes have small round nuclei with dense chromatin. Nuclei of astrocytes are larger, round or elongated and have less dense chromatin. Occasionally, astrocytic cytoplasm and fine cellular processes are visible (reactive astrocytes). Thick smears can be misconstrued as evidence of glioma. (**b**) Smear of normal Gray Matter (Cerebral Cortex) with neurons, glial cells and capillaries. Neurons (red arrow) have nuclei with smooth outlines, fine chromatin and prominent nucleoli. Nissl substance (red arrowhead) or lipofuscin can be identified in the cytoplasm of neuron. (**c**) Smear of normal cerebellum. Large Purkinje cells with extensive processes (black arrow) among abundant small neurons of granule cell layer (black arrowhead). (**d**) Touch imprint of anterior pituitary (adenohypophysis) shows the admixture of various cell types (basophilic, acidophilic and chromophobic) and delicate capillaries

Smear of normal cerebellum shows large Purkinje cells with extensive processes admixed with abundant small neurons of granule cell layer (Fig. 18.3c). Nuclei of neurons from normal granule cell layer may be misinterpreted as neoplastic medulloblastoma cells; however, cerebellar granule cells are smaller, round, and lack features of atypia. Touch imprint of anterior pituitary (adenohypophysis) shows the admixture of various cell types (basophilic, acidophilic, and chromophobic) and delicate capillaries (Fig. 18.3d). Mixed population of cytologically bland cells is evidence of normality. Consider inflammatory process (hypophysitis), pathogen-free granulomatous process, or atypical lymphoid proliferation in the presence of lymphocytic infiltrate.

Reactive Astrogliosis

Any neuropathological process, including infection, inflammation, vascular disease and infarct, neoplasms, can be associated with reactive astrogliosis which presents with increased number of evenly spaced slightly eosinophilic astrocytes with complex fine long cytoplasmic processes. The nuclei of astrocytes are large with delicate chromatin and smooth nuclear membrane. The presence of macrophages can be suggestive of a non-neoplastic process. Diffusely infiltrating low-grade glial neoplasm cannot be excluded.

Necrosis

Coagulative necrosis shows granular appearance and can be seen in tumor (malignant glioma, medulloblastoma, lymphoma (especially after steroid therapy)), but also in infectious process (toxoplasmosis, tuberculosis, aspergillosis, mucormycosis), in inflammatory disease (rheumatoid arthritis) and induced by treatment (radionecrosis). There is an increased number of macrophages in necrosis associated with demyelinating disease, progressive multifocal leukoencephalopathy, toxoplasmosis, leukoencephalopathy, inflammatory pseudotumor, Rosai-Dorfman disease and infarct. Presence of macrophages is an important feature of non-neoplastic lesion. Prominent neutrophils are suggestive of bacterial abscess.

Cerebrospinal Fluid Cytology

CSF

CSF is produced by modified ependymal cells in the choroid plexus, or *plica choroidea* in ventricles of the brain. CSF circulates in the ventricular system, in the subarachnoid space around the brain and in the central canal of the spinal cord. CSF is generated at the rate of approximately 500 mL per day, is constantly reabsorbed by arachnoid granulations and drained into vascular system of dural venous sinuses. Total volume of CSF at any one time is 125–150 mL in adults.

Clinical Indication of CSF Evaluation

CSF specimens are primarily obtained by lumbar puncture (LP). In some cases, CSF is sampled from ventricles or from Ommaya reservoir, an intraventricular catheter that can be used for the delivery of drugs. Urgent LP is indicated in neonates and immunocompromised patients with unexplained fever in evaluation of possible CNS infection [8, 9]. Urgent LP is considered as a gold standard for the diagnosis of subarachnoid hemorrhage (SAH) in setting of CT negative scan and high suspicion for hemorrhage [8]. Cytologic examination of CSF is useful in diagnosis of neoplastic diseases (primary and metastatic), lymphoma/leukemia and neuroimmunologic disorders. CSF cytology is helpful in posttreatment monitoring of tumors and infectious/inflammatory conditions.

CSF Collection

It is recommended to collect CSF in plastic tubes because cells adhere to glass. CSF specimen collected in the second or third tube is preferred to avoid possible blood contamination during LP. The specimen should be processed quickly to preserve integrity of cells. CSF can be refrigerated for up to 48 h. The addition of ethanol or commercial fixatives can promote longer preservation of cells; however, alcohol may induce cell shrinkage.

Macroscopic and Microscopic Features: Normal CSF

Normal CSF is a colorless and clear fluid. It should be considered as a potentially infectious specimen. It is recommended to use both Romanowsky and Pap stains. CSF specimen normally has low cellularity. Identification of a single well-preserved abnormal cell may have diagnostic implications. Acellular CSF specimens can be seen in cytospin preparations and are considered adequate for cytologic evaluation.

Normal cell count is 0–5/µL in adults. Cell count is higher in neonates, approaching 30/µL [10, 11]. Cells in CSF specimen are represented by lymphocytes (L) and monocytes (M) [8]. In adult CSF lymphocytes normally predominate with 2:1 ratio (L:M). CSF specimen is monocyte predominant in neonates.

Lymphocytes are normally presented in CSF (Fig. 18.4). Their number may increase in viral, fungal, and tuberculous infections of the CNS. Elevated white blood cell (WBC) counts also may occur in a variety of inflammatory conditions, granulomatous meningitis, and carcinomatosis. Large lymphocytes with irregular nuclear membranes and conspicuous nucleoli ("atypical" or reactive) can be detected in multiple sclerosis, meningitis, post chemotherapy, and radiation. A mixed polymorphous population of lymphoid cells is suggestive of benign reactive inflammatory process; however, differential diagnosis with lymphoproliferative disorder is required.

Monocytes are normally present in CSF (Fig. 18.4). Monocytosis is detected in conditions similar to lymphocytosis.

Fig. 18.4 Lymphocytes (arrow) and monocyte (arrowhead). Diff-Quick stain

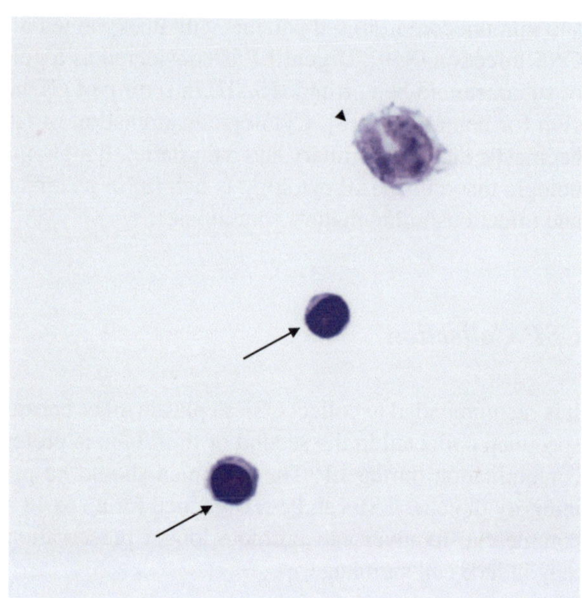

Fig. 18.5 Numerous red blood cells (arrow). Diff-Quick stain

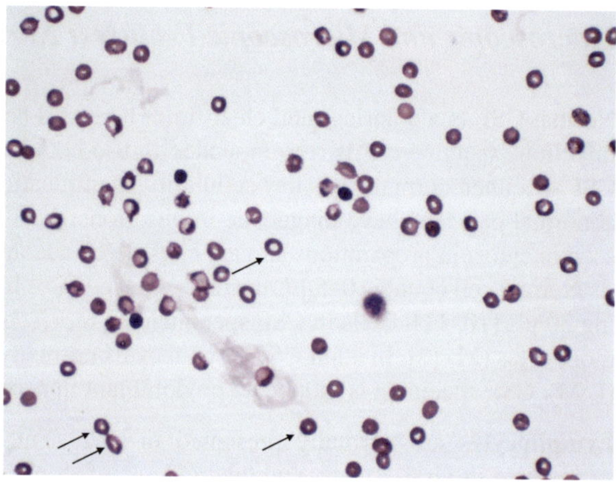

Red Blood Cells (RBS) are not present in CSF under normal conditions. Presence of numerous erythrocytes (Fig. 18.5) indicates abnormal bleeding/hemorrhage or a traumatic tap. In a traumatic tap, RBCs are usually well preserved. RBCs with degenerated change, siderophages and erythrophagocytosis are usually seen in abnormal bleeding.

Neutrophils are abnormal finding in CSF. Rare neutrophils may suggest blood contamination. The presence of large number of neutrophils indicates acute bacterial meningitis (Fig. 18.6). Neutrophils can be detected in early stages of viral infection of the CNS.

Fig. 18.6 Acute inflammation. Numerous neutrophils (arrow). Pap stain

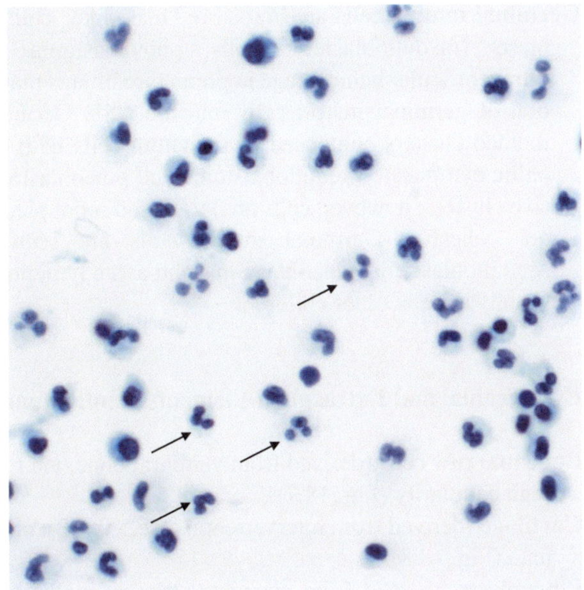

Macrophages are not present in CSF under normal conditions. They indicate tissue destruction which can be a result of infectious/inflammatory process, trauma, infarction, invasive procedure, foreign bodies, and neoplasm.

Plasma cells are abnormal finding in CSF. Plasma cells are characteristic for multiple sclerosis and neurosyphilis. They are associated with chronic inflammation, infectious diseases, and plasma cell malignancies which involve the CSF.

Eosinophils are not present in normal CSF. Their presence is associated with hypersensitivity/allergy, parasitic infections, foreign material, and lymphoproliferative disorders.

CNS cells. Ependymal cells, epithelioid cells of choroid plexus, neurons, glial cells (astrocytes and oligodendrocytes), pia-arachnoid (leptomeningeal) cells can be detected in CSF in hydrocephalus, trauma, infarction. and instrumentation.

Choroid plexus cells and ependymal cells are small and uniform, have epithelioid appearance, form small loose clusters or microacini. Individual cells have cilia, vacuolated cytoplasm, single round to oval nuclei with fine delicate chromatin.

Leptomeningeal cells may appear in CSF as a result of meningeal irritation. They have eccentric round to oval nuclei with fine chromatin, and moderately dense cytoplasm. Leptomeningeal cells often form small flat sheets.

Neurons and astrocytes usually are detected in CSF specimens obtained from ventricles, often associated with bleeding. Neurons are large cells with pyramidal or multipolar bodies, long processes, large nuclei with prominent central nucleoli. Astrocytes have multiple fine cytoplasmic processes and oval slightly hyperchromatic nuclei.

Germinal matrix cells are immature "blast-like" cells which resemble malignant blasts (medulloblastoma cells, pineoblastoma cells, and lymphoblasts). Intraventricular hemorrhage in premature infants may be associated with exfoliation of germinal matrix cells into the CSF. Germinal matrix cells form tight molded clusters composed of immature cells with oval nuclei and scant basophilic cytoplasm. Medulloblastoma and pineoblastoma cells form similar cohesive clusters; however, cells are larger and more pleomorphic. Lymphoblasts are not cohesive. Germinal matrix cells are seen exclusively in neonates. Medulloblastoma, pineoblastoma, and acute lymphoblastic lymphoma/leukemia usually arise in older children.

Extracranial and Extraspinal Elements/Contaminants

Bone marrow cells (derived from vertebral bone, via LP): hematopoietic elements, high cellularity (Fig. 18.7).
Cartilage (derived from intervertebral disc, via LP): chondrocytes with perinuclear halo (Fig. 18.8).
Fibroblasts (derived from connective tissue, including paraspinal and dural, via LP): bland elongated cells.

Immunocytochemical studies can be helpful in differential diagnosis.

Noncellular Elements in CSF

Proteinaceous material appears as an amorphous or fibrillar, gray blue precipitate in background of the slide. **Psammoma bodies** appear as PAS negative, laminated and calcified structures, often present in normal choroid plexus.

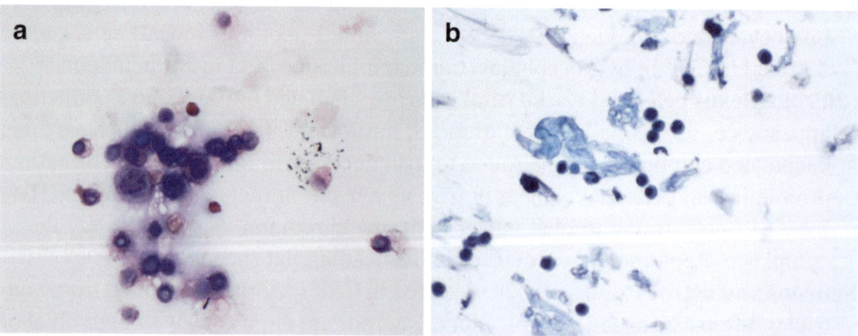

Fig. 18.7 CSF with bone marrow contamination: hematopoietic elements. (**a**) Diff-Quick stain. (**b**) Pap stain

Fig. 18.8 Chondrocyte

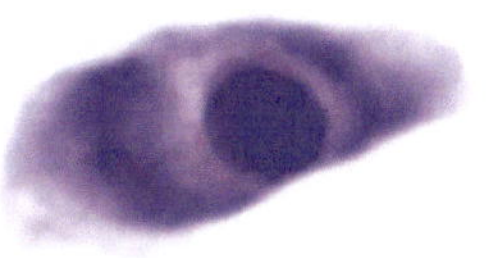

CSF in Benign CNS Conditions

Reactive conditions (hemorrhage, infarct, trauma): elevated numbers of normal
  cell types in CSF.

Meningitis
Bacterial meningitis: marked increase in number of neutrophils (Fig. 18.6), fibrin,
  cell debris, microorganisms (*E. coli* and *Listeria monocytogenes* in newborns;
  H. influenzae, *Neisseria meningitidis*, and *Streptococcus pneumoniae* in infants
  and kids; *Pneumococcus*, *Staphylococcus*, *Streptococcus* in adults).
Viral meningitis/encephalitis: an increase in the number of small lymphocytes and
  small macrophages. The presence of bleeding is suggestive of viral encephalitis.
Mollaret meningitis: associated with herpes simplex virus (most common). CSF
  shows marked pleocytosis, composed of lymphocytes and neutrophils, large
  "atypical" Mollaret cells (activated monocytes) with eccentric irregular bean-
  shaped nuclei and delicate finely vacuolated pale cytoplasm.
Fungal meningitis (*Cryptococcus neoformans*, *Blastomyces*, *Histoplasma*,
  Aspergillus, *Actinomyces*, *Phycomycetes (Mucor)*, *Coccidioides*): an increase in
  the number of predominantly small lymphocytes. Organisms can be identified by
  their cytomorphology. Microbiologic studies are required for confirmation. The
  most common fungal organism identified in CSF is cryptococcus (Fig. 18.9).
  Immunocompromised patients are usually affected by cryptococcal infection.
  The yeast form is approximately 5–15 μm in diameter, has mucoid capsule
  (highlighted by mucicarmine), is characterized by single, teardrop-shaped budding. Periodic acid-Schiff (PAS) and Gomori-methenamine silver (GMS) stains
  are used for detection of organisms.

Reporting
Negative for malignancy/benign
Atypical

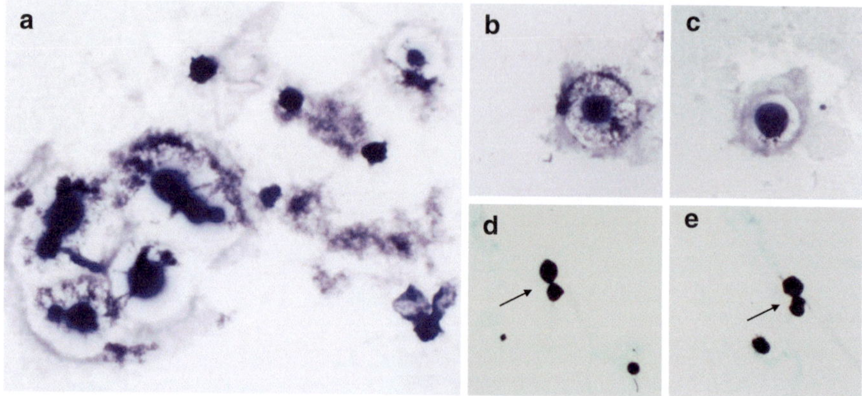

Fig. 18.9 *Cryptococcus.* (**a–c**) Diff-Quick stain. (**d, e**) GMS stain. Teardrop budding (arrow)

Suspicious for malignancy
Positive for malignancy
Nondiagnostic

References

1. Burger PC. Smears and frozen sections in surgical neuropathology: a manual. United States: PB Medical Publ; 2009.
2. Marshall L, Adams H, Graham D. The histologic accuracy of the smear technique for neurosurgical biopsies. J Neurosurg. 1973;39:82–8.
3. Silverman JF, Timmons RL, Leonard JR III, et al. Cytologic results of fine-needle aspiration biopsies of the central nervous system. Cancer. 1986;58:1117–21.
4. Silverman JF. Cytopathology of fine-needle aspiration biopsy of the brain and spinal cord. Diagn Cytopathol. 1986;2:312–9.
5. Deshpande AH, Munshi MM. Rhinocerebral mucormycosis diagnosis by aspiration cytology. Diagn Cytopathol. 2000;23:97–100.
6. Poon TP, Tchertkoff V, Win H. Subacute measles encephalitis with AIDS diagnosed by fine needle aspiration biopsy. A case report. Acta Cytol. 1998;42:729–33.
7. Seliem RM, Assaad MW, Gorombey SJ, Moral LA, Kirkwood JR, Otis CN. Fine-needle aspiration biopsy of the central nervous system performed freehand under computed tomography guidance without stereotactic instrumentation. Cancer. 2003;99(5):277–84.
8. Rahimi J, Woehrer A. Overview of cerebrospinal fluid cytology. Handb Clin Neurol. 2017;145:563–71.
9. Shahan B, Choi EY, Nieves G. Cerebrospinal fluid analysis. Am Fam Physician. 2021;103(7):422–8. Erratum in: Am Fam Physician. 2021 Jun 15;103(12):713.
10. Sarff LD, Platt LH, McCracken GH Jr. Cerebrospinal fluid evaluation in neonates: comparison of high-risk infants with and without meningitis. J Pediatr. 1976;88(3):473–7.
11. Srinivasan L, Shah SS, Padula MA, Abbasi S, McGowan KL, Harris MC. Cerebrospinal fluid reference ranges in term and preterm infants in the neonatal intensive care unit. J Pediatr. 2012;161(4):729–34.

Chapter 19
Quick Review

Khairya Fatouh and Syed M. Gilani

See Tables 19.1, 19.2, and 19.3.

Table 19.1 Immunohistochemical stains expression in normal and benign tissue cells [1–34]

Stains	Positive staining in benign or normal epithelium	Staining pattern
AFP	Fetal liver	Membranous, cytoplasmic
BAF47/INI-1	Normally expressed in all cells	Nuclear
BAP1	In most normal tissues	Nuclear
BCL-2	Mantle zone B-lymphocytes	Nuclear, cytoplasmic
BCL-6	Germinal center	Nuclear
Ber-Ep4	Epithelial cells	Membranous
CA-IX	Gastric mucosa, duodenum, intrahepatic bile ducts, and mesothelial lining	Membranous
Calcitonin	C-cell hyperplasia	Cytoplasmic
Caldesmin	Smooth muscle cells	Cytoplasmic
Calponin	Myoepithelial cells of the breast and the salivary gland, smooth muscle cells, and myofibroblasts	Cytoplasmic
Calretinin	Mesothelial cells, Leydig cells, adrenal cortical cells, and endometrial stromal cells	Nuclear and cytoplasmic

(continued)

K. Fatouh
St. John Hospital and Medical Center, Detroit, MI, USA
e-mail: khairya.fatouh@ascension.org

S. M. Gilani (✉)
Department of Pathology, Albany Medical Center, Albany Medical College, Albany, NY, USA
e-mail: gilanis@amc.edu

S. M. Gilani, G. Cai (eds.), *Non-Neoplastic Cytology*,
https://doi.org/10.1007/978-3-031-44289-6_19

Table 19.1 (continued)

Stains	Positive staining in benign or normal epithelium	Staining pattern
CD3	Thymic cells (thymocytes) and T-lymphocytes (mostly peripheral)	Membranous
CD5	Thymic cells (thymocytes) and T-lymphocytes	Membranous
CD10	Germinal center, small intestine, endometrial stroma, bile canaliculi	Membranous
CD19	Immature B-lymphocytes	Membranous
CD20	B-lymphocytes	Membranous
CD21	B-lymphocytes and follicular dendritic cells	Membranous
CD23	B-cells and follicular dendritic cells	Membranous
CD30	Activated B- and T-cells, immunoblasts, and decidual cells	Membranous
CD31	Endothelial cells, lymphatics, and megakaryocytes	Membranous
CD34	Hematolymphoid precursors, endothelium, and myofibroblasts	Membranous
CD56	NK cells, neuroendocrine cells	Membranous
CD68	Macrophages, Langerhans cells, osteoclasts, and multinucleated giant cells	Membranous
CD99	Endothelial cells, immature thymic T-cells and skin	Membranous
CD163	Macrophages and monocytes	Membranous
CEA	Epithelial cells, thyroid C-cells, granulocytes	Membranous and cytoplasmic
Chromogranin	Neuroendocrine and ganglion cells	Cytoplasmic
Claudin-4	Epithelial cells	Membranous
Cyclin D-1	Histiocytes, endothelial cells, skin	Nucleus
Cytokeratin	Epithelium	Membranous and cytoplasmic
D2-40	Lymphatics	Membranous
Desmin	Muscle cells, mesothelial cells, and endothelial cells	Cytoplasmic
DOG-1	Interstitial cells of Cajal, throughout the GI tract, and salivary gland (mostly in acini-apical luminal)	Membranous and cytoplasmic
E-Cadherin	Breast ductal epithelial cells	Membranous
Estrogen	Breast epithelium and endometrial stroma	Nuclear
FVIII	Endothelial cells, megakaryocytes	Cytoplasmic
GATA-3	Breast, parathyroid, epidermis, skin adnexal glands, kidney (collecting ducts), parotid (normal terminal ducts), T-lymphocytes	Nuclear
GCDFP-15	Breast parenchymal tissue, skin adnexal glands, and some minor salivary glands	Cytoplasmic
GFAP	Astrocytes, myoepithelial cells	Cytoplasmic
Glypican	Trophoblast, fetal liver, rarely in cirrhotic nodules	Membranous and cytoplasmic
Glutamine synthetase	Hepatocytes (perivenular pattern), focal nodular hyperplasia (map-like pattern)	Cytoplasmic
HBME	Mesothelial cells	Membranous
HMB-45	Melanocytes	Cytoplasmic

Table 19.1 (continued)

Stains	Positive staining in benign or normal epithelium	Staining pattern
Inhibin	Sertoli and Leydig cells, granulosa cells, adrenal cortical cells	Cytoplasmic
INSM-1	Neuroendocrine cells, adrenal cortical cells (rarely), Merkel cells in epidermis	Nuclear
LCA (CD45)	Pan WBCs marker, histiocytes	Membranous
Mammaglobin	Breast ductal epithelium, endocervical glands, eccrine glands	Cytoplasmic
Melan-A	Melanocytes and adrenal cortex	Cytoplasmic
MOC-31	Epithelial cells	Membranous
MTAP	Reactive mesothelial cells, inflammatory cells	Nuclear and cytoplasmic
MUM-1	Plasma cells, germinal center B-cells	Nuclear
Myb	Hematopoietic cells	Nuclear
MyoD-1	Skeletal muscle (fetal)	Nuclear
Myogenin	Skeletal muscle (fetal)	Nuclear
Napsin-A	Pneumocytes, renal cortex	Cytoplasmic granular
NKX3.1	Prostate, minor salivary gland	Nucleus
NUT (NUT midline carcinoma)	Testis	Nuclear
OCT-4	Embryonic germ cells	Nuclear
P16	Endometrial tissue or tubal metaplasia	Nuclear and cytoplasmic
P63 and p40	Breast myoepithelial cells, salivary gland myoepithelial/basal cells, skin basal layers, prostate basal cells, urothelial and squamous epithelium	Nuclear
P120 catenin	Epithelial cells	Membranous
P504s (AMACR)	Kidney tubules	Cytoplasmic
Parafibromin	Endothelial cells	Nuclear
PAX-5	B-lymphocytes	Nuclear
PAX-8 (polyclonal)	Renal, müllerian tract epithelium, thyroid follicles, B-lymphocytes, pancreatic islet cells, and seminal vesicle	Nuclear
PAX-8 (monoclonal)	Renal, thyroid, müllerian tract epithelium	Nuclear
PSA	Prostate, major salivary gland tissue	Cytoplasmic
PSAP	Prostate	Cytoplasmic
PLAP	Placental tissue	Membranous and cytoplasmic
Progesterone	Breast and endocervix	Nuclear
S100	Melanocytes, adipocytes, Schwann cells, nerve cells, myoepithelial cells	Nuclear and cytoplasmic
SALL-4	Adult germ cells	Nuclear
SATB2	Lower GI tract	Nuclear

(continued)

Table 19.1 (continued)

Stains	Positive staining in benign or normal epithelium	Staining pattern
SMA	Myoepithelial cells, smooth muscle	Cytoplasmic
SDHB	Most normal cells	Cytoplasmic
SF-1	Adrenal cortex and gonadotrophoblasts	Nuclear
SMAD4	Most normal cells	Nuclear
SMARCA4	Most normal cells	Nuclear
SOX-10	Melanocytes, nerve cells, myoepithelial cells, salivary gland	Nuclear
Synaptophysin	Neuroendocrine cells in different organs, islet cells, neuronal tissue	Cytoplasmic
TdT	Early T-cells, precursor B-cells, and thymic cells	Nuclear
TRPS1	Breast, salivary gland	Nuclear
TTF-1	Type 2 pneumocytes, alveolar cells, thyroid follicular cells	Nuclear
Thyroglobulin	Thyroid follicular cells	Cytoplasmic
WT-1	Mesothelial cells, ovarian granulosa cells	Nuclear

Table 19.2 Infections [35–48]

Fungi	
Blastomycosis	Large (8–15 μm), spherical thick walled (double contoured), single budding yeast cells with broad base. Cultures are helpful
Coccidioidomycosis	Necrotizing granulomatous inflammation, thick-walled spherules (20–100 μm) containing endospores (to 2–5 μm). Cultures and serology (IgM and IgG) may be helpful
Paracoccidioidomycosis	Necrotizing granulomatous inflammation, large, but thin-walled (as compared to blastomyces) rounded, single and multiple budding with narrow base (Mariner's wheel), cultures and serologic tests (antibodies) are also helpful
Histoplasma capsulatum	Small, oval, uniform yeast cells (2–4 μm) seen in macrophages and granulomas. Narrow based and oval single budding. Cultures, serology, and histoplasmin skin test may be helpful
Cryptococcus neoformans	Variably sized (5–10 μm in diameter), round to oval encapsulated budding yeasts with thin cell walls and narrow based budding. Cultures and serology (capsular antigen) are helpful
Aspergillus	Septate hyphae (3–6 μm), with regular, dichotomous branching at a 45° angle and may show fruiting bodies (Fig. 19.1) and calcium oxalate crystals (Fig. 19.2)
Mucormycosis	Broad hyphae (10–15 μm) mostly non-septate hyphae or may show sparse septation with branching (mostly 90°)
Candida	Pseudohyphae and yeast forms. Cultures, serology, and PCR (polymerase chain reaction) may be helpful
Pneumocystis jirovecii	Cyst and trophozoites, elliptical/or cup-shaped (Fig. 19.3) cysts with dark central area. Usually require cytology or histology confirmation
Viruses	
Herpes	Double-stranded DNA virus. Multinucleated cells with ground glass nuclei, nuclear molding, and margination (Fig. 19.4)

Table 19.2 (continued)

Cytomegalovirus (CMV)	Large DNA virus. Can affect endothelial cells, epithelial cells, and other cell types. CMV involved cell can show perinuclear cytoplasmic inclusion/or cytoplasmic granules and intranuclear inclusions. PCR testing is helpful
Epstein-Barr virus	Mostly affects B-lymphocytes. Cytology shows atypical/large lymphocytes with abundant cytoplasm and prominent nucleoli. Nuclei acid detection (PCR for EBV DNA)
Polyoma virus	Double-stranded DNA virus (JC and BK). Urine cytology shows infected urothelial cells with smudgy nuclei and basophilic nuclear inclusion (Fig. 19.5)
Adenovirus	Non-enveloped icosahedral DNA virus. Cells show intranuclear basophilic inclusions
Parasites	
Entamoeba histolytica	Cysts and trophozoite forms. Trophozoites (10–20 μm) can be seen on morphologic evaluation. They contain abundant cytoplasm with foamy, vacuolated, or granular appearance and can show red blood cells
Giardia lamblia	Trophozoite and cyst forms. Trophozoite (12–15 μm) consists of pair of nuclei and four pairs of flagella originate from the basal bodies
Leishmania	Transmitted by sandfly. Amastigote form (nucleus and rod-like kinetoplast) in cytoplasm (Fig. 19.6)
Cryptosporidium and Cyclospora	Oocysts in stool and stain positive for modified acid-fast stain
Enterobius vermicularis (pinworm)	Most common helminths in the US. Eggs are oval with a flattened side, 50 × 20 μm. Scotch tape test to detect eggs
Ascaris lumbricoides (roundworm)	Largest helminths to affect humans, can cause Loeffler's syndrome. Eggs are golden brown with knobs and bumps on both sides
Ancylostoma duodenale (hookworm)	Larvae enters through skin and involve intestine. Eggs are 60–75 μm, thin colorless shell with clear halo between shell and embryo
Schistosoma	*S. mansoni* (GI tract, liver, egg with lateral spine) *S. japonicum* (GI tract, liver, egg with small spine as compared to others) *S. haematobium* (urine, egg with terminal spine)
Echinococcus granulosus	Can involve liver (mostly) and spleen. Hydatid cyst (protoscolices within brood capsules)
Bacteria	
Gram-positive cocci	
Staphylococcus	Gram-positive cocci in clusters, all are catalase positive. Can be coagulase positive (*S. aureus*) or coagulase negative (such as *S. epidermidis*)
Streptococcus	Gram-positive cocci in chains and pairs. Further divided based on hemolytic reaction: *S. viridans* (mostly alpha hemolytic) *S. pyogenes* (local and systemic infection) are beta hemolytic *S. bovis* or group D (mostly non-hemolytic)
Gram-negative cocci	

(continued)

Table 19.2 (continued)

Neisseria meningitidis (meningococci) and gonorrhoeae (gonococci)	Mostly diplococcus and oxidase positive
Gram-positive rods	
Corynebacterium	Non-spore forming aerobic microorganisms (club-shaped rods)
Bacillus	Large, square-shaped, spore forming aerobic bacteria. Catalase positive. *Bacillus anthracis* are nonmotile (medusa head colonies), while *Bacillus cereus* are motile
Listeria monocytogenes	Non-spore forming, catalase positive (tumbling motility at 22–28 °C)
Gram-negative bacilli	
Helicobacter	Usually rod or spiral shaped, urease-positive microorganism. *H. pylori* is more common than *H. heilmannii* (which are corkscrew-shaped and longer than *H. pylori*)
Gram-positive anaerobes	
Actinomyces	Filamentous and branching bacteria (with sulfur granules)
Other bacteria	
Mycobacterium	Thin rods, acid fast bacilli (Ziehl-Neelsen), auramine-rhodamine stain, tuberculin test, PCR test/nucleic acid amplification
Nocardia	Filamentous and branching, gram-positive rods, modified acid fast

Table 19.3 Types of crystals [49–53]

Types of crystals	Conditions	Diagnostic clues
Monosodium urate	Gout	Needle shape, negatively birefringent, yellow when aligned parallel to polarized light and looks blue when aligned perpendicular to the polarized light
Calcium pyrophosphate dehydrogenase	Pseudogout	Rhomboid-shaped, positive birefringent, blue in color
Calcium oxalate	Increased oxalate intake, renal insufficiency, fungal infections (Aspergillus), nodular goiter (mostly in colloid)	Rhomboid, diamond shaped, rosettes of rods, translucent and positive birefringent
Tyrosine crystals	Tyrosinemia, liver disease, and some salivary gland tumors	Floret-shaped
Crystals in urine		
Calcium carbonate	Condition that increases urine pH	Round with lateral radiations, colorless to yellowish
Calcium oxalate	Kidney stones	Mono and dihydrate
Cystine	Cystinuria	Hexagonal
Ammonium biurate	Old specimens	Spherical with lateral spikes
Bilirubin	Liver disease	Needle like, yellowish in color
Cholesterol crystals	Renal tubular disease	Translucent rectangles

Table 19.3 (continued)

Types of crystals	Conditions	Diagnostic clues
Charcot-Leyden crystals	Asthma and atopy	Eosinophilic rhomboid shaped
Hematoidin crystals in sputum	Bronchiectasis, current smoking, hemoptysis, and malignancy	Golden/yellow to brown, can be positive or negative birefringent
Reinke crystals	Leydig cell tumors	Intracellular eosinophilic crystals
Apatite-like crystals	Osteoarthritis	Cuboidal to needle shaped

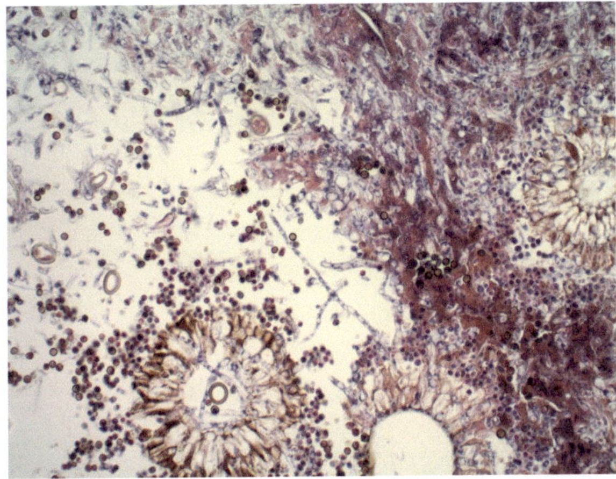

Fig. 19.1 Hyphae forms in a background of fruiting bodies (Aspergillus, H&E ×400)

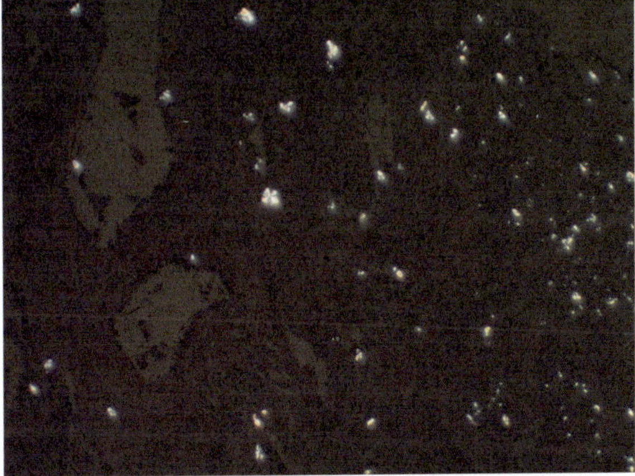

Fig. 19.2 Calcium oxalate crystals (case of aspergillus infection, polarized light ×100)

K. Fatouh and S. M. Gilani

Fig. 19.3 *Pneumocystis jirovecii*, cup-shaped organisms (GMS stain ×400)

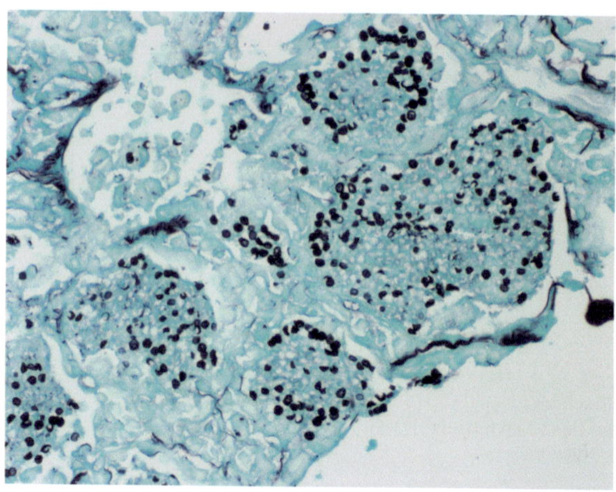

Fig. 19.4 Herpes viral cytopathic changes in a background of inflammation (Papanicolaou stain ×600)

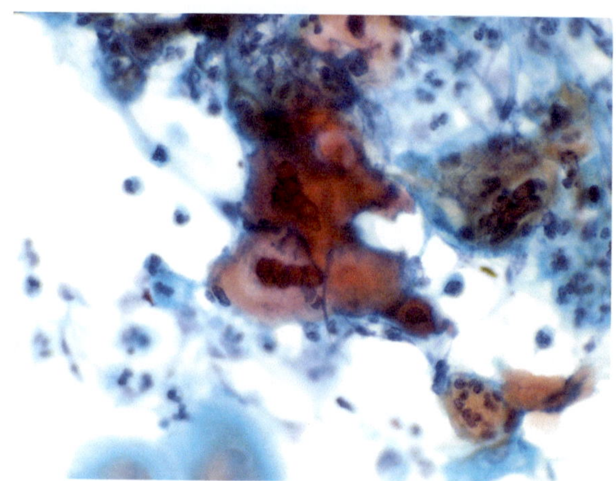

Fig. 19.5 Urine cytology with focal polyoma virus cytopathologic changes (ThinPrep ×400)

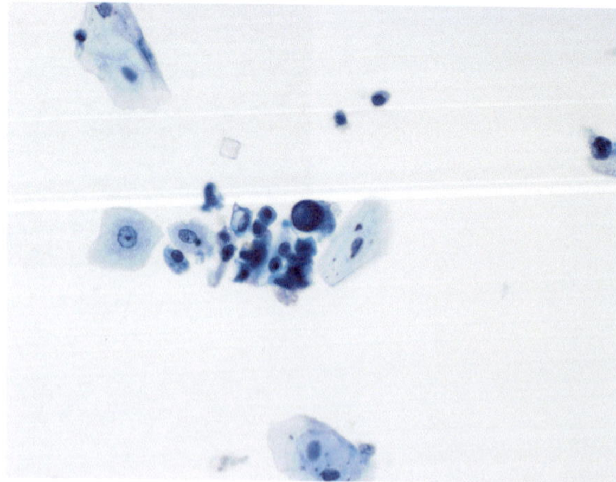

Fig. 19.6 Microorganisms within the cytoplasm with amastigote forms (Leishmania, H&E ×600)

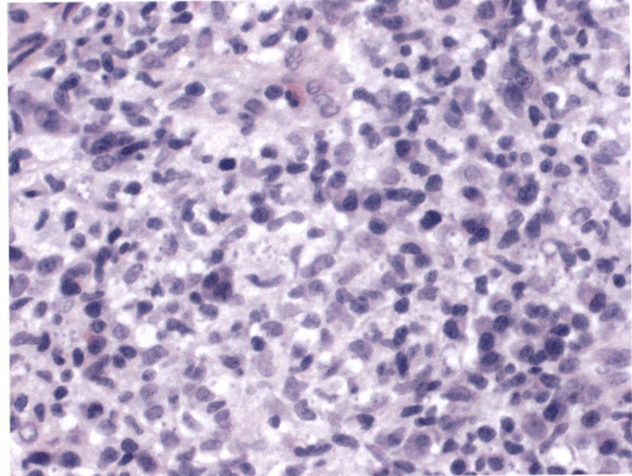

Acknowledgments None.

Conflict of Interest None.

References

1. Ivanov S, Liao SY, Ivanova A, et al. Expression of hypoxia-inducible cell-surface transmembrane carbonic anhydrases in human cancer. Am J Pathol. 2001;158(3):905–19.
2. Luong-Player A, Liu H, Wang HL, Lin F. Immunohistochemical reevaluation of carbonic anhydrase IX (CA IX) expression in tumors and normal tissues. Am J Clin Pathol. 2014;141(2):219–25.
3. Lloyd JM, Owens SR. CD10 immunohistochemistry stains enteric mucosa, but negative staining is unreliable in the setting of active enteritis. Mod Pathol. 2011;24(12):1627–32.
4. McCluggage WG, Sumathi VP, Maxwell P. CD10 is a sensitive and diagnostically useful immunohistochemical marker of normal endometrial stroma and of endometrial stromal neoplasms. Histopathology. 2001;39(3):273–8.
5. Shousha S, Gadir F, Peston D, Bansi D, Thillainaygam AV, Murray-Lyon IM. CD10 immunostaining of bile canaliculi in liver biopsies: change of staining pattern with the development of cirrhosis. Histopathology. 2004;45(4):335–42.
6. Craig CE, Quaglia A, Dhillon AP. Extramedullary haematopoiesis in massive hepatic necrosis. Histopathology. 2004;45(5):518–25.
7. Trovato M, Grosso M, Vitarelli E, Le Donne M, Barresi V, Trimarchi F, Barresi G. Immunoexpression of CD30 and CD30 ligand in deciduas from spontaneous abortions. Eur J Histochem. 2005;49(3):285–90.
8. Choi G, Roh J, Park CS. CD99 is strongly expressed in basal cells of the normal adult epidermis and some subpopulations of appendages: comparison with developing fetal skin. J Pathol Transl Med. 2016;50(5):361–8.
9. Nguyen TT, Schwartz EJ, West RB, Warnke RA, Arber DA, Natkunam Y. Expression of CD163 (hemoglobin scavenger receptor) in normal tissues, lymphomas, carcinomas, and sarcomas is largely restricted to the monocyte/macrophage lineage. Am J Surg Pathol. 2005;29(5):617–24.
10. Abdulla Z, Turley H, Gatter K, Pezzella F. Immunohistological recognition of cyclin D1 expression by non-lymphoid cells among lymphoid neoplastic cells. APMIS. 2014;122(3):183–91.

11. Truong LD, Rangdaeng S, Cagle P, Ro JY, Hawkins H, Font RL. The diagnostic utility of desmin. A study of 584 cases and review of the literature. Am J Clin Pathol. 1990;93(3):305–14.

12. Hasteh F, Lin GY, Weidner N, Michael CW. The use of immunohistochemistry to distinguish reactive mesothelial cells from malignant mesothelioma in cytologic effusions. Cancer Cytopathol. 2010;118(2):90–6.

13. Chênevert J, Duvvuri U, Chiosea S, Dacic S, Cieply K, Kim J, Shiwarski D, Seethala RR. DOG1: a novel marker of salivary acinar and intercalated duct differentiation. Mod Pathol. 2012;25(7):919–29.

14. Espinosa I, Lee CH, Kim MK, Rouse BT, Subramanian S, Montgomery K, Varma S, Corless CL, Heinrich MC, Smith KS, Wang Z, Rubin B, Nielsen TO, Seitz RS, Ross DT, West RB, Cleary ML, van de Rijn M. A novel monoclonal antibody against DOG1 is a sensitive and specific marker for gastrointestinal stromal tumors. Am J Surg Pathol. 2008;32(2):210–8.

15. Miettinen M, McCue PA, Sarlomo-Rikala M, Rys J, Czapiewski P, Wazny K, Langfort R, Waloszczyk P, Biernat W, Lasota J, Wang Z. GATA3: a multispecific but potentially useful marker in surgical pathology: a systematic analysis of 2500 epithelial and nonepithelial tumors. Am J Surg Pathol. 2014;38(1):13–22.

16. Stead RH, Qizilbash AH, Kontozoglou T, Daya AD, Riddell RH. An immunohistochemical study of pleomorphic adenomas of the salivary gland: glial fibrillary acidic protein-like immunoreactivity identifies a major myoepithelial component. Hum Pathol. 1988;19(1):32–40.

17. Shafizadeh N, Ferrell LD, Kakar S. Utility and limitations of glypican-3 expression for the diagnosis of hepatocellular carcinoma at both ends of the differentiation spectrum. Mod Pathol. 2008;21(8):1011–8.

18. Kim H, Park YN. Hepatocellular adenomas: recent updates. J Pathol Transl Med. 2021;55(3):171–80.

19. Rodriguez EF, Fite JJ, Chowsilpa S, Maleki Z. Insulinoma-associated protein 1 immunostaining on cytology specimens: an institutional experience. Hum Pathol. 2019;85:128–35.

20. Leblebici C, Yeni B, Savli TC, Aydın Ö, Güneş P, Cinel L, Şimşek BÇ, Yıldız P, Tuncel D, Kayahan S. A new immunohistochemical marker, insulinoma-associated protein 1 (INSM1), for Merkel cell carcinoma: evaluation of 24 cases. Ann Diagn Pathol. 2019;40:53–8.

21. Gorbokon N, Timm P, Dum D, Menz A, Büscheck F, Völkel C, Hinsch A, Lennartz M, Luebke AM, Hube-Magg C, Fraune C, Krech T, Lebok P, Clauditz TS, Jacobsen F, Sauter G, Uhlig R, Steurer S, Minner S, Marx AH, Simon R, Burandt E, Bernreuther C, Höflmayer D. Mammaglobin-A expression is highly specific for tumors derived from the breast, the female genital tract, and the salivary gland. Diagnostics (Basel). 2023;13(6):1202.

22. Kinoshita Y, Hida T, Hamasaki M, Matsumoto S, Sato A, Tsujimura T, Kawahara K, Hiroshima K, Oda Y, Nabeshima K. A combination of MTAP and BAP1 immunohistochemistry in pleural effusion cytology for the diagnosis of mesothelioma. Cancer Cytopathol. 2018;126(1):54–63.

23. Weidemann S, Böhle JL, Contreras H, Luebke AM, Kluth M, Büscheck F, Hube-Magg C, Höflmayer D, Möller K, Fraune C, Bernreuther C, Rink M, Simon R, Menz A, Hinsch A, Lebok P, Clauditz T, Sauter G, Uhlig R, Wilczak W, Steurer S, Burandt E, Krech R, Dum D, Krech T, Marx A, Minner S. Napsin A expression in human tumors and normal tissues. Pathol Oncol Res. 2021;27:613099.

24. Nakaguro M, Sadow PM, Hu R, Hattori H, Kuwabara K, Tsuzuki T, Urano M, Nagao T, Faquin WC. NKX3.1 expression in salivary gland "intraductal" papillary mucinous neoplasm: a low-grade subtype of salivary gland mucinous adenocarcinoma. Head Neck Pathol. 2022;16(4):1114–23.

25. Haack H, Johnson LA, Fry CJ, Crosby K, Polakiewicz RD, Stelow EB, Hong SM, Schwartz BE, Cameron MJ, Rubin MA, Chang MC, Aster JC, French CA. Diagnosis of NUT midline carcinoma using a NUT-specific monoclonal antibody. Am J Surg Pathol. 2009;33(7):984–91.

26. Hellquist H, French CA, Bishop JA, Coca-Pelaz A, Propst EJ, Paiva Correia A, Ngan BY, Grant R, Cipriani NA, Vokes D, Henrique R, Pardal F, Vizcaino JR, Rinaldo A, Ferlito A. NUT midline carcinoma of the larynx: an international series and review of the literature. Histopathology. 2017;70(6):861–8.

27. Jones TD, Ulbright TM, Eble JN, Baldridge LA, Cheng L. OCT4 staining in testicular tumors: a sensitive and specific marker for seminoma and embryonal carcinoma. Am J Surg Pathol. 2004;28(7):935–40.
28. Pereira Pinto P, Zanine RM. Diagnostic value of p16 and Ki-67 expression in cervical glandular intraepithelial disease: a review. Ann Diagn Pathol. 2023;62:152054.
29. Cetani F, Banti C, Pardi E, Borsari S, Viacava P, Miccoli P, Torregrossa L, Basolo F, Pelizzo MR, Rugge M, Pennelli G, Gasparri G, Papotti M, Volante M, Vignali E, Saponaro F, Marcocci C. CDC73 mutational status and loss of parafibromin in the outcome of parathyroid cancer. Endocr Connect. 2013;2(4):186–95.
30. Tazawa K, Kurihara Y, Kamoshida S, Tsukada K, Tsutsumi Y. Localization of prostate-specific antigen-like immunoreactivity in human salivary gland and salivary gland tumors. Pathol Int. 1999;49(6):500–5.
31. Miettinen M, Wang Z, McCue PA, Sarlomo-Rikala M, Rys J, Biernat W, Lasota J, Lee YS. SALL4 expression in germ cell and non-germ cell tumors: a systematic immunohistochemical study of 3215 cases. Am J Surg Pathol. 2014;38(3):410–20.
32. Tacha D, Qi W, Zhou D, Bremer R, Cheng L. PAX8 mouse monoclonal antibody [BC12] recognizes a restricted epitope and is highly sensitive in renal cell and ovarian cancers but does not cross-react with b cells and tumors of pancreatic origin. Appl Immunohistochem Mol Morphol. 2013;21(1):59–63.
33. Magnusson K, de Wit M, Brennan DJ, Johnson LB, McGee SF, Lundberg E, Naicker K, Klinger R, Kampf C, Asplund A, Wester K, Gry M, Bjartell A, Gallagher WM, Rexhepaj E, Kilpinen S, Kallioniemi OP, Belt E, Goos J, Meijer G, Birgisson H, Glimelius B, Borrebaeck CA, Navani S, Uhlén M, O'Connor DP, Jirström K, Pontén F. SATB2 in combination with cytokeratin 20 identifies over 95% of all colorectal carcinomas. Am J Surg Pathol. 2011;35(7):937–48.
34. Miettinen M, McCue PA, Sarlomo-Rikala M, Biernat W, Czapiewski P, Kopczynski J, Thompson LD, Lasota J, Wang Z, Fetsch JF. Sox10—a marker for not only schwannian and melanocytic neoplasms but also myoepithelial cell tumors of soft tissue: a systematic analysis of 5134 tumors. Am J Surg Pathol. 2015;39(6):826–35.
35. Crum NF. Coccidioidomycosis: a contemporary review. Infect Dis Ther. 2022;11(2):713–42.
36. Bradsher RW. Histoplasmosis and blastomycosis. Clin Infect Dis. 1996;22(Suppl 2):S102–11.
37. Mittal J, Ponce MG, Gendlina I, Nosanchuk JD. Histoplasma capsulatum: mechanisms for pathogenesis. Curr Top Microbiol Immunol. 2019;422:157–91.
38. Ibrahim AS, Spellberg B, Walsh TJ, Kontoyiannis DP. Pathogenesis of mucormycosis. Clin Infect Dis. 2012;54(Suppl 1):S16–22.
39. Kelly BT, Pennington KM, Limper AH. Advances in the diagnosis of fungal pneumonias. Expert Rev Respir Med. 2020;14(7):703–14.
40. Smith S, Reuven N, Mohni KN, Schumacher AJ, Weller SK. Structure of the herpes simplex virus 1 genome: manipulation of nicks and gaps can abrogate infectivity and alter the cellular DNA damage response. J Virol. 2014;88(17):10146–56.
41. de Melo Silva J, Pinheiro-Silva R, Dhyani A, Pontes GS. Cytomegalovirus and Epstein-Barr infections: prevalence and impact on patients with hematological diseases. Biomed Res Int. 2020;2020:1627824.
42. Mehraein Y, Lennerz C, Ehlhardt S, Remberger K, Ojak A, Zang KD. Latent Epstein-Barr virus (EBV) infection and cytomegalovirus (CMV) infection in synovial tissue of autoimmune chronic arthritis determined by RNA- and DNA-in situ hybridization. Mod Pathol. 2004;17(7):781–9.
43. Clark NJ, Owada K, Ruberanziza E, Ortu G, Umulisa I, Bayisenge U, Mbonigaba JB, Mucaca JB, Lancaster W, Fenwick A, Soares Magalhães RJ, Mbituyumuremyi A. Parasite associations predict infection risk: incorporating co-infections in predictive models for neglected tropical diseases. Parasit Vectors. 2020;13(1):138.
44. Hotez PJ, Bethony J, Bottazzi ME, Brooker S, Buss P. Hookworm: "the great infection of mankind". PLoS Med. 2005;2(3):e67.
45. Singhal AV, Sepulveda AR. Helicobacter heilmannii gastritis: a case study with review of literature. Am J Surg Pathol. 2005;29(11):1537–9.

46. Shah J, Shahidullah A. Ascaris lumbricoides: a startling discovery during screening colonoscopy. Case Rep Gastroenterol. 2018;12(2):224–9.
47. National Nosocomial Infections Surveillance (NNIS) system report, data summary from January 1992–April 2000, issued June 2000. Am J Infect Control. 2000;28(6):429–48.
48. Wang HY, Kim H, Kim S, Bang H, Kim DK, Lee H. Evaluation of PCR-reverse blot hybridization assay for the differentiation and identification of Mycobacterium species in liquid cultures. J Appl Microbiol. 2015;118(1):142–51.
49. Martinez-Giron R, van Woerden HC, Pantanowitz L. Hematoidin crystals in sputum smears: cytopathology and clinical associations. Ann Thorac Med. 2020;15(3):155–62.
50. Ali SY. Apatite-type crystal deposition in arthritic cartilage. Scan Electron Microsc. 1985;(Pt 4):1555–66.
51. Dieppe PA, Crocker PR, Corke CF, Doyle DV, Huskisson EC, Willoughby DA. Synovial fluid crystals. Q J Med. 1979;48(192):533–53.
52. Chaplin AJ. Histopathological occurrence and characterisation of calcium oxalate: a review. J Clin Pathol. 1977;30(9):800–11.
53. Schumacher HR Jr. Pathology of crystal deposition diseases. Rheum Dis Clin N Am. 1988;14(2):269–88. PMID: 3051152.

Index

A

Acini, 74
Actinomycin colony, 203
Acute inflammation
    and chronic inflammation, 27
    effusion, 63, 64
    in peritoneal fluid, 63
Acute mastitis, 170
Acute suppurative thyroiditis, 98
Adipose tissue, 75
Adrenal glands
    differential diagnosis, 271, 273
    endothelial lined cysts, 273
    epithelial cysts, 273
    neoplastic process, 273
    normal morphology, 271
    parasitic cyst, 273
    pseudocysts, 273
Alternaria, 29
Alveolar macrophages, 195
Amastigote forms, 349
Amyloid goiter, 92
Ancillary Tests for Detecting Common
    Organisms in Cervix, 46–49
Apocrine cells, 146
Artifacts and contaminants, 88
Ascites, 57
Aspirates of acute mastitis and breast
    abscesses, 171
Atrophic changes, 38
Autosomal dominant polycystic kidney
    disease, 270

B

Bacillus Calmette-Guerin (BCG) treatment, 29
Bacteria in urine samples, 29
Bacterial infections, 28, 345–346
Bacterial meningitis, 336, 339
Bacterial overgrowth, 25
Basal cells, 37, 75
Basal urothelial cells, 20
B-cell lymphoma, 121
Benign and reactive conditions and differential
    diagnosis, 93–94
Benign appearing endometrial cells, 37
Benign cystic lesion, 77–79
Benign ductal epithelial cells, 149
Benign epithelial breast lesions, 145
Benign follicular cells with histiocytes, 86
Benign lymphadenopathy, 113
Benign salivary gland,
    immunohistochemistry, 76
Bethesda system, 35
Bile duct epithelium, 259, 260, 262
    cells, 251
Bladder wash specimen, 16
Body cavity fluid cytology, 66
Bone, 301
    acellular irregular fragments, 303
    adequacy and reporting, 302
    bursitis, 321
    CPP crystals, 320–321
    CPPD, 320–321
    crystal arthropathies, 318–321
    cystic lesions, 306–307, 321–323

Bone (*cont.*)
  elements, 305, 306
  evaluation of, 301
  fractures, 308
  ganglion cysts, 322–323
  gout, 318–320
  ground substance, 303
  hyperparathyroidism, 307–308
  joint replacement surgery, 316–317
  joints, 310–311
  metabolic bone disease, 307–308
  osteoarthritis (OA), 314–316
  osteoclasts, 303–305
  osteomyelitis, 309–310
  rheumatoid arthritis (RA), 313–314
  septic arthritis, 312, 313
  synovial cyst, 322–323
  synovial fluid, 310–323
  technical considerations, 302–303
Brain
  anterior pituitary, 333
  cytologic examination, 330
    advantages, 331
    disadvantages, 331
  necrosis, 334
  normal white matter glial cells, 332
  Purkinje cells, 333
  reactive astrogliosis, 334
  smears/squash preparation, 332, 333
  touch imprints, 331–332
Branchial cleft cysts, 107
BRCA1 associated protein (BAP1), 60
Bronchogenic cysts, 110
Brush specimen, 17

C
Calcium oxalate crystals, 85, 97, 347
Calcium pyrophosphate deposition disease
        (CPPD), 320–321
Calcium pyrophosphate disease, 320–321
Candida, 29
  in urine samples, 30
Castleman disease (CD), 122–124
Catheterized urine
  with reactive changes, 16
  sample, 14
Cat scratch disease, 119, 120
Cell block, 7
Cellular degeneration, 25
Cerebrospinal fluid (CSF) cytology
  choroid plexus, 334
  clinical Indication, 334–335
  CNS conditions, 339, 340

collection, 335
  extracranial and extraspinal elements, 338
  lymphocytes, 335, 336
  macroscopic and microscopic
        features, 335–338
  noncellular elements, 338
Cervical Cancer Screening Guidance in United
        States, 36
Cervical cytology specimens, 35
Cervical lymph node enlargement, 111
Cervical pap specimens, cytomorphologic
        features, 44, 49
Cervical thymic cysts, 107, 108
Chemotherapy and radiation, 30
Choroid plexus cells, 337
Chronic follicular cervicitis, 42
Chronic inflammation, salivary gland acini, 80
Chylous effusion, 66
Ciliated hepatic foregut cyst (CHFC), 257
Classic Hodgkin lymphoma (CHL), 117,
        120, 130
Claudin-4, 62
Clustered urothelial groups with true
        fibrovascular core, 31
CMV lymphadenitis, 117, 118
Coccidioidomycosis, 207
Collagen ball, 52
Contaminants, 67–68
  hematopoietic cells, 68
Core needle biopsy (CNB), 302
Cryptococcal granulomatous
        osteomyelitis, 310
Crystals, 346–347
Cystic lesions
  infectious etiology/abscess, 111
  neck, 105, 107, 109, 111, 112
  in salivary gland, 76
Cystic liver disorders, 256
Cystic neck lesion FNA, 108
Cystic thyroid nodules, 94
Cytologic atypia, 100
Cytology specimen, 6
Cytoplasmic/membraneous staining
        interpretation on ThinPrep/direct
        smear slides, 9

D
Degenerated cells in ileal conduit
        specimen, 27
Degenerated urothelial cells, 26
Dendritic cells, 130
De Quervain (sub-acute granulomatous)
        thyroiditis, 90, 91

Dermatopathic lymphadenopathy, 127,
    128, 130
Dermoid cyst, 109–110
Desmin immunostaining, 58
Diffuse large B-cell lymphoma
    (DLBCL), 124
Direct smears, 5, 6
Distal tubular cells, 267
Ductal cells, 74, 75
    epithelial cells, 261
Dystrophic calcification, 97

E
EBV lymphadenitis (infectious
        mononucleosis)
    differential diagnosis, 117
    histological findings, 116
    lymph node aspirates, 116
Effusions, 57
Elevated angiotensin-converting enzyme
        (ACE) serum levels, 135
Empyema, 66
Endocervical cells, 37
Endometrial pathology, 37
Endosalpingiosis: bland columnar epithelial
        cells, 54
Endoscopic retrograde
        cholangiopancreatography
        (ERCP), 259
Eosinophils, 66
    effusion, 66
Epidermoid cysts, 106, 109
    with anucleated squamous cells and rare
            multinucleated giant cells, 110
    and dermoid cyst, 109–110
Epithelial markers, 60
Epithelioid histocytes, 26
Epstein Barr virus (EBV) status, 117
Erdheim-Chester disease (ECD), 132
Esophagus, 217–220
    Barrett's esophagus, 220
    contaminants, 218
    duplication cyst, 219
    heterotopic tissue, 220
    microorganisms, 218–219
    normal epithelial cells, 217–218
    radiation and chemotherapy induced
            changes, 218
    reactive and reparative changes, 218
Exfoliated endometrial cells, 37
Exfoliative cytology, 5
Exodus, 37

F
Fat necrosis, 162–165
Fibrinous bursitis, 321
Fibrocystic change (FCC), 143–145
    with atypia, 151
    proliferative, 148
Fine needle aspiration (FNA) cytology,
        5, 99, 248
    induced changes in thyroid gland and
            differential diagnosis, 99
    of non-neoplastic breast disease (*see*
            Non-neoplastic breast disease fine
            needle aspiration)
    of salivary gland, 82
Fluid lactate dehydrogenase (LDH)/serum
        LDH level, 57
Fluid protein/serum protein level, 57
Fluorescence in situ hybridization
        (FISH), 65, 296
Focal nodular hyperplasia, 253
Follicular cells, 86
Follicular hyperplasia (FH), progressive
        transformation of germinal center
        (PTGC), 121, 122
Fracture healing, 308
Free silicone, 167
Fungal infections, 29, 344
Fungal lymphadenitis, 120
Fungal meningitis, 339

G
Galactocele, 154–156
Ganglion cyst, 322–323
Gastrointestinal (GI) tract
    esophagus, 217–220
    large intestine, 226–227
        abscess, 227
        endometriosis, 227
        inflammatory bowel disease, 226–227
        normal epithelial cells, 226
        polyps, 227
        reactive and reparative changes, 226
    lymph node, 227
    small intestine, 224–225
        contaminants, 224
        normal epithelial cells, 224
        pathogens, 225
        reactive and reparative changes, 225
    stomach, 220–224
Germinal matrix cells, 338
Glandular cells post-hysterectomy, 43
Goblet cells, 194

Granulomas, 113
Granulomatous inflammation, 26–27
Granulomatous mastitis, 177
Granulomatous thyroiditis, 98
Graves' disease, 89
Gynecologic (non-neoplastic)
      cytology, 5
    differential diagnosis of benign
        findings, 39
Gynecomastia, 177–180

H
Hashimoto's thyroiditis (HT), 89
Hematoxylin and eosin (H&E)
      staining, 7
Hemosiderin-laden histiocytes, 53
Hemosiderin pigment, 96
Hepatocellular carcinoma, 254
Herpes simplex virus (HSV) lymphadenitis,
      118–119, 133
Herpes viral cytopathic changes, 348
HHV8 positive diffuse large B-cell lymphoma
      (DLBCL), 124
HHV8-positive plasmablasts, 124
    malignancy, 124
High-grade urothelial carcinoma, 25
Histiocytes, 62, 63, 111
    necrotizing lymphadenitis, 132, 133
Hormone related changes, 41
Human papillomavirus, 46
Hyaline cartilage, 310–311
Hypercalcemia, 135
Hyperchromasia, 60
Hyperkeratosis, 38
Hyphae forms, 347

I
IAC Yokohama System for Reporting Breast
      Cytopathology, 142
Idiopathic granulomatous lobular mastitis
      mastitis, 173–175
IgG4-related disease, 133
IgG4-related lymphadenopathy, 133–135
IgG4-related salivary gland disease
      (IgG4-RSGD), 79
Ileal conduit urine, 14, 15
Immunohistochemical staining (IHC)
      techniques, 9
    expression, 341–344
Infections, 98
    effusions, 66

Infectious mononucleosis (IM), 118
Inflammatory/infectious renal diseases
    differential diagnosis, 271
    non-neoplastic lesions, 269
    renal abscess, 271
    xanthogranulomatous
        pyelonephritis, 270–271
INSM1, 65
Instrumentation procedures, 31
Interlobular ducts, 75
Intermediate cells, 37
    urothelial cells, 19
International Academy of Cytology (IAC), 142
Intralobular ducts, 74
Intranuclear pseudoinclusions, 100
Intra-parenchymal lymph node, 75
Intraparotid lymph node, 75
Intra-vesicular administration of BCG, 29
IUD related changes, 40

K
Kikuchi-Fujimoto disease (KFD), 127,
      132, 133
Kimura disease (KD), 125, 126

L
Lactating adenoma, 156–158
Lactational mastitis/abscess, 170–172
Langerhans cell histiocytosis (LCH),
      129, 131–132
Large intestine, 226–227
Laryngocele, 107
Lipofuscin, 97
Liquid-based cytology, 36
Liver, 247–259
    anatomy and histology, 247
    ancillary testing, 262
    bile duct brushing cytology, 260
    bile duct cells, 251
    biliary tract
        anatomy and histology, 259
        normal cytology, 259–260
    cirrhosis, 254, 255
    cystic lesions, 254–258
        amebic liver abscess, 257
        caroli disease, 258
        CHFC, 257
        echinococcal cyst, 254–257
        liver pseudocysts, 258
        noninfectious cysts, 257–258
        PCLD, 257

pyogenic abscesses, 258
        simple cysts, 257
    diagnosis, 248
    focal nodular hyperplasia (FNH), 252
    granulomas, 259
    hepatocellular adenoma (HCA), 252
    histopathology, 248
    normal and reactive hepatocytes, 248
    pigments in hepatocytes, 249, 250
        bile pigment, 249
        copper, 251
        hemosiderin, 249
        lipofuscin, 249
        melanin, 251
    primary sclerosing cholangitis, 261–263
    sinusoidal endothelial cells, 251
    stenting, 263
    stricture, 260–261
Low grade urothelial neoplasm, 31
Lung parenchyma, 189
Lymphadenopathy, 111
Lymphocele with scattered lymphocyte sand
        macrophages, 108
Lymphocytic effusion, 63–65
Lymphoepithelial cyst with scattered
        lymphocytes, salivary gland acini
        and histiocytes, 79

M
Mammary duct ectasia (MDE), 159–161
Mammary fat necrosis, 162, 165
Mammary tuberculosis, 175
Marginal zone lymphoma, 124
Maturation index, 41
Megakaryocytes, 68
    in pleural fluid, 68
Melanin, 97
Menstrual cycle changes, 37
Mesothelial cells, 52, 58
Mesothelial markers, 60
Mesothelioma, 60
Metaplastic changes, 75
Metaplastic squamous cells, 200
Metastatic carcinomas in fluids, 60
Metastatic lobular carcinoma from breast
        primary, 61
Metastatic small cell carcinoma in pleural
        fluid, 65
Methylthioadenosine phosphorylase
        (MTAP), 60
    cytoplasmic expression, 60
Microfollicular and macrofollicular cells, 86

Minocycline, 96
Minor salivary gland, 73
Mollaret meningitis, 339
Monoclonal antibodies, 9
Monocytosis, 335
Monomorphic small lymphocytes, 64
Monosodium urate (MSU) crystals, 282
Multicentric Castleman disease in HIV
        infected patient, 123
Multicystic kidney disease, 270
Multilocular cyst, 270
Multinucleated cells, 67
Mycobacterial lymphadenitis, 120
Mycosis fungoides (MF), 129–130
Myoepithelial cells, 75, 148

N
Neck cystic lesions, 105, 106, 109, 111
    differential diagnosis, 105–106
Necrotizing lymphadenopathy, 133
Necrotizing Sialometaplasia, 81
Neoplastic lymphocytes, 64
Non-neoplastic breast disease fine needle
        aspiration
    advantages, 142
    complications, 142
    inter-observer reproducibility, 142
    pregnancy and lactation, 153, 154
    radiologic imaging studies and cytologic
        results, 142
    risk of malignancy, 143
    ultrasound guidance, 142
Non-neoplastic lymph node fine needle
        aspiration
    classification, 115
    cytopathologic evaluation, 113
    flow cytometry, 115
    limitation, 114
    lymphoproliferative disorders or metastatic
        malignancy, 113
Non-proliferative fibrocystic change, 145–147
Normal flora and cytolysis, 43
Normal urine cytology, 17–24

O
Oncocytic epithelium, 75
Osteoblasts, 303, 304
Ovarian benign non-neoplastic cysts and
        differential diagnosis, 55
Ovarian cystic lesion FNA, 55
Ovary, 55

 Index

P

Pancreas
  accessary spleen, 238
  acinar cells, 230
  acute pancreatitis, 234
  adequacy, 230
  anatomy and histology, 229
  ancillary tests, 242
  autoimmune pancreatitis (AIP), 236–237
  chronic pancreatitis, 234, 236
  contaminants, 232
  cystic lesions, 238
    autosomal dominant polycystic kidney
      disease (ADPKD)., 242
    characteristics, 239
    cystic lymphangiomas, 241
    dermoid cyst, 241
    duplication cysts, 242
    epidermoid cyst, 241
    lymphoepithelial cyst (LEC), 240–241
    pseudocyst, 239–240
    retention cysts, 240
  cytomorphologic features, 231
    cytomorphologic features
    chronic pancreatitis, 235
    reactive conditions, 235
    well-differentiated
      adenocarcinoma, 235
  ductal adenocarcinoma (Papanicolaou
    stain), 236
  ductal epithelial cells, 231
  duodenal epithelial contaminant (Diff-Quik
    stain), 233
  ectopic splenic tissue, 238
  groove pancreatitis, 237
  histopathology, 230
  islet cells, 231
  mimics, 232
  mucinous background, 243
  necrotic background, 243
  nesidioblastosis, 238
  organs/contaminants, 232
  sampling methods, 230
Pap smears
  artifacts, 47
  contaminates, 47
  cytomorphologic features, 44
  cytomorphologic mimics, 44
  Miscellaneous Findings Features, 47
  molecular studies, 44
Papanicolaou (Pap) staining, 6, 249
Parabasal cells, 37
Parakeratosis, benign reactive change, 38
Parapneumonic effusion, 66
Parasites infections, 345

Parathyroid cysts, 95, 110
Parotid gland, 73
Periarticular tissue and pitfalls, 305, 306
Pericardial cavity (pericardiocentesis), 57
Pericardial transudates, 57
Peritoneal cavity (abdominal paracentesis), 57
Peritoneal effusions, 57
Peritoneal washing, 51, 54
Pigmented material, 96
Plasma cells, 65, 337
Plasmacytoid dendritic cells (PDCs), 132
Pleomorphic lymphocytes, 63
Pleural fluid (Thinprep), 59
Pneumocystis jirovecii, 348
Pneumocystis jirocevi pneumonia (PJP), 208
Polyclonal antibodies, 9
Polycystic liver disease (PCLD), 257
Polymerase chain reaction (PCR), 65
Polyomavirus, 28
  cytopathic effects, 28
  infection, 25
Pregnancy-related changes, 38
  secretory changes, 154
Primary biliary cirrhosis (PBC), 251
Primary effusion lymphoma (PEL), 124
Progressive transformation of germinal center
    (PTGC), 121, 122
Proliferative myositis (PM), 288–290
Proliferative fasciitis (PF), 288–290
Proliferative fibrocystic changes, 147–150
  with epithelial atypia, 151–153
Proteomics assays, 324
Proximal tubular cells, 267
Psammoma bodies, 97
  with surrounding bland epithelial cells, 54
Pseudogynecomastia, 177
Pulmonary fungi, 205
Pyknotic nuclei and apoptotic bodies, 30

R

Radial scar, 150
Radiation atypia, 152, 153
Radiation-related changes, 42
Rapid on-site evaluation (ROSE), 142, 303,
    323, 324
Reactive bronchial cells, 213
Reactive changes related to urolithiasis, 31
Reactive endocervical cells, 37
Reactive immunoblasts, 117
Reactive mesothelial cells, 58–60
  vs. adenocarcinoma, 60, 61
Red blood cells (RBS), 336
Renal cystic lesions
  cytology and cytologic diagnosis, 269

overview, 268–269
simple cysts, 269
Respiratory epithelium, 189
Respiratory system
  anatomy, 189
  bacterial infections, 201–203
    nocardiosis, 203
    tuberculosis, 201
  cellular elements
    alveolar macrophage, 195
    basal or reserve cells, 194
    goblet cells, 194
    mesothelial cells, 196
    squamous cells, 195
  histology of, 189
  lung disorders, 209–213
    Langerhans cell histiocytosis, 212
    lipid pneumonia, 209
    rheumatoid arthritis, 212
    sarcoidosis, 211
  non-cellular material, 196–198
    amyloid, 197
    cytomorphology and diagnostic
      implications, 196
    pseudoamyloid, 197
  pulmonary mycoses, 205–209
    coccidiomycosis im, 206–207
    cryptococcus neoformans, 205–206
    morphologic characteristics, 205
  reactive cellular changes, 198–201
    bronchial cells, 198
    ciliocytophthoria, 198
    diagnostic pitfalls, 199
    differential diagnosis, 199
  specimens, 190
    bronchial brushings, 192
    bronchial washing, 192
    bronchioalveolar lavage, 192
    fine needle aspiration biopsy, 192
    sampling techniques, 191
    sputum specimen, 190
  subepithelial seromucinous glands, 190
  viral Infections, 203–205
    CMV infection, 204
    cytopathic effects, 204
    herpes infection, 203
Rheumatoid effusion, 67
Rosai-Dorfman disease (RDD), 80, 130–132

S
Salivary gland
  acini and crystalline material, 81
  acini in lobular architecture, 74
  locations, 73–74
  morphology, 74–76
  origin, 73–74
  reactive and inflammatory
    conditions, 79, 82
  types, 73–74
Sampling methods, 12–17
Sarcoidosis, 135, 136
Schistosoma hematobium, 29
Sebaceous glands, 75
Seminal vesicle epithelial cells, 21
Septic arthritis, 312, 313
Serous effusion, 57
Sialadenitis, 81
Silicone granuloma, 166, 167
Sinus histiocytosis with massive
  lymphadenopathy, 130
Skeletal muscle in pleural fluid, 68
SLE lymphadenopathy, 133
Small cell carcinoma, 64, 65
Small intestine, 224–225
Small lymphocytic lymphoma/chronic
  lymphocytic leukemia (SLL/
  CLL), 64
Soft tissue cytology, 323
Soft tissue lesions
  abdominal fat pad fine needle
    aspiration, 280
  abscess, 290–291
  brown adipose tissue, 294–295
  epidermal inclusion cyst, 292–293
  fat necrosis, 285, 286
  foreign body granuloma (FBG), 286, 287
  granulomatous infection, 292
  hematomas, 283–284
  ischemic fasciitis, 288
  metabolic conditions, 278
    abdominal fat pad fine needle aspiration
      (AFP-FNA), 280
    amyloidoma, 278–279
    extracellular material, 279
    tophaceous gout, 282–283
    tumoral calcinosis, 280–282
  necrotizing soft tissue infections, 291–292
  non-neoplastic lesions., 278, 288, 296
  overview, 277
  PF/PM lesions, 288–290
  postoperative seroma, 284–285
  pseudosarcomatous lesions, 288, 289, 296
  rheumatoid nodules, 294
  sarcoidosis, 293–294
  tumoral calcinosis, 280–282
Special stains, 7, 8
Specimen collection techniques1, 1–5
Specimen preparation, 6, 7
Spermatozoa, 21

Squamous cell contaminants, 20
Squamous epithelial lining in the urethra, 12
Squamous epithelium, 11
Staining technique, 6
Stomach, 220–224
    atypical mycobacteria, 222
    contaminants, 221
    duplication cyst, 222
    gastritis, 223
    helicobacter pylori, 222
    heterotopic tissue, 222
    normal epithelial cells, 220–221
    reactive and reparative changes, 222–223
    ulcer, 223–224
Subareolar abscess (SA), 168–170
Sublingual gland, 73
Submandibular gland, 73
Superficial cells, 37
Swiss cheese-like pattern, 287
Systemic lupus erythematosus (SLE)
            lymphadenopathy, 67, 124, 126,
            127, 133

T
Therapy-related reactive changes, 30
Thin colloid with background histiocytes, 87
Thymic cyst, 109
Thyroglossal duct cysts (TGDC), 94, 106
Thyroid cystic lesions, 94–96
Thyroid FNA cytology specimens, 86
    artifacts, 87
Thyroid follicular cells
    and histiocytes, 107
    in neck region, 98–99
Thyroid gland
    demographics and nutritional factors, 85
    fine needle aspiration (FNA)
            examination, 85
Tophaceous gout, 319

Touch imprint cytology, 6
Transudates vs exudates, 58
Tubal metaplasia, 42
Tuberculosis, 175
Tuberculous effusion, 67
Tuberculous mastitis, 175, 176
Tumor clusters with nuclear molding, 65

U
Umbrella cells, 19
Ureteral brush specimen, 17
Urinary system, 11
Urinary tract
    acute and chronic inflammation, 26
    anatomy, 11–12
    colored crystals, 21
    colorless crystals, 22
    histopathology, 11–12
    lubricant gel material, 24
    reactive changes, 24, 26
Urine cytology, 348
Urine sample collection methods, 13, 17
Urolithiasis, 30
Urolithiasis-associated changes, 31
Urolithiasis-associated cytological atypia, 30
Urothelial cell clusters, 31, 32
Urothelial cell degeneration, 25, 31
Urothelial lining in urinary bladder, 12
Urothelium, 11

V
Viral meningitis/encephalitis, 339
Virus infections, 344–345
Voided urine, 14, 15

W
Wash specimen, 16–17

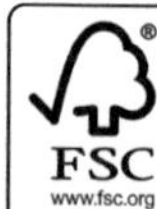

MIX
Papier aus verantwortungsvollen Quellen
Paper from responsible sources
FSC® C105338

FSC
www.fsc.org

If you have any concerns about our products,
you can contact us on
ProductSafety@springernature.com

In case Publisher is established outside the EU,
the EU authorized representative is:
Springer Nature Customer Service Center GmbH
Europaplatz 3, 69115 Heidelberg, Germany

Printed by Libri Plureos GmbH
in Hamburg, Germany